Fierce Medicines, Fragile Socialities

Series: Epistemologies of Healing
General Editors: David Parkin and Elisabeth Hsu, University of Oxford

This series publishes monographs and edited volumes on indigenous (so-called traditional) medical knowledge and practice, alternative and complementary medicine, and ethnobiological studies that relate to health and illness. The emphasis of the series is on the way indigenous epistemologies inform healing, against a background of comparison with other practices, and in recognition of the fluidity between them.

For a full volume listing, please see the series page on our website:
https://www.berghahnbooks.com/series/epistemologies-of-healing

Fierce Medicines, Fragile Socialities
Grounding Global HIV Treatment in Tanzania

Dominik Mattes

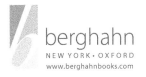

berghahn
NEW YORK · OXFORD
www.berghahnbooks.com

First published in 2019 by
Berghahn Books
www.berghahnbooks.com

Library of Congress Cataloging-in-Publication Data
Names: Mattes, Dominik, 1978- author.
Title: Fierce medicines, fragile socialities : grounding global HIV treatment
in Tanzania / Dominik Mattes.
Description: New York : Berghahn Books, 2019. | Series: Epistemologies of
healing ; v. 18 | Includes bibliographical references and index.
Identifiers: LCCN 2019014380 (print) | LCCN 2019015677 (ebook) | ISBN
9781789203226 (ebook) | ISBN 9781789203219 (hardback : alk. paper)
Subjects: LCSH: HIV-positive persons--Tanzania--Social conditions. | AIDS
(Disease)--Treatment--Tanzania. | AIDS (Disease)--Alternative
treatment--Tanzania. | Antiretroviral agents--Social aspects--Tanzania.
Classification: LCC RA643.86.T34 (ebook) | LCC RA643.86.T34 M38 2019 (print) |
DDC 362.19697/92009678--dc23
LC record available at https://lccn.loc.gov/2019014380

British Library Cataloguing in Publication Data
A catalogue record for this book is available from the British Library

ISBN 978-1-78920-321-9 hardback
ISBN 978-1-78920-322-6 ebook

Contents

Contents

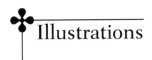

Illustrations

Figures

Table

Acknowledgments

This book marks the end of a journey that would not have been possible without the varying forms of support that I received throughout the years from friends, colleagues, and family. First of all, I want to thank Hansjörg Dilger for his close accompaniment and exceptional guidance throughout the research project on which this book is based. I have benefitted immensely from his always insightful comments and his continual academic support. Most importantly, however, I sincerely thank him for significantly widening my (medical) anthropological field of vision.

I would also like to express my gratitude to Tom Bonnington and Caroline Kuhtz at Berghahn Books for their very helpful and reliable guidance in preparing this manuscript. My particular thanks, further, go to the editors of this book series, David Parkin and Elisabeth Hsu, as well as the anonymous reviewer for their very constructive and useful comments on previous versions of the text.

In Tanzania, I am immensely grateful to the medical professionals who so generously provided me with the opportunity to get to know their daily work routines and so patiently answered all of my questions, notwithstanding the manifold demands and scarcity of time they faced every day. I am also highly indebted to the hospitality of the many people living with HIV/AIDS and ARVs in Tanga who granted me entry into their local moral worlds and open-heartedly shared even their most intimate concerns with me. A step that was anything but self-evident considering what it could mean for them to have their health status exposed to others.

I also thank the Tanga AIDS Working Group for functioning as my local research partner and facilitating my research by connecting me with patients, healers, and HIV (self-)support groups. I am grateful to Haruna and Fatuma Rashidi as well as Rama and Zahara Ramadhani and their children for offering their company and assistance in the manifold everyday practicalities that would have hopelessly overwhelmed me without them. A great thank you also goes to Ismail Shemdea for having been a most valuable and reliable provider of daily news from Tanzania to this very day. I owe special thanks to Uta Gleichmann for her friendship and for providing shelter, and Michael Nyangusi for enabling me to move in and around Tanga in a motorized way and for helping me find a research assistant for my second stint of fieldwork. Thank you to Jemimah van Rouijen for her assistance in transcribing. I am also most indebted to Edna Sichalwe for having been such an inestimable research assistant and cultural broker.

In Berlin, I am very indebted to the Working Group (Arbeitskreis) Medical Anthropology at the Institute of Social and Cultural Anthropology at Freie Universität Berlin. Discussing my work with the group has been invaluable in straightening out my thoughts and always provided me with inspiration to keep going. My greatest gratitude, however, goes to Susann Huschke, Caroline Meier zu Biesen, Britta Rutert, Hanspeter Reihling, and Claire Beaudevin for being the greatest crew not only to count on in an academic sense, but also, even more importantly, when it came to spending timeless and weightless nights in Berlin and other places that helped to clear my mind.

I am also indebted to Eva Grotenhuis and Christoph Pörksen, who made the stay in Tanga so much more rewarding and have become the greatest friends one could wish for, while often helping in practical ways too. A sincere thank you also goes to my sister Heidrun Mattes, Anita and Florian Fischer, and Theodor von Hippel for being there in every imaginable emergency and beyond. My sincere appreciation furthermore goes to Zoe Goldstein and Mary Hardegree for their extraordinarily precise, careful, and reliable language editing of this work.

A lot of life has "happened" since the first draft of my research proposal back in 2007. My children Alma and Lian have come into the world, turned everything upside down, and become the source of my most profound joy and inspiration. I want to thank them for that. And this, finally, brings me to their mother and my life companion, Sandra von Hippel, to whom I am indebted more than anyone else. I benefitted tremendously from her company in the field, from her emotional, psychological, and practical support, and her critical appraisals of my attempts to make sense of my observations in the hospitals and beyond. Her immense self-sacrifice and unconditional support throughout this book's extended coming into being, which coincided with the formation of our family, cannot be put into words. While being most grateful for the likewise unconditional and invaluable lifelong support of my parents, Uta and Winfried Mattes, it is Sandra to whom I dedicate this book.

Notes on Transliteration

I translated the Swahili quotes into English. Single English expressions that my interlocutors integrated into conversations otherwise held in Swahili are marked by "[English expression in original Swahili quote]."

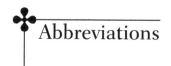
Abbreviations

AFRIWAG	The African Women AIDS Working Group
AIDS	Acquired Immune Deficiency Syndrome
AMREF	African Medical and Research Foundation
ART	Antiretroviral Therapy
ARVs	Antiretroviral Medicines
CHAC	Council HIV and AIDS Control Coordinator
CHICC	Community Health, Information, and Care Center
COSTECH	Tanzania Commission for Science and Technology
CTC	HIV Care and Treatment Center
EED	Evangelischer Entwicklungsdienst (German Evangelical Development Service)
Global Fund	The Global Fund to Fight AIDS, Tuberculosis and Malaria (GFATM)
HBC	Home-Based Care
HIV	Human Immunodeficiency Virus
IMF	International Monetary Fund
LTFU	Loss to Follow-Up
MoH	Ministry of Health and Social Welfare
MSF	Médecins Sans Frontières (Doctors Without Borders)
NACOPHA	National Council of People Living with HIV and AIDS
NACP	National Care and Treatment Program
NGO	Nongovernmental Organization
NIMR	National Institute for Medical Research
OXFAM	Oxford Committee for Famine Relief
PASADIT	Pastoral Activities and Services for AIDS of the Roman Catholic Diocese
PEPFAR	The US President's Emergency Plan for AIDS Relief
PLHA	People Living with HIV/AIDS

PMTCT	Prevention of Mother-to-Child Transmission
SAP	Structural Adjustment Programs/Policies
TACAIDS	Tanzania Commission for AIDS
TALPHA	Tanga People Living with HIV/AIDS
TANOPHA	Tanzania Network of Organizations of People Living with HIV/AIDS
TASAF	Tanzania Social Action Fund
TAWG	Tanga AIDS Working Group
TRC	Tanzanian Redcross Society
TRIPS	Trade-Related Intellectual Property Rights
UNAIDS	Joint United Nations Programme on HIV/AIDS
URT	United Republic of Tanzania
WHO	World Health Organization
WTO	World Trade Organization

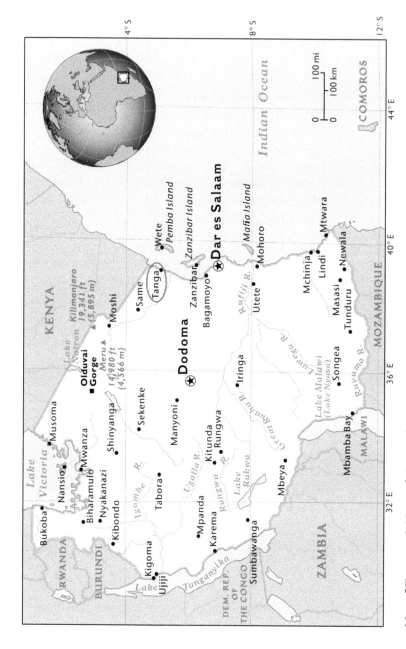

Map of Tanzania © National Geographic Image Collection. Published with permission.

Introduction

"'Willing to start ARVs'[1]: Do I tick it or *not*?!" the nurse almost shouted, while pointing to the "adherence counseling checklist" laying on the large office desk in front of her.[2] All prospective recipients of antiretroviral treatment (ART) in public health centers in Tanga, Tanzania, during the time of my research (2008–2011) were required to answer the sixteen questions on this list before being provided with the pharmaceuticals that would potentially return them to health and extend their lives for years. Did the client come on the appointed date? Spouse's serostatus known and treated accordingly? Disclosure to at least one relative/friend? Client understands what ART does: improve immunity/less opportunistic infections/ART not a cure? Client understands treatment as continuous and lifelong treatment? So read the list of questions, at the end of which the health professionals were asked to estimate whether their clients' "commitment/readiness to adhere to treatment" was (1) Good, (2) Indeterminate, or (3) Poor.

"I ask you *not* to tick it, so I can investigate the other medicine," replied Haruna,[3] the patient sitting on the other side of the office desk, shyly staring at the ground. The atmosphere in the small room was tense. It was difficult to tell if the vague smile on the nurse's face was meant to express disdain or compassion. A moment later, she seemed to decide for the latter. "I won't take you to the doctor, because I feel pity for you." After a short discussion, she conceded that, after all, the treatment was voluntary, yet she strongly recommended that Haruna come back after some time in order to verify the effect of the herbal medicines that he wanted to try instead of ARVs. "Patient not willing to start ART," she noted on the checklist and— loudly reading out what she was writing as a warning—added that he had been fully informed about the possible negative consequences of his decision for his health. "We're finished!" she concluded and called in the next client.

This scene occurred at the HIV Care and Treatment Center (CTC) of the Bombo Regional Hospital in Tanga, a city with approximately 250,000 inhabitants on the shore of the Indian Ocean in northeastern Tanzania. The treatment center operates under the Tanzanian National HIV/AIDS Treatment Program, which began providing cost-free ARVs in November 2004. It is one of the numerous health facilities for the treatment of HIV/AIDS that opened their doors in Tanzania and many other African countries within the last one and a half decades, and which form part of a health intervention of an unprecedented scale: the global rollout of antiretroviral treatment.

Since the early 2000s, global HIV/AIDS treatment has been pushed forward by a heterogeneous assemblage of international policymaking bodies, national development agencies, private philanthropic foundations, transnational nongovernmental organizations, and, mainly, North American global health and research departments. Two well-heeled funding programs were established and have since provided the largest part of the financial support to the global intervention: the Global Fund to Fight AIDS, Tuberculosis and Malaria (Global Fund)—a multisectoral public-private partnership—and the United States President's Emergency Plan for AIDS Relief (PEPFAR)—a program that is administered by the US Department of State and is considered to be the largest disease-specific governmental health intervention of all time. The progress that has been made during roughly a decade and a half is immense. In mid-2017, some 20.9 million people living with HIV across the globe had access to ART (UNAIDS 2017b, 1), a 30-fold increase in comparison to the year 2000 (cf. UNAIDS 2015, 13).

The logic behind this worldwide spread of a biomedical technology is part of what can be called a large-scale process of "epistemological standardization—a standard set of solutions, responding to a standardized set of framings of the problem that link biomedical notions to what have become globalized received wisdoms about HIV and AIDS" (Cassidy and Leach 2009, 15). With respect to treatment (that exists alongside—and in a competitive relationship with—other forms of HIV intervention such as social modes of HIV prevention, impact mitigation, and care and support), standardization targets not only the technical management of HIV through pharmaceuticals and clinical protocols. It also seeks to govern the domain of the social in prescribing—for instance, the nature of

2

an effective relationship between health professionals and patients. More than that, it interferes in the moral sphere by meticulously stipulating patients' desirable conduct and subjectivities.

The respective directives find their expression in international health policies and treatment guidelines issued by major global health institutions like the World Health Organization (WHO). They are adopted by transnational programs such as PEPFAR and are translated into national guidelines, which provide the protocols for clinical HIV management in countless health facilities on the ground and guide counseling processes that reach deep into patients' private lives. In defining patients' rights and responsibilities, and ultimately determining who will be granted access to life saving technologies, these directives and guidelines become instruments of "social triage" (Kalofonos 2008, 9; see also Nguyen 2010) that are an exemplar of the functioning of standards "as central sites of power—organizing and channeling flows of knowledge, capital, and resources in specific directions, and blocking others" (Petryna and Kleinman 2006, 12).

Through standardized, "universal" treatment regimes, ART patients are subjected to the "therapeutic sovereignty" (Nguyen 2010, 6) of a global health apparatus that assumes the regulation and management of the health of entire populations in territories where eroded state treasuries and deficient infrastructures prevent national governments from meeting this responsibility. These regimes aim to transform the targeted patients' bodies through biomedical technologies, but also to fashion their subjectivities by propagating "more intimate technologies" that "target the way in which [they] care for [their] bodies, constitute families, talk to [their] lovers, raise [their] children, and live out [their] sexuality" (Nguyen 2010, 186). Thus, in HIV treatment centers—the sites of the global HIV treatment's local materialization—it is not only therapeutic technologies that are transferred and offered in the form of blood tests, pharmaceuticals, and laboratory equipment. Simultaneously, the health facilities are also places where a globalized form of AIDS knowledge, and the corresponding rationalities and moral regimes, are transmitted (cf. Hardon and Dilger 2011).

In Tanga, I got to know many people who signed onto ART and readily submitted themselves to the treatment regime in a technical and moral sense. Many of them fared well. They bore witness to the pharmaceuticals' power to restore health and induce dramatic changes in their shattered biographies. I visited one man at his workshop where he repaired electronic devices for several hours a day; this was just a few months after his treatment uptake, at which point he had barely been able to walk. Another woman who had been too weak to feed herself was, after taking the drugs, able to prepare chai tea and *chapatis* (flatbread made of wheat flower) for her children before walking them to school and selling fruits at the local market for the rest of the day. ARVs enabled many people who had been excluded from social life to resume their roles as family and community members, to reconstitute their disrupted relationships, and to continue their work or studies, while those living with HIV who had not yet experienced the destructive effects of full-blown AIDS had a good chance of avoiding this devastating experience altogether. But there were also cases like Haruna, which complicated the narrative of positive transformation.

Haruna had heard about the transformative power of ARVs at length during the educational sessions provided at the CTC, and to which all patients who were eligible to start treatment were required to attend. Why then, I wondered, would he refuse to receive this promise of life, in the form of tiny, multicolored capsules, despite the nurse's insistent warnings and opt for taking a local healer's herbal medicines instead? In order to better grasp what was at stake for Haruna, his story requires further elaboration.

Haruna and Zahra: Navigating Local Moral Economies

When my research assistant, Edna, and I first met Haruna at his HIV test at one of Tanga's CTCs shortly before Christmas 2008, he was forty years old and earned his living as a freelance construction worker, struggling his way from one short-term contract to the next. Unfortunately, the test turned out positive. His CD4 count of 68 cells/μl indicated that his immune system had already been severely affected by the virus, and he was therefore scheduled for ART initiation.[4] Throughout the procedure of treatment preparation, Haruna was attentive and understood everything that the nurse explained to him about the therapy and how to live with it. But the discussion took an unexpected turn when, during his "adherence assessment," she finally asked him, "So, are you ready to take these medicines for your whole life as long as you are in this world?" Instead of responding directly, Haruna started to talk about his wife Zahra, who had tested HIV-positive two years before. With a CD4 count of just above 200 cells/µl, she had not started ART, but had been told to get it checked again after a few months. Haruna had consulted a "traditional healer"[5] well known to his family and had administered the herbal medicines he obtained to Zahra. She kept doing well, had become pregnant, and had given birth to an HIV-negative girl. When, after a while, she had her CD4 count tested again, she happily registered that it had risen to above 600 cells/µl. Therefore, Haruna told the nurse that rather than initiating ART, he intended to start taking the same herbal medicines as Zahra. As indicated above, however, the nurse simply insisted, this time in a louder voice: "Are you ready to take the medicines?!" A short discussion evolved, the nurse grew increasingly annoyed, and—her finger pointing to the question on the checklist—she raised her voice once more: "'Willing to start ARVs': Do I tick it or *not*?!"

Two months later, I rode my bicycle along the dusty roads of a neighborhood in Tanga's expanded outskirts where Edna and I were to visit Haruna and Zahra in their modest home, a mud house with two bedrooms separated by a tiny kitchen. When we arrived, they introduced us to Zahra's parents who were visiting, asked us to follow them into their bedroom, and closed the thin wooden door behind them. As the room was too small to accommodate any other furniture, we all took a seat on their bed. After they had shown me a large pile of family pictures and Haruna had told us at length about the additional income he had once made with the rental of a PA system, I hesitantly asked them if we could talk about their health condition. They smiled politely—and remained silent. Obviously, they felt too uncomfortable to talk about the issue while Zahra's parents were sitting next door, but they had been too respectful to call me and postpone the interview date.

A few days later, we met again in the patio of a school in the city center, where a friend of Haruna's was a teacher. The distance between us and the few students who were studying on the other side of the patio and the droning noise of a TV somewhere in the background gave Haruna and Zahra enough confidence to talk about their health situation, albeit in very low voices. Haruna told us that they were still carrying on with their "experiment": Zahra continued taking the therapeutic mixture from the family's herbalist, while Haruna resorted to a self-made herbal concoction. Neither considered ARVs an alternative. While Zahra pointed to the positive effects of the herbal medicine she was taking, Haruna explained that his unstable work situation required a high degree of mobility. At times, he had to spend several weeks out of town, and he worried about forgetting to take the pills regularly in such a situation. In contrast to what he was warned about with regard to ARVs, he reported that there were neither any preconditions to nor adverse effects of taking his herbal medicines. Strongly convinced of their potency, he even had plans to combat his family's constant financial precariousness by producing these on a commercial basis. Even some nurses at one of Tanga's health centers had secretly expressed their interest in his concoction, he proudly revealed.

Zahra and Haruna had not told anyone about their infection in order to mobilize social support—as suggested by the nurses at the hospital. Instead, they told me stories of heavily stigmatized HIV-positive people in their neighborhood, where HIV was still considered a shameful disease and a death sentence. During a second interview some ten weeks later, Haruna reported his latest laboratory results: his hemoglobin level had risen and he had gained four kg of weight. Zahra remained quiet, but Haruna explained that she was also doing well. They had not yet had time to go back to the CTC to get another CD4 count, Haruna claimed, before reaffirming their decision not to commence ART as long as the herbal medicines were effective.

One afternoon about four months later, Edna received a phone call. Haruna delivered the sad news that Zahra had died two days earlier. One week after giving birth to a baby boy, she had succumbed to what was, according to Haruna's speculations, a severe malaria attack. A few hours later, still shocked, Edna and I attended the mourning ceremonies at Haruna and Zahra's crowded house. Amid the loud lamentations of the women present, Haruna sat in the bedroom, his newborn son in his arms. Absentmindedly, he received our contribution to the costs of Zahra's burial and mumbled something about where his children would be accommodated so that he could continue to work. Then he was summoned by the group of elder men reciting prayers for the deceased in the shade of a tree in the front yard.

The following week, we met Haruna again in the school patio. Staring at the table in front of him, he calmly explained to us—and maybe to himself as well—what had happened. Together with Zahra, he had gone to the CTC to check the advance of their immune systems' recovery. Fortunately, his CD4 count had risen to more than 200 cells/µl, so the nurses had instructed him to come back after three months for the next follow-up. Zahra's CD4 level had also increased, and they happily returned home. Zahra finally gave birth to their son in their neighborhood's health center and soon after returned home. One week later, however, she suddenly caught a high fever and fell into a coma. At the hospital, she received several drips and blood transfusions, but nothing would ameliorate her condition. After three days, she died without ever having regained consciousness. As was often the case when people died in hospital in Tanga, the ultimate cause of Zahra's death remained unknown.

After Zahra's passing, her sister and brother-in-law took four of Zahra and Haruna's seven children, including the newborn, with them to the capital of Dar es Salaam, so that Haruna could continue to work and take care of the eldest children. When I asked Haruna if any measures had been taken to prevent perinatal HIV transmission to his newborn, he was not sure if Zahra had been enrolled on a program for the Prevention of Mother-to-Child Transmission (PMTCT). Apparently, they had never talked about it. I recommended that he inform his brother-in-law and ask him to take the baby to a hospital in Dar es Salaam, but Haruna hesitated. On the one hand, he repeatedly expressed his anxieties about being stigmatized and did not want to risk a rupture with his in-laws. On the other hand, he wanted to ensure the appropriate care for his baby. Only after further explanations about the risks of perinatal HIV transmission did he consider asking his brother-in-law to take the baby to hospital. Due to Haruna's frequent work-related absences, however, I never managed to follow up on him throughout the rest of my fieldwork.

The Rationale of Refusal

Haruna's insistence on using herbal medications instead of ARVs, his decision to remain silent about his and his wife's HIV status, his ignorance of whether or not she had enrolled in a PMTCT program, and his hesitance about informing his brother-in-law about the possible HIV infection of his newborn son may be read as "a refusal of assuming an AIDS identity, of becoming that biological being that the virus and the regimen of its treatment determine its host to become" (Kistner 2009, 11). Clearly, this case exemplifies the collision between the "rules" and implicit moral exigencies of a global health intervention, and the concerns of local "beneficiaries" situated in webs of social solidarity that face the danger of disruption through their association with HIV. While many ART patients' practices of self-fashioning seemed to develop in accordance with the treatment regime's moral requirements, in Haruna's and several other patients' cases, frictions emerged.

Whether these frictions resulted from scientific ignorance and irrationality—as local health professionals often assumed—is, however, a matter of perspective. In Haruna's eyes, his and Zarah's conduct was the result of a well-considered decision. Aside from anticipating that he would not be able to harmonize the rigid treatment regime with his working conditions, he judged the drugs' prospective consequences on the basis of previous negative experiences with biomedical pharmaceuticals. Instead, he opted for herbal medicines from a well-known local healer, which in his experience were highly effective, had no negative side effects, and did not require lifelong intake.

Haruna and Zahra's refusal to disclose their health status can, in turn, be understood as an equally reasonable decision in consideration of the HIV-related stigmatization that they had repeatedly witnessed in their community where knowledge about ARVs was scarce. Given this environment and their fragile financial situation, it later seemed self-evident to Haruna not to disclose to his brother-in-law and so risk the proper care for his children. Indeed, the case shows how Haruna had to negotiate "conflicting moral economies" (Nguyen et al. 2007, 31). On the one hand, health professionals encouraged patients to develop a positive attitude, to disclose to others, and not to stigmatize themselves (see Chapter 4). On the other hand, his dependency on kinship-based networks of social support required the careful maintenance of secrecy around his health status. Haruna's dilemma thus tellingly confirms that "the ways people deal with HIV/AIDS are based not *exclusively* on knowledge . . . and technologies of the self that are derived from . . . AIDS campaigns but . . . have become embedded simultaneously in . . . the social and moral priorities formulated by communities and families in relation to the disease" (Dilger 2012, 76).

From the Global Health Intervention to the Individual Lifeworld: Making Sense of What Is at Stake

In this book, I explore the articulation and effects of the encounter of standardized material and sociomoral technologies that are transported around the world under the umbrella of global HIV/AIDS treatment with local forms of knowledge, infrastructures, and moral economies. I address processes of convergence but also of conflict and friction (cf. Tsing 2005) that evolve through this encounter, seeking to contribute to an understanding of "the disconnects between public health notions of responsible behaviors, including moral ways of thinking and acting, and the situated ethics of the everyday struggles of men and women in Africa" (Langwick, Dilger, and Kane 2012, 2). The unfolding of global ART in Tanga is thereby examined based on the premise that "pharmaceuticals affect the human body as a site of control and creative experience," but that "drugs and treatment strategies also go beyond the body, affecting and potentially reshaping interpersonal, family, and community domains" (Petryna and Kleinman 2006, 8).

When carrying out the research this book is based on, I was interested in understanding the financial and political parameters of Tanzania's national HIV treatment program in relation to larger scale developments in the realm of global health politics and activism. What particularly caught my attention, though, was the specific social and (infra)structural concretization of patient enrollment and surveillance in Tanga's treatment centers. Taking on the perspective of hospital ethnography (Van der Geest and Finkler 2004; Long, Hunter, and Van der Geest 2008), I explored what kinds of relations were established between "target populations" and the "global health apparatus" within these sites of mass HIV treatment. I focused on the power dynamics involved in treatment preparation, the transmission of biomedical knowledge to patients, and the long-term control of the therapy's effects in Tanga's health facilities. This included an examination of how far these processes engendered "empowered" and self-responsible patients, as called for in international and national guidelines (e.g., NACP 2012).

Beyond such institutional settings, however, I wanted to learn about the therapy's inscription in patients' life worlds: the ways in which the ARVs affected their bodily well-being; their sense of a return to "normalcy" after treatment initiation; and their anxieties and aspirations with regard to their long-term use of these pharmaceuticals. Furthermore, I wished to explore how ART was managed in patients' social environs, and what transformations it provoked therein. I placed particular emphasis on the treatment's effects on diverse forms of sociality, ranging from the interactions and communication among friends, couples, and within families to the organization of care and support within more institutionalized contexts like HIV (self-)support groups. How does ART enable processes of reconstructing patients' formerly disrupted social relations, I wondered? Who is informed to what extent about the everyday implications of living with ART in patients' social surroundings, and what kinds of support structures are mobilized or disrupted? What effect do treatment uptake and resulting physical transformations have on families' and friends' readiness to get tested for HIV? What dynamics, necessities, and discourses does ART evoke within (self-) support groups, whose focus prior to the advent of treatment had been the mutual provision of social and moral support?

Considering that Tanga is particularly well-known for its density of "traditional healers" (McMillen 2004; Scheinman 2002), I set my third larger focus on the emplacement of ART within the region's highly pluralistic therapeutic landscape (Feierman 1985; Giles 1995; Langwick 2011; Parkin 2014). I explored the varying ways in which Christian and Muslim religious leaders, as well as traditional healers, integrated ART into their conceptual frameworks of disease causation, theological and moral reasoning, and therapeutic practices. Of particular interest was the question of whether and to what extent patients' engagement in discourses and practices of traditional and religious healing interfered with their adherence to their biomedical therapy.

Through these thematic foci, I sought to gain a deeper understanding of how "global ART" was transferred, appropriated, "lived," and conceptualized by a multitude of actors at the local level, ranging from clinicians to patients, from policymakers to specialists in spirit possession. A central concern, thereby, centered on achieving a sense of the extent to which the availability of ART has indeed actuated the "normalization" (and medicalization) of HIV/AIDS that was envisaged by activists, medical professionals, and health policy-makers as coming along with the drugs' increasing availability in all regions of the world (Moyer and Hardon 2014).

Throughout the entire project, I was guided by the "biographi-cal life course perspective" (Van der Geest and Chamberlain 2011, 236). Building on the idea of "the social life of things" (Appadurai 1988), this approach traces the social lives of medicines (Whyte, Van der Geest, and Hardon 2002). It thereby draws attention not only to the different levels of social organization that pharmaceuti-cals pass through in their global trajectories, but also to the varying "regimes of values" they traverse and the distinctive meanings they are ascribed in particular stages of their "'life cycle' from production, marketing, and prescription to distribution, purchasing, consump-tion, and finally their efficacy" (Appadurai 1988, 4; see also Hardon and Sanabria 2017; Van der Geest and Chamberlain 2011; Van der Geest, Whyte, and Hardon 1996, 153; and Whyte et al. 2002). Applying this to the matter of this book, I trace the life trajectory of ARVs. This begins with what could be viewed as their "prenatal" phase in terms of the political-economic framework that shapes the conditions of their production, and ends with their "life after death" in terms of their efficacy—both physical, in the sense of individual patients' (possibly) relieved bodily suffering, and sociocultural, in the sense of the effects (or lack thereof) that these recoveries have within patients' social surroundings and beyond (cf. Van der Geest and Hardon 2006).

The biographical life course perspective serves as a useful analyt-ical tool to account for the multitude of levels of social organization, actors, and complexes of meaning/values that shape and are affected by the global circulation of pharmaceuticals. However, it does not imply any specific way to *theoretically* grasp the multifarious work-ings of power within and across these levels and entities. To this purpose, I additionally draw on the notion of "governmentality," as coined by Michel Foucault (1991). It designates a specific political rationality, according to which government not only includes admin-istrational forms of domination and disciplining but also more subtle kinds of guidance through which subjects, perhaps even unwittingly, are steered toward particular forms of self-control. Government, in this sense, is understood as "the conduct of conduct" (Foucault 1982, 220–21) and as "a continuum, which extends from political government right through to forms of self-regulation" (Lemke 2002, 59). Such self-regulation, in turn, is to be achieved through the fostering and application of particular "technologies of the self, which permit individuals to effect by their own means or with the help of others a certain number of operations on their own bodies and souls, thoughts, conduct, and way of being," (Foucault 1988, 18) so as to achieve, not least, desired states of optimized health and well-being. In the domain of health and welfare, the fostering of such technologies constitutes a mode of governing through which individuals are to be motivated and enabled to modify their own conduct in such a way that the sum of these practices of self-management are convenient for the population as a whole (cf. Bunton and Petersen 2002; Miller and Rose 2008; Rose 2007). The inducement of proper self-regulation is to complement other, perhaps more overt biopolitical activities of registering and regulating the population and its biological processes, be this in the form of "collecting, collating and calculating data on [its] characteristics . . . (births, deaths, rates of disease, levels and types of employment etc.)" (Nettleton 1997, 210), or establishing, designing, and implementing health institutions, policies, and interventions to the end of its positive development.

Against this background, I view biomedicine and public health as institutions that exercise power through the acquisition of a particular kind of knowledge and correlated practices of disciplining and surveillance, normalization and standardization, inclusion and exclusion. But simultaneously, both biomedicine and public health intervene deeply in the vital matter of populations and the individuals that compose them through less imposing, more horizontal forms of power including the subtle and suggestive promotion of particular, presumably appropriate forms of risk-assessment and self-care that are to be internalized by the subjects of their interventions. As will be shown in the course of this book, these characteristics apply particularly well to the apparatus of global HIV treatment.

Notwithstanding the enormous analytical potential of governmentality, the critique has been formulated that in his elaborations on the notion, Foucault preoccupied himself too much with processes occurring *within* sovereign states rather than studying "power relations between polities" (Kelly 2010, 1; see also Ingram 2009). In the "post-Foucauldian" era, scholars working on governmentality made efforts to rectify this shortcoming. Taking this further development into account is particularly important for the attempt to apply the governmentality perspective to the analysis of health care provision in Africa, which throughout the past two to three decades has increasingly been privatized and transnationalized.

To begin with, it is important to note that a crucial characteristic of Foucault's notion of modern political power represented by "governmentality" is its

> refusal to reduce political power to the activities of the state. Indeed, for Foucault, governing . . . is not merely a matter of *the* government and its institutions but involves a multitude of heterogeneous entities: from politicians, philanthropists, and state bureaucrats to academics, clerics, and medics. What thus counts in thinking about governmental power is not simply the state but also all these other actors, organizations, and agencies concerned with exercising authority over the conduct of human beings. (Inda 2005, 6)

In support of this argument, shifting the focus from the state to the multitude of nonstate actors involved in the governing of health and well-being is essential for the analysis of public health interventions in Tanzania and elsewhere in Africa. The examination of the "proliferating global institutional ecology of pharmaceuticals" (Petryna and Kleinman 2006, 6) in the case of HIV treatment, for instance, reveals a staggering number of heterogeneous actors involved in global ART provision: governmental institutions and nongovernmental (transnational and domestic) organizations, multiple constellations of private-public partnerships, university departments and research institutes, pharmaceutical companies, churches, and even the military (cf. Nguyen 2009a, 196). Mass HIV treatment programs are thus an example par excellence of how to transfer national governments' sovereignty and responsibilities to "transnationally constituted conglomerates, which have come to perform statelike functions all across Africa" (Dilger 2009, 102).

This has much to do with the stringent structural adjustment programs (SAPs) that the World Bank and International Monetary Fund (IMF) began prescribing for destitute African governments in the wake of the world economic recession of the 1970s as a precondition for receiving financial loans. Reflecting the fundamental tenets of neoliberalism, these programs were based on the premise that "development" and social welfare were best achieved through the engagement of market-based, private, and nongovernmental actors rather than state interference. They imposed "a steep reduction in governmental expenditure for health care, education, and housing programs, including a significant reduction of salary expenses for public sector employees" (Dilger 2012, 64; see also Ferguson 2006; for analyses of the negative impact of these structural reforms on health care provision in Tanzania, see Lugalla 1995; and Turshen 1999). The consequence of such massively interventional international politics was the deepening of mass poverty, not least due to the rapidly increasing stratification of the African wage labor market and the entrenchment of large subpopulations in conditions of long-term unemployment and informal petty trade (cf. Mbembe 2001, 55ff). This has left numerous contemporary African governments in a state of economic stagnation, if not downturn, and massively diminished their capacities to reliably provide even basic social welfare.

The SAP-supported reorientation toward nongovernmental actors as the major drivers of development led to an increasing fragmentation of the Tanzanian and other African public health sectors, a process that has been referred to as "NGOization" (Hearn 1998) and "projectification" (Whyte 2013). While this yielded some positive effects in terms of improved health care provided by often transnationally financed and powerful nonstate entities, the desired results remained territorially delimitated to islands of "medical prosperity" with vast areas of continuing under-provision in between (cf. also Ferguson 2006; Geissler 2015, 14f; Sullivan 2011a). Furthermore, it has been critically observed that the innumerable newly emerging projects in the area of health care "enact unequal relations of power, reinforced in the discourse of 'donor' and 'recipient,' and . . . are unstable, driven by short-term funding cycles and working through a variety of often-precarious institutional 'partnerships'" (Prince 2014a, 209).

The proliferation of nonstate actors and the increasing reliance of health care sectors on external donor funds is particularly pervasive in the context of HIV/AIDS. The disease's framing as an "exceptional humanitarian emergency with security implications" (Ingram 2013,

6) provided humanitarian agencies with a powerful legitimization to move into sub-Saharan Africa in order to ameliorate its inhabitants' suffering and secure their survival. The resulting configurations of the "government" of African (sub)populations' health by transnational entities constitute a striking example of the contemporary shifts in power relations that prompted Gupta and Ferguson to extend Foucault's notion of governmentality

> to modes of government that are being set up on a global scale. These include not only new strategies of discipline and regulation, exemplified by the WTO [World Trade Organization] and the structural adjustment programs implemented by the IMF, but also transnational alliances forged by activists and grassroots organizations and the proliferation of voluntary organizations supported by complex networks of international and transnational funding and personnel. The outsourcing of the functions of the state to NGOs and other ostensibly nonstate agencies, we argue, is a key feature, not only of the operation of national states, but of an emerging system of transnational governmentality. (Ferguson and Gupta 2002, 990)

Placing the focus on the transnational governmentality at play in the global response to HIV/AIDS has helped identify dynamics that have been referred to as "therapeutic sovereignty" (Nguyen 2010, 6) and "therapeutic domination" (Rottenburg 2009). Critical observers have argued that these forms of exercising power largely reduce social agents to mere passive human bodies (McFalls 2010, 322f), inasmuch as

> people's lives are constructed according to the medical priorities of HIV interventions independent of their actual lived experiences within their context [and] the framing of the disease together with proposed solutions to many problems it articulates is referenced to the agency of external experts. (Seckinelgin 2012, 454)

While this attests to the analytical purchase of viewing the global ART rollout through the lens of transnational governmentality, a further theoretical approach is needed in order to extend the analysis to the realm of affected people's social, cultural, and moral contexts of everyday life. "The high-profile 'global' regimes shaping health-care provision such as transnational HIV treatment programs are important objects of anthropological analysis," Ruth Prince argues similarly. "Yet . . . we must be careful not to privilege the agency of the global and overlook how local interests, actors, sensibilities, and social forms are often what anchor externally planned interventions in a meaningful way (Prince 2014b, 14f; cf. also Dilger 2012).

This resonates with other critiques of the interpretations of biomedical health interventions in Africa as instruments of biopolitical subjection that have burgeoned within the last two decades or so. "Tak[ing] issue with . . . the idea that medical practices and interventions simply produce disciplined subjects, simply work," these studies foreground "moments of *resistance and creativity*", as well as "the inevitable *incompleteness* of any disciplining project especially in Africa . . . and even . . . the outright failure that is built into the biopolitical endeavor" (Geissler, Rottenburg, and Zenker 2012, 11—emphasis in original).

What is needed, then, for a comprehensive understanding of how people respond to strategies of medical power is a "phenomenology of everyday life and subjectivity" (Lupton 1997, 104) that is capable of accounting for "the ways [global] configurations are constantly constructed, un-done, and re-done by the desires and becomings of actual people—caught up in the messiness, the desperation, and aspiration, of life in idiosyncratic milieus" (Biehl 2011, 115).

People's ways of dealing with ART in their day-to-day lives— including their (non)compliance with medical professionals' instructions, their ideas and practices concerning sexuality and reproduction, their ability to reconstruct their damaged self-image, and their capacity to resume social roles and economic activities— are profoundly shaped by their sociomoral entanglements in their lifeworlds. In my attempt to adequately account for the fundamental importance of often highly contingent and rapidly transforming social relations, as well as people's multiple moral longings, I found inspiration in the "local moral world." Arthur and Joan Kleinman first introduced this concept in a coauthored article in which they propose that the ethnographer take a particular orientation, one that closely attends to "*the overbearing practical relevance* in the processes and forms of experience. That is to say, *something is at stake* for all of us in the daily round of happenings and transactions" (Kleinman and Kleinman 1991, 277—emphases in original). Eliciting what is locally (and morally) most at stake for people afflicted by illness, pain, and other forms of suffering, the Kleinmans argue, should form a central concern for the ethnographer. In fact, a few years later,

Arthur Kleinman delineated the pursuit of an "ethnography of experience" as a core task of (medical) anthropology (Kleinman 1994, 190). Yet it is important to note that he does not propose restricting analytical attention to the level of the particular and idiographic. Notwithstanding the emphasis on the (inter)subjective sphere in which moral stakes are claimed and suffering is experienced in the form of instantaneous incidents or prolonged periods of felt resistance to one's fundamental moral aspirations, he does not argue for a complete disengagement of individual experiences from the social processes by which they are shaped. After a person's "microcontext of experience" has been explored, he rather suggests that it "can be further contextualized by a view from afar that relates this highly focused perspective to the larger-scale political, socioeconomic, and cultural forces that impinge on the local world" (Kleinman 1992, 131).

I hold the notion of the local moral world to be particularly fertile for the analysis of the experiences of people living with ARVs in Tanga. The first benefit I see concerns the special emphasis the concept places on the *pragmatic* aspect and contingency inherent to individual ART patients' moral concerns and on the inseparability of these concerns with the moral longings of other persons within their social surroundings or networks, no matter how restricted these might be. The focus on people's "everyday pragmatics" and lived experience serves as an effective measure against too hasty abstraction and the attribution of particular individual practices, conceptions, and conduct to the impact of structural forces and social characteristics like gender, class, political position, and ethnicity. It also precludes viewing individual practices as entirely determined by power dynamics such as the transnational governmentality exerted by the global HIV treatment apparatus. Without denying the imprint that these dynamics and collectivized experiences leave on individual subjectivities—that is, individual persons' "inner life processes and affective states" (Biehl and Kleinman 2007, 3)—I believe that such a moment of analytical deceleration is expedient in order to take adequate account of the complexity and vicissitudes of affected people's lifeworlds and fundamental moral concerns. Only in this way, I argue, can we gain a profound understanding of people's conceptualization of and attitudes toward HIV treatment and correlated social technologies like HIV disclosure.

A further merit I see in using local moral worlds as an analytical lens is related to the specific idea of experience evolving in the intersubjective sphere, as was proposed by Kleinman and other phenomenologically oriented anthropologists (e.g., Crapanzano 2010; Csordas 2008; Jackson 1989, 1998). Understanding experience "as an interpersonal, intersubjective, realm of engagements, transactions, communications, and other social activities" (Kleinman 1992, 128) inevitably implies the need for the researcher to render her/himself visible, at least as a temporary constituent of the research participants' local moral worlds. "The ethnographer," Kleinman notes, "is 'called' into the stories and lives by the moral process of engaged listening and by the commitment to listening. That call to take account of what is at stake for people becomes an instructive aspect of the ethnographer's sensibility" (1999, 89).

As will be seen in the case studies provided in this book, what Kleinman designates as following a "call" could just as well materialize as a process of "blundering into" particular research participants' lifeworlds. No matter how this process may be conceived of, however, I fully agree that trying to understand and make these local moral worlds intelligible to others, without reflecting on and revealing how the researcher her/himself has participated in and shaped these worlds, would constitute a flawed process of anthropological knowledge production (cf. Stoczkowski 2008). I therefore attempt to make my relationships, at least with the protagonists among my research participants, and the ways in which I became involved in their navigations of the quandaries of life on ART, equally as transparent as their social relations with other persons who coconstituted their central moral concerns.

The focus on the local moral worlds of ART patients further has consequences, both with regard to the methodology of the present study as well as to the representation of its results. In order to provide profound insight into "what was at stake" for people living with ARVs in Tanga, I present my ethnographic material predominantly in the form of extended case studies. On the one hand, this accommodates the understanding of anthropological research and knowledge production as an intersubjective endeavor, inasmuch as "the extended case method emulates a reflexive model of science that takes as its premise the intersubjectivity of scientist and subject of study" (Burawoy 1998, 4). On the other hand, a central aim of the extended case method centers on applying "reflexive science to ethnography in order to extract the general from the unique, to move from the 'micro' to the 'macro'" (Burawoy 1998, 5). As outlined above, this is an analytical move that will not be disregarded, but only be accomplished after a thorough immersion into the particular life circumstances of people living with ARVs and their struggles to arrange with the chronicity of their health status with all its economic, social, and moral implications.

Taking inspiration, finally, from the idea of "slow research" (Adams, Burke, and Whitmarsh 2014), in this book, I wish to illustrate the close entanglement of ART as a globally circulating biomedical technology with the lived economic, social, and moral realities of its recipients in a specific African locality. This runs counter to the tendency in the global health arena "to dismiss local specificities because they get in the way of large-scale comparisons and scaled-up implementations" (Adams et al. 2014, 180). The resulting complexity may be daunting when it comes to deciding on the design of future interventions in the field of HIV/AIDS, since it points to the shortcomings of the currently dominating top-down and technocratic "magic bullet" approach that is narrowly focused on "treating our way out of the epidemic" (cf. Merson et al. 2008; see also Pfeiffer 2013) through the scaled up provision of pharmaceuticals (Biehl 2007). But it is my hope that this book sheds some additional light on "the trial and error, the endless tinkering, of real people in specific circumstances trying to figure out what works for them" (Biehl and Petryna 2013, 9) and potentially contributes to a closer alignment of future HIV interventions with the needs of the people they target.

Outline of the Book

The book consists of this introduction, eight chapters, and a conclusion. Chapter 1 provides a historical and demographic overview of Tanga, followed by an outline of the local therapeutic economy and the landscape of social support for people living with HIV/AIDS. It then offers a detailed description of the research sample and the methods I utilized, including some reflections on research ethics as well as my own positionality and emotional engagement in the field. Chapter 2 outlines the historical and political-economic background of the global ART rollout before it turns to the history of HIV/AIDS and the efforts to respond to the disease in Tanzania, including the country's National Care and Treatment Program.

Chapter 3 focuses on the translation of (inter)national HIV treatment policies and guidelines into daily clinical practice in Tanga. Exploring the concrete articulation of treatment expansion from the Bombo Regional Hospital to several smaller health centers across the city, it accentuates the challenges and constraints that health workers perceived in their attempts to provide high quality care to rapidly increasing numbers of patients. In a further step, it offers a description of a workshop for health workers and voluntary community care providers that aimed to establish an effective continuum of treatment surveillance from health facilities to patients' domestic and private lives. Attending to the uncertain sustainability of Tanzania's treatment program in consideration of donor phase-outs and funding flatlining in the wake of the global financial crisis of 2008, finally, it binds the local materialization of ART provision back to the global political economy.

Chapter 4 elaborates on the micro-politics of ART enrollment and monitoring in Tanga's HIV clinics. Giving attention to the power relations shaping the organization, performance, and supervision of the processes involved in producing treatment literacy and surveilling patients' treatment adherence, it analyzes whether these engendered the actualization of the well-informed, empowered, and self-responsible ART patient that has been called for and indeed observed to be constructed in other African settings at the dawn of the era of HIV mass treatment (Nguyen 2010; Robins 2006).

In Chapter 5, the focus of attention shifts from the routines and power dynamics within biomedical institutions to the inscription of ARVs in patients' local moral worlds beyond the treatment centers. The chapter takes a close look at the physical, social, and moral aspects of the process of reconstitution after ART uptake, primarily from the perspective of individual patients, and explores their strategies for, and difficulties with, restoring a sense of normalcy to their lives. Thereby, particular attention is paid to processes of bodily transformation, to the reconstitution of patients' positive sense of self, to the moral implications of their (re)engagement in sexual and reproductive activities, and finally to their anxieties as well as aspirations concerning their future as long-term ARV users.

The question of whether ART implicates a normalization of people's lives is further pursued in Chapter 6, with a focus on the context of the kin-based networks in which patients live their everyday lives with ARVs, rather than patients' inner affective states and individual attitudes toward their medicines. The predominant issues of interest here are the forms, scope, and effects of patients' communication about their health status and therapy within their social environment; the quotidian management of ART, as well as the (limitations of the) provision of care and support within mostly familial solidarity networks; and the dynamics of HIV-related stigmatization and discrimination that shaped the social interactions within these networks.

In Chapter 7, I turn to HIV (self-)support groups, which constitute a further important social domain for people living with ARVs. Drawing on the observations made during numerous meetings of such groups in the city, the chapter examines the extent to which these biosocial collectives serve as platforms of modeling patient subjectivities, much in the same fashion as the CTCs. It further highlights the particular forms of care and support that group members actually receive (and mutually provide) in practice, the difficulties the groups face in coping with state bureaucracies and navigating Tanga's confined economy of social support for people living with HIV/AIDS, as well as the limitations of biosociality as a factor of the groups' social cohesion.

Chapter 8, finally, takes the Tanzanian mass-healing phenomenon that became internationally known as the Wonder of Loliondo as a prism for exploring the interrelations of HIV/AIDS and ART with religious and traditional healing practices. The Wonder of Loliondo serves as a particularly illustrative example of the contested nature of therapeutic and interpretive authority in relation to HIV/AIDS in Tanzania's highly heterogeneous landscape of healing traditions. The first part of the chapter differentiates the political, social, economic, and moral dimensions and implications of this large-scale phenomenon. Drawing on the comments of religious leaders and traditional healers in Tanga on the Wonder of Loliondo, as well as the narratives of two patients who were simultaneously undergoing ART in Tanga and setting their hopes on the herbal medicine they had received in Loliondo, I will then return to the local context and elaborate on these actors' varying forms of conceptual boundary-making and pragmatic transgression of the epistemological divide between science and religious and "traditional" healing.

Notes

1. Antiretroviral drugs for the treatment of Human Immunodeficiency Virus (HIV) and Acquired Immune Deficiency Syndrome (AIDS).
2. Parts of this introduction have been published in Dominik Mattes, "'We Are Just Supposed to Be Quiet:' The Production of Adherence to Antiretroviral Treatment in Urban Tanzania," *Medical Anthropology* 30, no. 2: 158–82.
3. All names of research participants appearing in this book are pseudonyms. In some cases, additionally their gender or other personal details were changed in order to protect their identities.
4. The decrease of CD4 cells—the main targets of HIV—indicates the disease's progress. Based on WHO recommendations (WHO 2006, 14), the national guidelines in force during my first field stay in Tanga in 2008/2009 prescribed ART initiation at a CD4 level below 200 cells/μl, irrespective of the patient's clinically observable symptoms (NACP 2008, 134). Throughout the following years, this limiting value was first raised to 350 cells/μl (WHO 2010) and then to 500 cells/μl (WHO 2013). In 2015, the WHO finally recommended: "ART should be initiated among all adults with HIV regardless of WHO clinical stage and at any CD4 cell count" (WHO 2015, 24). The implementation of these changing recommendations each time implied a massive increase in the number of patients eligible for treatment, which in turn significantly enhanced the challenges facing the national health care infrastructure. To date, the Tanzanian Ministry of Health has adopted the respective latest recommendations only after a delay of two years. The "treatment for all" policy was thus adopted in 2017 (NACP 2017).
5. The terms "traditional healers" and "traditional medicine" bracket together a wide variety of medical practices and imply equally heterogeneous— often politically instrumentalized—assumptions of what "the traditional" is meant to designate (see Feierman 1985, 100). This diversity also applies for Tanga, where *waganga wa kienyeji* (local healers) are engaged in spirit possession and exorcism, witchcraft (*uchawi*), herbalism, Quranic healing, bone-setting, and ancestor veneration (Mackenrodt 2011). Clear-cut boundaries between the "main types of traditional healers" (Mshiu and Chabra cited in Gessler et al. 1995, 146) were difficult to identify, since the majority of the healers flexibly combined several diagnostic and therapeutic practices.

Chapter 1
Exploring ART in Tanga

Tanga—Swahili Commerce, Colonial Seaport, and Postcolonial Decline

The city of Tanga is situated in the northeastern part of Tanzania on the shores of the Indian Ocean, near the Kenyan border. It serves as the administrative center of both Tanga Region and District.[1] With its roughly 273,000 inhabitants, Tanga ranks seventh among the most populous cities in Tanzania (The United Republic of Tanzania 2013, 48). Walking through the city center close to the seaport, however, does not evoke the impression of a thriving commercial hotspot. On the contrary, the old colonial style buildings that dominate the streets of its rather calm center, which are slowly molding away in the heat and humidity of the nearby ocean, lend it an ambience of somnolence and oblivion, as if the city has slid into obscurity after once having been an urban center of national importance.

Indeed, a look into history confirms that over the course of several centuries, Tanga was once a location of great economic and political relevance. Archeological findings dating back to the year 1600 suggest that the settlements that would later conflate into the city long constituted an important hub in the network of trade relations between Bantu-speaking African fishermen and farmers, and Arabic, Persian, and Indian merchants and immigrants (cf. Becher 1997, 51), a circumstance that led to the peculiar cultural amalgam that to this day characterizes the societies of the Swahili coast from southern Somalia to northern Mozambique. As Patricia Caplan argues, "It is precisely the role of coastal dwellers as intermediaries, traders, merchants and cultural brokers which has given this area its distinctive quality" (Caplan 2004, 3f).

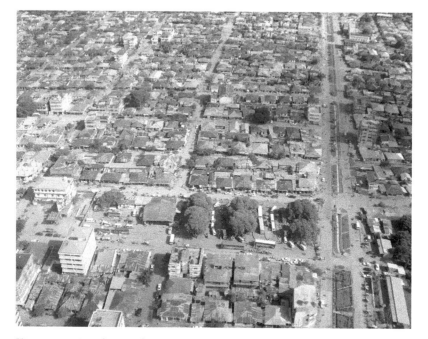

Figure 1.1. Aerial view of Tanga Center © Dominik Mattes 2009.

During the seventeenth and eighteenth centuries, Tanga gained economic importance—particularly due to its location on the sea, which made it an ideal starting and end point for the caravan routes extending into the interior until reaching the Lake Victoria region. By the beginning of the nineteenth century, Tanga had become one of the main transshipment points for ivory and slaves (Becher 1997, 53). These were highly lucrative "goods" for the Omani rulers who had wrought power from the Portuguese in 1698, moved their capital from Muscat to Stone Town (Zanzibar) in 1837, and from there executed control over Tanga (and the largest part of the Swahili coast) until German colonial rule manifested itself in the region in 1888 (Becher 1997, 54).

During the thirty-three year period when present mainland Tanzania formed part of German East Africa (1885–1918), Tanga was particularly important to the German colonial administration as it served as an entry point to the exceedingly fertile hinterland of the Usambara mountains, where by the early 1890s, large trade companies like the German East Africa Company had established coffee, tea, rubber, cotton, and sisal plantations (Becher 1997, 72). In order to transport these crops from the hinterland to the sea, the construction of the Usambara Railway, Tanzania's first railway line, was begun in 1891 (Iliffe 1969, 14). By 1912, it stretched 352 km from the seaport in Tanga to Moshi in the interior (Becher 1997, 71). This infrastructural development led to Tanga, by 1906, evolving into the colony's main port of export (Becher 1997, 74).

The period of German colonial rule was defining for Tanga, and not only economically. Corresponding to the city's steady growth during the first years of German administration, construction regulations restructured the city's topography in a way that led to the segregation of its inhabitants according to broad ethnic categories. The African, Indian, and Arabic inhabitants were ousted to the southern and western densely built-up areas of the city's periphery, part of whose visible boundary is still constituted to this day by a railway line (cf. Van de Bruinhorst 2007, 92f). The Germans and other European settlers, in turn, claimed the central and eastern part of the city, including the Raskazone peninsula that stretches some 2.5 km northeast from Tanga's center to a cape of the same name and served as an exclusive residential area for Europeans who built extensive mansions on plots of up to 9,000 m² (Becher 1997, 65).

This settlement pattern to some extent still influences the spatial ordering of Tanga's population to this day, even though the boundaries between the different areas have become a lot more permissive, and inhabitants' socioeconomic status has replaced ethnicity as the predominant differentiating factor. The Raskazone peninsula is thus predominantly inhabited by the local political and economic elite and a handful of European and North American expatriates, most of whom are involved in development cooperation and medical research projects in the region. Tanga Central is where many entrepreneurial lower middle class families have their homes and run small-scale businesses. Many of these have Arab and Indian ancestry and maintain close ties with relatives in the home countries of their forefathers (Grube 2008). The largest and least well-off portion of Tanga's populace, finally, resides in the densely populated and extended periphery surrounding the former "European central area." While in the neighborhoods immediately adjacent to the city center the houses are mostly made of bricks and concrete and have corrugated iron roofs, the further one leaves the center behind,

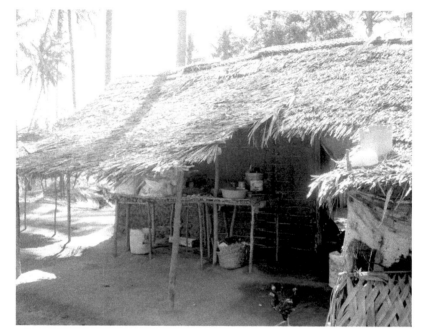

Figure 1.2. Mud-walled house in Tanga's periphery © Dominik Mattes 2009.

the more mud-walled constructions thatched with mats of woven coconut leaves shape the appearance of the roads, which, in contrast to those in the more centrally situated areas, are unpaved.

On 2 November 1914, Tanga became the sad scene of the first major event in the proxy war of European warring parties in East Africa. Indian marine troops attacked Tanga following British orders "to bring the whole of German East Africa under British authority" (Iliffe 1979, 242). In a two-day battle against outnumbered companies of *askaris* (Swahili: guard, soldier; a term that was used to refer to the African soldiers serving in the German colonial army) who were fighting under the order of Colonel Paul von Lettow-Vorbeck, however, the Indian forces were resoundingly defeated. Tanga remained under German control and its bay was left littered with dead Indian soldiers. Only two years later, however, the city finally fell under British control. In 1919, after Germany's defeat and the end of World War I, German East Africa was redistributed by the League of Nations. While parts of it were subjected to Belgian and Portuguese authority, the largest proportion of the territory became a British mandate and was shortly thereafter renamed Tanganyika Territory. As the colony was not particularly attractive for the British authorities in comparison to economically much more profitable ones, "Britain's economic interest in Tanganyika was confined to imperial firms which took the pickings of the old regime" (Iliffe 1979, 261), one of which was the sisal estates in Tanga, the largest of their kind in the colony.

Throughout the following decades, sisal production remained one of the main drivers of Tanganyika's economy and sustained the development of Tanga, which grew into the main site of the production of the fiber. Under the leadership of Julius Nyerere (1964–1985) and his unity party Tanganyika African National Union (TANU, which later became the Chama Cha Mapinduzi [CCM], the party that has ruled Tanzania ever since), however, the country's sisal production decreased significantly after the base of the industry was affected by the nationalization of sisal estates in 1967 (Tenga 2008, 36)—the year when the signing of the Arusha Declaration rang in Tanzania's socialist era—and the prices for the fiber on the world market dropped significantly due to competition with synthetic fibers (Hartemink and Wienk 1995, 93). This global development heralded the decline of Tanga too. While "the sisal industry attracted labor movement from other upcountry regions" to the city, and during the period of large-scale exports "Tanga ranked second from Dar es Salaam in terms of population and economic activities," the decline of the industry "influenced the decline of harbor activities and growth of the city economy" (Tanga City Council 2007, 20). This negative development correlated with a decrease in Tanga's population size, as many people who had been working in the sisal industry and who had lost their jobs migrated to other parts of the country in search of wage labor, or returned to their rural homes (Tanga City Council 2007, 32). Tanga's population growth rate of 4.8 percent between 1988 and 2002 was the lowest "since the pre-independence period" (Tanga City Council 2007, 27).

At the time of my research, Tanga was still struggling to regain some of its former economic importance. A report by the Tanga City Council states that in 2007, there were some twenty small- to large-scale industrial companies (engaged in mineral exploitation and cement production, milk processing, agriculture, fishing, and manufacturing), some of which had been publicly owned during

Tanzania's socialist era and had later been privatized (Tanga City Council 2007, xv). However, large parts of Tanga's population were unable to find regular employment and unavoidably turned to the informal sector. In the mid-2000s, it was estimated that nearly half of Tanga's labor force was earning their livelihood through informal economic activities, while the per capita income of a citizen living in Tanga leveled at 270,000 TSH[2] (Tanga City Council 2007, 36).

There are no official statistics available on the composition of Tanga's population with regard to ethnicity and religious affiliation. This is attributable to the socialist and postsocialist governments' attempts to create a unified body of national citizens, which included the deliberate omission of the citizens' religious and ethnic affiliation in the five national censuses conducted between 1967 and 2012. The above cited report by the Tanga City Council thus simply claims that Tanga is "inhabited by ethnic groups of mixed tribes and religions," that "socially there is no discrimination among them despite a wide difference in dialects and clans," and that "economically they share smoothly all business opportunities and development utilities that are offered and availed by the City" (Tanga City Council 2007, 27). A report of the National Bureau of Statistics and Regional Commissioner's Office dating from 2008 provides only slightly more precise information, by listing the Wadigo, Wasambaa, Wabondei, Wazigua, and Wasegeju as the dominant ethnic groups in the Tanga region, while several others "from up-country Regions have moved and settled in the Region in search of employment" (National Bureau of Statistics and Tanga Regional Commissioner's Office 2008, 4).

My own research sample confirms that the ethnic composition of Tanga's population is highly diverse. While many of the research participants identified as Msambaa (singular of Wasambaa, an ethnic group living in the Usambara mountains) and Mdigo (one of the groups indigenous to the area), many others claimed ethnic affiliation to groups from all over Tanzania and even Kenya and the Democratic Republic of Congo.[3] In many cases, the parents of these respondents had migrated to Tanga during the 1950s and 1960s; that is, at a time when the city's economy had been flourishing and a large number of wage laborers were hired by the many local industries.

In light of Tanga's ethnic heterogeneity, it would be oversimplifying to refer to the city's inhabitants merely as "Swahili." Many of my interlocutors whose parents had migrated to Tanga over the course of three to four decades identified themselves with their parents' ethnic group rather than with "Swahili culture" and were proficient in their parents' home language in addition to Swahili. Even those with long-term genealogical ties to ethnic groups indigenous to Tanga predominantly self-identified as, for instance, Mdigo or Mzigua rather than Mswahili. This did not prevent them, however, from referring to themselves as Waswahili in *particular* contexts or in reference to *particular* cultural characteristics such as food or music, while discursively utilizing "Swahiliness" as a marker of moral inferiority in *other* contexts and at *other* times. This speaks for the necessity of conceiving of Swahili (as any other ethnic) identity as the outcome of often politically contested processes of (self-) ascription, as well as a flexibly and strategically deployable social construct. While some scholars of East African societies thus define "the Swahili" through their common features of the use of Swahili as a first language, a specific internal social structure and stratification, and a distinctive Islamic coastal culture (Caplan 2004; Horton and Middleton 2000), this does not necessarily mean that the people who are classified as Swahili according to such criteria solely and consistently self-define as such.

With regard to Tanga's religious demography, only rough estimations can be made. While for Tanzania as a whole, the estimates on the breakdown of religious affiliation have varied widely over the past decades (Otiso 2013, 46), a survey in 2010 with a sample of 1,500 participants concluded that 60 percent of Tanzanian citizens were Christian, 36 percent Muslim (Pew Forum on Religion and Public Life 2010, 12), and the remaining 4 percent, by implication, belonged to other religious denominations, adhered to "African traditional religious practices," or were atheists.[4] As for Tanga, I can only assume on the basis of my personal impressions that Muslims outnumber Christians and the members of other, notably smaller Hindu and Sikh religious communities. This impression is in accordance with accounts on Islam in East Africa, which state that the majority of Tanzania's Muslim population resides in Zanzibar (more than 90 percent of the archipelago's population are claimed to be Muslim—see Van de Bruinhorst 2007, 94) and the coastal area of the mainland.

Finally, it is important to note that, as in other Tanzanian coastal areas, Tanga's Muslim and Christian communities are highly heterogeneous. While many moderate Muslim groups form part of the government-endorsed Central Muslim Council of Tanzania (*Baraza Kuu la Waislamu Tanzania*, BAKWATA), other revivalist or reformist groups such as the *Ansuari Sunna* have also emerged, particularly in the context of postindependence economic decline since the 1970s. These various revivalist groups, often externally financed and inspired by reformists in Egypt, Kuwait, and Saudi Arabia, "combine a religious and political agenda, with very varying emphases" (Becker 2007, 25). Yet they are largely unified in their proposition of "purifying religious practice from anything they consider 'innovation' (*bid'a*), that is, additions made after the Prophet's lifetime" (Becker 2007, 25), and thus in their "deep concern with the promotion of 'true faith' and the spiritual and moral integrity of fellow Muslims" (Dilger 2014, 60). Tanga's Christian community is similarly diverse. It comprises long-established Catholic, Lutheran, and Anglican mission churches but also so-called African-initiated and (neo-)Pentecostal churches, some of which were only founded in the past two decades and exhibit revivalist tendencies similar to their Muslim counterparts with whom they engage in a "competition . . . for resources and moral and spiritual hegemony in the urban setting" (Dilger 2014, 55).

Tanga's Therapeutic Economy

The Biomedical Health Care Sector

During the early years of the twentieth century, Tanga was not only an important mainstay of German East Africa's economy, but also one of the main locations of the establishment of biomedical research and preventive and curative services in the colony. Around the turn of the nineteenth century into the twentieth, Tanga was a significant site of malaria research conducted by German scientists, including Dr. Robert Koch who made essential contributions to the discovery of the disease (Beck 1977, 14f). Around the same time, a three-story building was constructed to house one of the largest government-run hospitals of the German colony at the time. The imposing structure, widely referred to as "the Cliff Block"— presumably due to its prominent position on top of the cliff coast of the Tanga Bay—still stands in the compound of the Bombo Regional

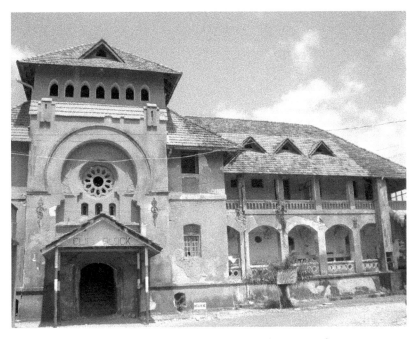

Figure 1.3. "Cliff Block," Bombo Regional Hospital © Dominik Mattes 2008.

Hospital, though it has been out of use for many years and is in an advanced state of disrepair (Figure 1.3).

Since the period of German colonial rule, various new hospital buildings have been built next to the Cliff Block (Figure 1.4). Together, they form the Bombo Regional Hospital, which has a capacity of approximately four hundred beds and comprises a dental clinic as well as surgical, internal, gynecological and obstetrics, and pediatric wards. Moreover, several smaller health centers and dispensaries have been erected to cater to Tanga's population.[5] The extension of the city's infrastructure of public health care delivery was particularly promoted during the 1970s. Aiming at a general elevation of living standards in Tanzania, not least through improving citizens' access to primary health care across the country, the socialist regime governing at the time adopted a new health policy of "treat[ing] people as close to their homes as possible in the smallest, cheapest, and most simply equipped rural health units," which meant shifting "expenditure from hospitals and doctors to health centres, dispensaries, village health posts, and auxiliaries" (Iliffe 1998, 203).

31

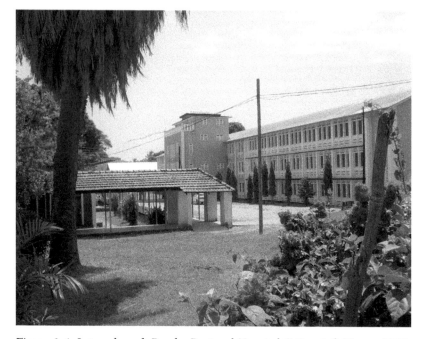

Figure 1.4. Internal ward, Bombo Regional Hospital © Dominik Mattes 2008.

While there had therefore been a steady increase in biomedical facilities in Tanga during the colonial and socialist eras, as elsewhere in the country, the government regimes, nevertheless, consistently struggled to provide adequate quality in terms of the health care that was provided in these facilities. Under German and British colonial rule, a major challenge consisted of recruiting and training a sufficient number of medical professionals to fill the positions in the newly established hospitals, health centers, and dispensaries, not least because for a long time, Africans were deemed incapable of filling the higher positions in the medical sector and were only used as "auxiliaries [who were] allocated purely menial functions and learned by practical apprenticeship" (Iliffe 1998, 2; see also Bruchhausen 2006). Even when colonial authorities became increasingly aware that adequate health care provision in their territory could only be achieved by qualifying local personnel, the efforts to install the necessary training facilities remained limited. Only after Tanzania had gained independence were government approved medical degree courses established, which would finally allow larger numbers of Tanzanians to enter the higher cadres of the medical profession (cf. Bruchhausen 2006, 123f). Yet it still remained difficult to staff the increasing number of health facilities with sufficient and adequately trained personnel, whose services were in increasing demand due to rapid population growth in the country.

The socialist government's priority to invest in preventive health services in rural areas, at the cost of further development and adequately equipping existing urban-based health facilities, left large parts of the state's public health care infrastructure in a desolate state. "By the late 1980s the socialist medical experiment was close to failure," concludes historian John Iliffe.

> Health facilities had multiplied, as had staff at all levels, but the facilities were often dilapidated and the staff demoralized, chiefly for lack of money. . . . Poverty explained why the main complaint against health facilities was lack of drugs, for poverty not only prevented their procurement and distribution but corrupted the medical staff who sold them for their own profit. (Iliffe 1998, 212)

After 1992, when an amendment of the constitution allowed for multiple political parties for the first time since the adoption of the Arusha Declaration in 1967, the situation remained critical despite increasing international development assistance to Tanzania. In order to counter a grave economic crisis that seized the country during the late 1970s and early 1980s as a consequence of a global oil and energy crisis, the government had self-imposed the first structural adjustment measures in an attempt to reinvigorate the national economy. In 1986, the World Bank and IMF tied the grant of loans to Tanzania to the accomplishment of more extensive SAPs, laid out by the government in the Economic Recovery Program (Rösch 1995, 95ff). The austerity measures that were applied over the following years in accordance to this and its successor program had particularly far reaching consequences for the country's health sector. An employment freeze between 1993 and 1996 in the public sector left government health institutions deprived of one third of their workforce (Kwesigabo et al. 2012, S39); cuts in government expenditure resulted in deteriorating health infrastructure and a lack of drugs and other medical equipment; and the introduction of cost-sharing programs "placed heavy burdens on patients and their families, who, in addition to hospital and clinic charges, had to cover costs for transports, food, (admission) bribes, drugs, and other medical supplies" (for further critical analyses of the consequences of SAPs in Tanzania, see Benson 2001; Dilger 2012, 65; Lugalla 1995; and Turshen 1999).

The long-term consequences of self- and externally imposed austerity politics during the 1980s and 1990s are still being felt in the health sector to this day. As Kwesigabo and colleagues (2012, S40) argue, "Of all the cuts in the Tanzanian health workforce in the 1990s, it was training institutions, the cornerstone of skills development for human resources that were most adversely affected." This led to the fact that as late as 2008, the government lamented "a severe [65 percent] shortage of human resource[s] at all levels [of health care delivery, which is] exacerbated by the expanded population, HIV/AIDS pandemic, malaria, tuberculosis and others" (The United Republic of Tanzania 2008, 7).

At the time of my research, a considerable number of biomedical facilities were providing health care in Tanga. These included the Bombo Regional Hospital, three public and three private health centers, nineteen dispensaries, and two private medical practices. Additionally, there were two private pharmacies and a handful of private medical laboratories. However, public health facilities were routinely overcrowded with large numbers of patients, which stretched the personnel to the limits of their capacities. Positions for specialized physicians often remained vacant for extended periods of time. Technological equipment was often malfunctioning, if it was available at all, and supplies of basic medical consumables were often interrupted, obliging patients to turn to private facilities to receive the services they needed. Finally, for highly specialized care, such as cancer treatment, patients had to seek treatment in consultant hospitals or private specialized care units in faraway places, such as Dar es Salaam or Arusha, which often exceeded their financial and logistical capacities.

Biomedical health care provision, in short, was often experienced as highly deficient and difficult to access, which might explain why many people resorted to other healing traditions in situations of impaired health. But this was not the only reason. So-called traditional medical practices have never lost their appeal, because they accommodated people's need to make sense of their suffering in accordance with locally specific understandings of health, illness, and healing, which also accommodate social, moral, and spiritual-religious dimensions. Rather than leading to the successive abandonment of nonbiomedical healing practices, the advent of colonial biomedicine in Africa thus instigated processes of medical hybridization, in the sense that African healing systems "tended rather to absorb and internalize, to 'indigenize,' those elements of biomedical practice which seemed most effective and most impressive" (Vaughan 1991, 24). In many ways, biomedicine thus fell in line with many other "external" healing practices, which had been flexibly and pragmatically incorporated into East African therapeutic knowledge and practice over the previous centuries.

Nonbiomedical Therapeutic Options

Across Tanzania, Tanga has the reputation of being a hotspot for traditional healers, and indeed during my research, I encountered countless people, including patients undergoing ART, who in one way or another resorted to the use of traditional medicine, as well as nonbiomedical healers who treated people living with HIV/ AIDS (see especially Chapter 8). Before I provide an outline of the traditional medical practices prevalent in Tanzania in general, and in Tanga in particular, however, a short note on terminology is in order.

As mentioned above, an essential problem when using the term "traditional" in combination with nonbiomedical practices and practitioners lies in the fact that this brackets together an enormous variety of nonbiomedical healing traditions and their representatives, and thus implies a nonexistent homogeneity in an often politically instrumentalizing way (Bruchhausen 2010, 262; see Feierman 1985, 100). Furthermore, denoting indigenous healing practices as "traditional" is problematic, because the notion often serves as a euphemistic substitute for "static, irrational, unconscious, collective, and ineffectual; the opposite of 'modern,' euphemistic for dynamic, rational, conscious, individualistic, and effectual" (Feierman and Janzen 1992, xvi) that are held to be the exclusive attributes of "Western" scientific biomedicine (see also Marsland 2007). Nonetheless, I hold on to the terms "traditional medicine/healer/healing," not least because healers in Tanga defined themselves in English as "traditional healers" and placed great emphasis on the distinctions between their therapeutic practices and underlying epistemological assumptions and those of biomedicine. This, in turn, once more emphasizes the need

> to distinguish between "traditional medicine" as a failed analytical category and "traditional medicine" as a resilient, polyvalent "folk category" that is deployed by a multiplicity of folk, including social scientists, representatives of international health organizations and development institutions, biomedical practitioners, and state officials as well as, revealingly, healers and their patients. (West and Luedke 2006, 5)

With this in mind, let me briefly circumscribe the disease etiologies and therapeutic approaches that have commonly been denoted as "traditional medicine" in Tanzania and that significantly shaped many of my interlocutors' way of thinking about their illness and possible routes to healing. Under the premise that every "historiography of African medical practice is simultaneously a historiography of European imaginations about and attitudes toward these ways of dealing with illness and healing" (Bruchhausen 2006, 141—translation mine), I follow medical historian Walter Bruchhausen's distinction between three major areas of disease causation that define the healing approaches of traditional healers in the country: God/nature, witchcraft, and spirits (Bruchhausen 2006, 143). According to this distinction, the origins of ill health are viewed as being found in the realms of the natural, social, and spiritual respectively, a distinction that in turn denotes "herbalists," "ritualists," and "spiritualists" as the corresponding traditional medical specialists (Bruchhausen 2006, 144). Herbalists, it is assumed, are experts in medicinal plants, of local *materia medica*. From a scientific vantage point, their practice is rational and effective as it is presumably based on a long tradition of acquiring knowledge about the therapeutic effectiveness of a particular plant through processes of trial and error. This explains why local herbalists throughout the past decades have received the greatest attention from government authorities, with the intention of complementing deficient biomedical health care delivery with standardized, scientifically approved traditional medicine, and with medical scientists who aim to discover and market new plant-based biomedical pharmaceuticals.

A closer look, however, reveals that the implicit comparison of traditional Tanzanian healers working with plant-based medicines with Western phytotherapists applying therapeutic herbal substances is, in many cases, misguided. Healers' precise choice of plants, Bruchhausen points out, is often explained as being a matter of spirits showing these plants to them in their dreams, rather than being based on previous empirical trials, which thus renders these practices highly idiosyncratic (Bruchhausen 2006, 57). Moreover, traditional healers often deliver their plant-based substances to patients in the form of cremated and pulverized leaves or highly watered-down brews. While, from a scientific perspective, such practices cannot be effective, since they destroy the plant material's biochemical potential, healers do not consider this to be paradoxical, because they ascribe their medicines' effectiveness to the rituals that go along with the application of the herbal medicines through oral ingestion or incisions in the body. While this already points to an overlap and blend of categories in terms of disease causation, which will be addressed further below, let me turn to the next category of healers, namely witchcraft specialists.

The essential point about illness and other kinds of misfortune that are associated with witchcraft is that they are viewed as result-ing from malevolent *human* influence by way of the application of evil magic and malicious medicine. Witchcraft victims as well as the healing experts to whom they turn for help are thereby less concerned with the possibility of supernatural interference per se, but rather with the motives of the persons who have applied black magic, or commissioned others to do so, in order to make a person sick (cf. Bruchhausen 2010, 187). This means that witchcraft is essentially a matter of impaired social relations and moral judgment (cf. Stroeken 2012).

Ideas regarding the particular manifestations of witchcraft, the way in which the respective knowledge and practical expertise is acquired, and what kinds of persons predominantly practice it vary widely from one place and community to another. In order to analytically structure this diversity, early anthropologists suggested distinguishing between witchcraft—as an innate capacity to bring affliction upon someone (sometimes even unconsciously) by way of a "mystical power inherent in [one's] personality" (Marwick 1990, 12)—and sorcery—as a learned expertise in harming others illicitly through the use of black magic and pernicious material objects and substances that are also called "medicines" (Evans-Pritchard 1987; Middleton 1992, 182; Middleton and Winter 1963, 2f). Yet ethnographic examples from various parts of East Africa, including Tanzania, have revealed this categorization to be too rigid and often inapplicable (Bruchhausen 2006, 285; cf. Middleton and Winter 1963). As the following quote demonstrates, this does not mean, however, that the discursive and practical manifestations of witchcraft in different geographical locations have nothing in common.

> Whether witches are said to be elderly women . . . or young children who have inherited witchcraft paraphernalia from their parents, whether witchcraft powers derive from a physical site within the body or from [purchased] substances . . . discourses on witchcraft in Tanzania consistently address themes of envy, greed, consumption, cannibalism and death. They are, then, firmly implicated in local and national debates about poverty and development . . . at the same time that they demand strategies for dealing with witchcraft and those alleged to practice it. (Green and Mesaki 2005, 373)

The latter part of this quote points to the fact that witchcraft is by no means merely a negligible remnant of African "premodern" beliefs, irrationality, and superstition that will gradually vanish in correlation with stricter legal prosecution and increasing Western education, as colonial authorities once expected (cf. Englund 1996, 257). To the contrary, if one takes into account the fact that witchcraft allegations and their respective counter-activities are articulated as a commentary on and reaction to increasing social distortions and inequalities precipitated by transnational capitalism and global market liberalization, the phenomenon needs to be viewed as "an integral aspect of contemporary disparate modernities" (see also Green and Mesaki 2005, 372; Comaroff and Comaroff 1993; Geschiere and Roitman 1997). Not surprisingly then, collective witchcraft finding movements and cleansing rituals occur consistently to this day in Tanzania and many other parts of Africa (Bruchhausen 2006, 207; Mesaki 1993; Yamba 1997).

While witchcraft is a framework that shapes people's thoughts and practices in relation to illness, affliction, and healing all over Tanzania, the same applies for the matter of spirit possession, which brings us to the third category of traditional healers, the "spiritualist," who deals with impaired health and other kinds of misfortune inflicted on people as the consequence of spirit possession. Bearing

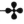

in mind "the Islamization of African cults and Africanization of Islam" (Behrend and Luig 1999, xv), a process of mutual borrowing, influence, and convergence that has taken place in a particularly intense way along the Swahili coast over the course of many centuries, a first step in approaching the phenomenon of spirit possession consists of distinguishing between two larger traditions of spirit possession that often merge in the discourse and practice of Swahili spirit specialists and their clients. The first is a wide range of pre-Islamic rituals and cults of affliction, which are widespread across sub-Saharan Africa and are based on "the interpretation of misfortune in terms of domination by a specific non-human agent and the attempt to come to terms with the misfortune by having the afflicted individual, under the guidance of a 'doctor' of that mode, join the cult association venerating that specific agent" (Turner 1968, 15f). Such cults of affliction have been observed in all parts of sub-Saharan Africa; and despite a myriad of regional differences in terms of the exact implementation of the respective healing rituals, they have been observed to feature many commonalities. These are, for instance, the importance of the "patterned rhythm of words, the use of performance dance, and the invocations or the songs that articulate the affliction and the therapeutic rite" (Feierman and Janzen 1992, 108), but, most of all, the central role of drumming, which is why, also in reference to the colloquial emic term for such rituals, they are referred to as *ngoma* (Swahili: drum). "The drumming," states John Janzen, "is considered to be the voice or influence of the ancestral shades or other spirits that visit the sufferer and offer the treatment" (Janzen 1992, 1).

Ngoma entails the idea that the spirits of ancestors or other supernatural entities take possession of people and thus exert a negative influence on their well-being and affairs of everyday life, at least as long as they are not properly venerated and respected. These afflictive forms of possession need to be countered by healing rituals that may take several days. They are often attended by many members of the respective possession cult and the wider community, and are guided by a specialist healer who has expertise with regard to the specific malicious spirit and is thus able to induce him or her to release the possessed person.

Throughout the previous centuries, *ngoma* cults of affliction have entered into reciprocal relations with other religious traditions, for instance, in the context of African Independent Churches (Janzen 1992, 1). Along the Swahili coast, they have coalesced with conceptions of different types of spiritual beings that are mentioned in the Qu'ran (cf. Bruchhausen 2006, 268), and have thus formed a bricolage that is distinctive for the Swahili coast and comprises a large pantheon of spirits (*majini*, Singular: *jini*)[6] that can potentially take possession of humans. While they are supernatural, the spirits are ascribed remarkably human characteristics. "They can be male or female, Muslim, Christian, Jewish or pagan, evil or benign; they can be of low or high status, willing or not willing to marry, hungry or thirsty, ugly or attractive, greedy or satisfied" (Mackenrodt 2011, 91). Some are categorized according to their ethnicity, geographic origin, and religiosity, so that people speak, for instance, of the Maasai, Arabic, and even European spirits (respectively *majini ya kimasai*, *majini ya kiarabu*, *majini ya kizungu*), spirits of the coast (*pwani*) and of the African interior (*bara*), and pagan (*kafiri*) and Muslim (*kiislamu*) spirits (Bruchhausen 2006, 266f; Giles 1995, 90).

A central element of spirit possession on the Swahili coast is the spirits' ambivalence. They can be a nuisance and inflict serious pain and illness on their victims. But, when regularly appeased through the right means, they can also "protect and assist in all manner of endeavors and may bring supernatural gifts of divining and curing (*uganga*)" (Giles 1987, 241). The rituals evolving around spirit possession (*kilinge*),[7] therefore, predominantly serve the aim of establishing beneficial and peaceful relationships with spirits by properly revering them and making offers such as food, incense, or an animal sacrifice, rather than confronting and exorcising them from the possessed person's body, which serves as their "vehicle" (Bruchhausen 2006, 291f; see also Giles 1995, 90). People who are troubled by a particular spirit often consult a diviner in order to receive a diagnosis of which spirit exactly is causing their disturbance before they are referred to a healer who, through her/his own experience (usually in the form of periodically being possessed by this spirit her/himself), has acquired special expertise on how to deal with this particular supernatural entity (cf. Giles 1987, 240).

It is important to note that in the practice of traditional healers, the three above-presented disease etiologies and correlated modes of diagnosis and therapy overlap, influence, and depend on one another (Bruchhausen 2006, 143f). During my research in Tanga, I met *waganga wa kienyeji* (lit. local healers)[8] whose services included spirit veneration and exorcism, protection from witchcraft and treatment of related afflictions, herbalism, Qu'ranic healing, bone-setting, and ancestor veneration. None of the six healers (all of whom were Muslim) whom I interviewed and in whose healing consultations I participated could be clearly classified as "herbalist," "ritualist," or "spiritualist." They all conceptually and practically combined particular elements of the different domains of traditional healing, and, in some cases, integrated additional components from entirely different therapeutic traditions. While four concurrently offered herbalism, divination, and spirit exorcism, a fifth additionally engaged in antiwitchcraft practices, and a sixth claimed also to offer homeopathy and *reiki* treatment (a form of energy healing through the laying-on of hands originating from Japan) as part of his therapeutic portfolio.

In order to complete the overview of Tanga's therapeutic economy, finally, the matter of faith healing within Christian churches has to be mentioned. As will be explored in greater depth in Chapter 8, at the time of my research, there was a range of Christian denominations, particularly (neo-)Pentecostal churches, that offered collective prayer sessions for congregants suffering from illness, including HIV/AIDS, as well as individual spirit deliverance ceremonies, which held out the promise of cure from chronic and acute health conditions inflicted through satanic influence and spirit possession. In contrast to the *ngoma* rituals and more Islamic-oriented approaches to the phenomenon of spirit possession, in this context, spirits were exclusively conceptualized as malicious and dangerous entities from which affected persons needed to be delivered through the power of prayer and the reciting of the "word of God." Even though Christian pastors at times tended to dismiss traditional healing practices, such as *ngoma* cults, as backward and pagan customs, the attractiveness of their own activities of religious healing may be associated to the very "integration of African ecstatic religiosity and African conceptions of spiritual and moral disease causation" (Bruchhausen 2010, 257—translation mine) into their own healing framework, which once more speaks to people's refusal to deal with illness in an exclusively secular manner.

Social Support for People Living with HIV/ AIDS

The Tanga AIDS Working Group

The most relevant institution providing assistance to people living with HIV/AIDS in several districts of the Tanga Region during the time of my research was the Tanga AIDS Working Group (TAWG), which had its headquarters on the compound of the Bombo Regional Hospital and was well-known far beyond the city's confines. In 1990, the TAWG had evolved from the initiative of traditional healers and clinicians working in Pangani (a small coastal town some 35 km south of Tanga) "with the overall goals of bridging the gap between traditional and hospital medicine for the benefit of people living with AIDS and reducing the HIV transmission in the region" (King 2002, 19). In 1994, the group was officially registered as an NGO. Since then, it has established an impressively wide range of working areas, ranging from HIV-prevention and stigma reduction campaigns to advocacy work and networking, voluntary counseling and testing (VCT), nutritional support, and the provision of home-based care and medical treatment. By the end of December 2008, the organization employed forty-four staff members, including clinicians, professional counselors, nurses, home-based care (HBC) providers, a secretary, and two drivers.

Since its beginning, cooperating with traditional healers has constituted an important pillar of the TAWG. It regularly conducted trainings for traditional healers in the region in order to provide them with comprehensive biomedical information on HIV/AIDS; enable them to safely treat HIV-positive patients; and establish reliable referral structures so as to ensure that patients in need find their way from healers' practices to the hospital where they can be enrolled on ART or receive other biomedical treatment.

Additionally, long before the advent of ART in Tanga, the TAWG established a collaboration with healers whose herbal medicines proved to be highly effective in the treatment of opportunistic infections (cf. McMillen 2004). In the absence of biomedical treatment, these medicines significantly contributed to clients' well-being by helping them "increase appetite ... gain weight, stop diarrhea, reduce fever, clear up oral thrush, resolve skin rashes and fungal infections, treat herpes zoster, and clear ulcers" (Scheinman 2002, 3f). Until early 2009 (see Chapter 7), the TAWG provided the medicines gratis to those who were not yet eligible for ART, with the result that many patients' health conditions improved significantly within a short period of time. In fact, I met a number of people who had been taking the herbs for several years and whose health status had remained stable enough to obviate the necessity of initiating ART. This can certainly be taken as evidence for the mutually fruitful and highly successful collaboration of biomedical health workers and traditional healers, which makes the TAWG "an outstanding example of how positive results can be achieved in the fight against AIDS by using local, culturally relevant expertise and resources to provide low-cost care and prevention for people living with AIDS" (King 2002, 19).

Aside from the provision of herbal medicines, a large number of people living with HIV/AIDS in Tanga benefited from the TAWG's HBC program. The organization's staff included several trained nurses holding certificates in HBC and HIV counseling who regularly visited patients (many of whom were living with ARVs) in their homes in order to check on their progress, provide them with medications and/or emergency medical treatment such as infusions, initiate referrals to the hospital if needed, provide psychological assistance in difficult life situations, and at times provide education to family and household members on how to appropriately care for HIV patients. In 2008, the organization conducted a total of 7,519 home care visits, with an average of four visits per household (Mtullu et al. 2009, 7). The large number of patients requiring HBC services could only be managed with the help of nearly one hundred volunteers (in the following referred to as community HBC providers), most of whom had no professional medical background and had only completed basic HBC training. While they were thus unable to provide medical care at their clients' homes, they nevertheless constituted an important connecting link between ART patients and CTCs; and aside from providing psychological support, they organized help in case of medical and other emergencies.

A further important institution of the TAWG were the Community Health, Information, and Care Centers (CHICCs), which at the time of my research, it had established in Tanga, Muheza, Pangani, Lushoto, and Korogwe. In these centers, HIV testing and counseling was provided, information material on HIV/AIDS was made available to the public, and—at least at the center in Tanga—educational films on HIV and other health issues were regularly screened for groups of mostly young adults who squeezed together into the small TV room. Moreover, Tanga's CHICC served as a venue for the meetings of the (self-)support groups belonging to an association called Tanga People Living with HIV/AIDS (TALPHA [sic]). As will be explored in greater detail in Chapter 7, these groups constituted an important source of information as well as material and psychological support for a large number of HIV-positive people in Tanga, many of whom were living with ARVs.

Other Institutions Working in the Field of HIV/AIDS

The second important NGO providing social services to people living with HIV/AIDS in Tanga was the Tanzania Red Cross Society Tanga Branch (in the following referred to as TRC), which had started to provide HBC in 2006. The program was predominantly financed with funds from the US Center for Disease Control, which were channeled through the transnational NGO Pathfinder International. In August 2011, the TRC was supervising ninety-eight community HBC providers who, similar to their colleagues from the TAWG, had received basic training in HBC and related matters such as "food and nutrition" and "HIV stigma and discrimination." Some of these providers catered to upward of one hundred clients, each of whom was supposed to be visited at least twice a month, which meant that their voluntary engagement took on the dimension of a full-time job. For this work, they received a monthly allowance, which during the fiscal year 2009–2010 amounted to 20,000 TSH. Aside from providing psychological support and counseling to their clients, these providers also distributed so-called HBC kits containing first aid material, some basic medications, and small quantities of soap to their clients. In emergency cases, they accompanied them to the nearest health center and assisted them in receiving adequate care and treatment. Like their colleagues from the TAWG, the TRC community HBC providers served as an important instrument to counter the problem of patients undergoing ART who were lost-to-follow-up.

An HIV testing and counseling program named *Angaza* (Swahili: shed light), an initiative funded by PEPFAR and led by the Anglican Church Tanga Deanery (in the following referred to as the Anglican

Church), in turn provided services to the public and people living with HIV/AIDS in Tanga in the form of a VCT center and materials, as well as moderate financial support for seventeen (self-)support groups (as of mid-September 2009) for ART patients in the city who had established small-scale income generating projects or intended to do so. While the Anglican Church did not provide any HBC services, members of the (self-)support groups under its supervision were regularly referred to the TAWG or TRC in order to receive services from these organizations. With funds from the Oxford Committee for Famine Relief (OXFAM), the Anglican Church also ran a small sisal farm whose profits were channeled into the Anglican Church's activities to support people living with HIV/AIDS.

The focus of two further organizations in Tanga was directed toward the support of AIDS orphans. The first, Pastoral Activities and Services for AIDS of the Roman Catholic Diocese in Tanga (PASADIT), predominantly supported the work of a local orphanage for HIV-positive children by covering their school fees. The African Women AIDS Working Group (AFRIWAG) equally enabled children who had lost their parents to AIDS to go to school by paying fees and for school materials.

Finally, it has to be mentioned that according to an oral report of Tanga Councils' HIV/AIDS Coordinator (25 May 2009), the City of Tanga was also providing some financial and material support for groups of people living with HIV as well as for AIDS orphans and widows and widowers. This support, however, seemed to be so marginal that throughout my entire research, I did not come across a single person infected with or affected by HIV/AIDS who mentioned the city council as a source of assistance. Even the PASADIT and AFRIWAG were hardly ever mentioned by those in need of support, implying that the TAWG and TRC were by far the most relevant institutions in this respect.

Research Methodology

I am drawing on fifteen months of ethnographic fieldwork in Tanzania carried out between September 2008 and September 2011. Throughout my research, I spent several weeks in Dar es Salaam in order to conduct interviews with relevant health officials and representatives of nationally operating NGOs and patient associations.

The largest part of my fieldwork, however, I spent in Tanga, where I stayed in an apartment just off the Bombo Regional Hospital, which housed the region's largest CTC.

In order to gain a comprehensive picture of what it means to provide and live with ARVs in the city, I drew on a range of research methods. I took extensive fieldnotes while conducting participant observation in biomedical facilities offering ART, VCT centers, (self-) support groups for people living with HIV/AIDS, patients' private homes, orphanages for children living with HIV,[9] the consultation sessions of traditional healers, and Pentecostal Sunday services. Additionally, I conducted semistructured interviews with forty-two ART patients, seventeen relatives and caretakers, thirty-two medical professionals, eight health officials, eleven traditional healers, and four religious leaders, as well as four focus group discussions with patients and one with a group of Muslim religious leaders (for further details, see Table 1.1).

Informal conversations with research participants, however, often proved to be more instructive than formal interviews or group discussions. Clinicians and nurses, for instance, spoke more freely

Table 1.1. Overview of research participants.

Category of interlocutors	Number of individuals interviewed	Number of focus group discussions
Patients	42 (22f, 20m; 9–55 years); 13 of them children and adolescents aged 9–19 years	4 (2 f/m, 1f, 1m)
Relatives/Caretakers	17 (15f, 2m)	–
Health care providers	32 (15 nurses, 11 clinicians, 2 pharmacists, 3 HBC providers, 1 laboratory technician)	–
Traditional healers	11 (all male)	–
Religious leaders	4 (2 Christian, 2 Muslim; 1f, 3m)	1 (Muslim, all male)
Health officials	3 NACP, 2 TACAIDS, 1 regional health management, 1 district health management, 1 council health management	–
NGOs	4 AIDS Relief, 4 TAWG, 1 TANOPHA, 1 NACOPHA	–

about their work constraints and partly tense relationships with colleagues or superiors over a cup of tea during their work break. And patients felt more at ease in revealing their skepticism and anxieties about their therapy or addressing emotionally fraught topics when they chatted with me while doing their daily household chores in their backyard.

Moreover, meeting and interviewing people undergoing ART once in one specific site—be it the hospital or private home—would have forestalled a more profound appreciation of the processual nature of a life with ARVs. It would also have prevented the development of a more nuanced sense of the articulation of patients' different illness- and treatment-related experiences in the wide range of microsocial contexts that formed their local moral worlds. In order to avoid this methodological (and epistemological) blind spot, I followed nine of the twenty-nine adult patients of my sample more closely throughout the entire research. I frequently visited them at home, participated in burials of their relatives, and accompanied them to their support-group meetings. I got to know their partners, families, neighbors, and friends. I gained insight into the social composition of their households and a sense for the material and economic bases and constraints of their existence, the organization and activities of their everyday lives, and the immediate social relations in which their lives on ART were embedded and which were crucial for securing their livelihood. In this way, I was able to witness the fluctuating health states that many of them went through during the months following their treatment uptake, as well as incidents and processes of conflict and the (re)negotiation of social relationships within their predominantly kin-based social networks.

Getting Access and Sampling Strategies

Access to research participants was established in multiple ways. The TAWG formed a first "entry gate." This organization functioned as my local research partner, which every researcher who intends to conduct research related to medical issues in Tanzania has to have in order to receive research permission and ethical clearance from the Tanzania Commission for Science and Technology (COSTECH) and the National Institute for Medical Research (NIMR). As a very first step, I thus participated in several VCT sessions at the TAWG headquarters. This not only provided me with first impressions of the positioning of patients, or rather clients, vis-à-vis professional health care providers and the delicacy of speaking about HIV and related topics such as sexuality and domestic power relations, but also with my first interview partners, who declared themselves willing to talk about their experiences and to be accompanied through the extended procedure of being enrolled on ART after their positive test outcome. These participants were first asked by the counselor if they agreed to my being present during the counseling session, and I explained the purpose of my research to them only after they had received adequate post-test counseling.

Initially, I proceeded in the same way at the VCT center of the Bombo Regional Hospital. Nevertheless, after approximately six weeks, I shifted to the HIV (self-)support groups run by the TAWG in order to recruit further patient participants for the study. Contrary to my expectations, the response of group members to my request was mostly overwhelmingly positive. Almost after every group meeting, I had a further list of ten to twenty names and contact details of group members who had invited me to visit them in their homes, would let me accompany them to their hospital appointments, and were willing to share their experiences of living with HIV and ARVs with me.

Only two of the twenty-nine interviewed adults had completed secondary school and received higher education. The remainder had completed primary school, and some had only rudimentary reading and writing capabilities. Correspondingly, the largest proportion of patients (twenty-four out of twenty-nine) did not have regular work contracts in the formal sector, but instead relied on a wide range of activities in the informal economy and with subsistence farming to secure their livelihoods. The generally low income and educational level of most of the patients who participated in the study reflects the clientele of the public HIV treatment centers in Tanga. Evidently, better-off people in need of ART received treatment at private facilities. Finally, I aimed to achieve a sample of patient participants with the greatest possible diversity with regard to the duration of their therapy. This information will be provided consistently each time a case study or quote of a particular patient is presented throughout the book.

Entry to the biomedical facilities providing ART was obtained via the Regional and District Medical Officers as well as the director of the Bombo Regional Hospital. With their permission, I approached the clinicians and nurses working at Tanga's CTCs. Most of the professionals quickly accepted my regular presence at their workplace, and throughout the months to follow, many of them went out of their way to support my research, share their views on the successes and challenges of ART provision, and grant me generous and detailed insight into their daily routines. I aimed to interview at least one nurse and one clinician per treatment center. Ultimately, however, I ended up interviewing almost the entire clinical staff at the Bombo Regional Hospital's CTC and a significant proportion of the personnel of five smaller centers, which will be described in more detail in Chapters 3 and 4.

As for the traditional healers, I tried to largely avoid resorting to the wide network of healers established by the TAWG, assuming that these healers might consider me to be a staff member of the organization and thus be reluctant to openly articulate ideas that did not correspond to a biomedical understanding of HIV/AIDS and its treatment. I rather relied, therefore, on people living with HIV/AIDS, who showed me the way to the homesteads of traditional healers residing in their neighborhoods.

Patients also helped me get access to religious leaders inasmuch as I approached two neo-Pentecostal churches that were reported to conduct healing sessions and services for people living with HIV/AIDS rather than, for instance, other mainline churches that were said not to offer any study relevant services. After I had conducted a focus group discussion with Muslim leaders of a liberal, government-near Muslim organization that had an official branch office in the city, I also established contact, through the knowledge of Muslim patients, with two sheikhs of Muslim communities who were more revivalist in orientation.

Doing Hospital Ethnography

An extended phase of participant observation at Tanga's governmental CTCs constituted a significant part of my research. These institutions included the Bombo Regional Hospital and three government health centers. The study also included two private medical institutions (one hospital of a size equivalent to the government health centers and one smaller private doctor's practice). Information on the articulation of ART provision at these facilities (see Chapter 4), however, was predominantly gained through semistructured interviews with their health staff.

For a four month period from December 2008 onward, I spent each day at one of the public CTCs in order to examine in detail the material conditions, work flows, and power dynamics involved in the enrollment of new patients in the treatment programs and the subsequent procedures of treatment monitoring and patient follow-up. I thus conducted a rather intense form of hospital ethnography (Van der Geest and Finkler 2004; Long et al. 2008). Doing participant observation in a specialized clinic space may include the assumption of diverse roles for the researcher (Van der Geest and Finkler 2004, 1998; Wind 2008), which is why I will specify in more detail what exactly I observed during my prolonged stays in Tanga's CTCs, the ways in which I actually participated in particular practices, and the nature of my relationships with the medical professionals working in these facilities.

The aim of doing participant observation in the CTCs was to gain a profound understanding of the procedures for patient enrollment and surveillance and the social and material factors that shaped this process, as well as the involved interactions between medical professionals and patients. To this purpose, I spent several hours per day (mostly the entire working day from around 7 a.m. to 5 p.m.) at one of the CTCs, where I observed the interactions going on at each "station" of the itinerary of treatment enrollment and patients' control visits (for a detailed description and analysis of these routines, see Chapter 4). These stations included the VCT sessions, the patients' registration at the CTC, treatment education sessions, doctor consultations, and the handing over of drugs at the pharmacies. Additionally, I accompanied many patients through the entire or parts of the enrollment procedure until they finally started to take their first doses of ARVs.

The innumerous hours I spent sitting, watching, chatting, and taking notes in various subspaces of the clinics proved to be invaluable for gaining an understanding of the micropolitics involved in treatment provision in terms of the particular power dynamics that shaped the interactions between clinic staff and their supervisors, among nurses and clinicians, and between medical professionals and patients. The CTC personnel quickly became accustomed to my daily presence and let me move more or less freely across the clinic spaces. As far as I noted, they had no difficulties in comprehending the purpose of my regular presence and my curiosity as a researcher, nor did they have any objections to my seemingly pointless habit of "just sitting around and taking notes," as has been reported from other hospital ethnography contexts (Wind 2008). It would be an exaggeration to designate my relationship with these staff as a form of friendship, as our encounters and interactions remained limited to the work context.

Many of the patients, in turn, evidently regarded me as a medical professional (even though I did not wear a white coat like the rest of the staff), which often found its expression in their addressing me with the title "doctor." Alternately, they saw me as a representative of the donor organizations supervising the CTCs, perhaps due to my constant note taking. One effect of this was that my relationship with some of the patients whom I recruited for the study on the hospital floors was initially characterized by a stark power imbalance. The deconstruction of this asymmetry, which was crucial for achieving a trusting relationship that would make patients feel comfortable enough to voice critical views of the CTC routines as well as to openly speak about treatment-related practices that, from a biomedical perspective, were considered noncompliant, subsequently took quite some time. The fact that some patients considered me a part of the CTC staff, who often displayed an authoritarian style when dealing with patients, may also be ascribed to the fact that the clinicians and nurses regularly asked me to assist them in encouraging new treatment enrollees and fostering their treatment adherence through spontaneous "pep talks" addressed to large crowds of waiting patients, which were usually delivered by nurses or "expert patients."

This leads me to the question of the "participant" part of my participant observation in the clinics and whether it really is the case that "in a hospital, participant observation in the true sense is an oxymoron" (Van der Geest and Finkler 2004, 1999). Obviously, this is a matter of how one defines "participation." I did not undergo any medical consultation or treatment myself, nor did I provide any treatment-related services at the CTCs in the fashion of the nurses and clinicians, and so it could be argued that my role was mostly confined to that of an observer. And yet, in addition to the "pep talks" that the medical professionals demanded I engage in, there were also other occasions where I took on a more active involvement, as, for example, when I explained to individual patients the details of the complex and at times incomprehensible procedures that they were expected to go through; when I tried to negotiate between health staff and patients in order to accelerate the processing of particularly weakened patients and save them from unbearably long waiting times; when I attempted to assist patients in accessing medical services that were temporarily unavailable at their regular treatment center in other institutions; or when I helped nurses to sort and distribute large piles of laboratory result slips to the waiting patients. Apart from this, my more passive presence at the CTCs carried a profound sense of "participation" too. For ultimately, it was the long and exhausting hours of sitting on the hospital floors with patients who were waiting for their doctor consultation or laboratory results, or, on the other side, spending tiring work days in small and stifling consultation rooms with clinicians until they had finally seen the last patient of the day, that gave me a sense of how physically and psychologically challenging, and often frustrating, mass ART provision can be, both for providers and receivers.

The above notwithstanding, it is important to note the limitations of understanding "the Other" in the hospital through such (or any other) forms of participation. As Gitte Wind argues in regard to the role of intersubjectivity in anthropological research on illness and suffering, "the best we can do is 'sharing of relevant experience' and remaining constantly reflective; but we should never forget that we are not committed in the same way as the people whose experience and world we are trying to grasp" (Wind 2008, 85f). In this vein, despite my prolonged and intense observations in Tanga's CTCs, my understanding of what it really felt like to work day after day in these constrained environments and to navigate the tiring procedures of treatment enrollment in the hope of finally being provided with urgently needed life-prolonging medications necessarily remains partial.

A Note on Language and Working with a Research Assistant

Even though, in addition to Swahili, English counts as the official language in Tanzania, most of my research participants' proficiency in English was marginal. It was predominantly the health officials at the national level who had a sufficient command of the language to the extent that enabled me to conduct the interviews with them in English. The majority of health care providers were not fluent enough to converse freely, and neither were the patients, their relatives and caretakers, religious leaders, and traditional healers. Consequently, I conducted the largest part of the interviews in Swahili. I had acquired basic Swahili skills before starting my fieldwork by way of self-study and regular conversation practice with a Tanzanian, and I completed a three-week intensive language course upon arriving in Tanga. This enabled me to understand most of the conversations going on at the treatment centers, for instance during the treatment education sessions. Nevertheless, throughout the first months of the research, my Swahili skills were insufficient to conduct one-on-one interviews in a satisfactory way.

I therefore hired a research assistant whose translation help was invaluable, particularly during the first research phase. Edna was in her early twenties and fluent in Swahili and English. Additionally, she held a BA degree in Cultural Anthropology and Tourism from the University of Iringa and was thus familiar with qualitative research methods, including ethnographic interviewing. The collaboration with Edna was not only highly useful in the sense that she helped me translate and transcribe interviews. Moving through the different research settings in her company was also very conducive to establishing rapport with research participants. I often had the impression that Edna's high capacity to quickly establish emotional ties, especially with female research participants, contributed significantly to the decrease of participants' reservations, particularly those of younger women, toward me as a male European researcher, and that her presence (as a fellow Tanzanian) generally facilitated the development of mutual trust between me and both female and male participants.

Moreover, I often discussed my first impressions with Edna, for instance after we had participated in the meeting of a (self-)support group, and more than once, our interpretations of the observed events differed in particular ways. In this way, she not only widened my perspective by bringing things into view that otherwise would have gone unnoticed, but she also constituted an important element in the process of data analysis, in the sense that she constantly challenged me to reflect on my own implicit assumptions that shaped my interpretations. Even though after some months I felt secure enough in speaking Swahili to conduct interviews without her help, I still often asked her to accompany me to interviews and meetings that I wished to attend. Edna also served as a great conversation partner in psychologically challenging situations, such as after the death of research participants, and she helped me to navigate particularly delicate situations in which my lack of cultural competency left me with a sense of uncertainty about how to adequately behave myself in the face of, for instance, conflictive relationships with research participants or particularly emotionally laden situations such as funerals.

Emotional and Practical Involvement in the Field

Conducting research in a field as delicate and morally and emotionally loaded as HIV/AIDS implicates a host of questions concerning the researcher's ethical responsibilities, engagement, and emotionality. I often found it difficult to find and sustain an ethically appropriate mode of interaction with research participants, and, just as frequently, I wondered how to deal with my own emotionality, positioning, and particular ways of engaging in the field. At various occasions throughout the research, I experienced a "crise de conscience," that is "a sense of responsibility for real or imagined disruptions that [my] interventions have effected" (Crapanzano 2010, 62). These were moments that exacted a decision about how much I was ready to get emotionally and practically involved in patients' day-to-day struggles to obtain appropriate health care, social support, and an income that would secure their survival. Yet I often felt that getting involved was not a matter of choice but of meeting an inevitable moral obligation.

Furthermore, conducting research as an empathic human being in a field of illness and suffering, where the social and biological existence of the Other—that is one's interlocutors and research participants—is not uncommonly endangered, raises the question of the extent to which it is possible (and desirable) to sustain a stance of "professional" detachment, distance, or abstraction, and to produce accounts that are "not influenced by personal feelings or opinions in considering and representing [the] facts" (Hegelund 2005, 648). When conducting research on illness, violence, death, and suffering, immersion can be a deeply moving and painful experience. "In a discipline where immersion in the field is essential to the generation of our disciplinary knowledge, we must enquire how far the human consequences of such immersion affect these very processes of production," deduces Davies (2010, 79). Immersion, he continues, "invariably involves some sort of ethical, cognitive, or emotional transformation, no matter how perfunctory or short-lived. In other words, fieldwork affects the very instrument, the anthropologist, through which data is gathered and represented" (Davies 2010, 80).

Coinciding with this thought, I hold it to be important to make my own affective situatedness transparent, particularly in relation to those instances and moments of the research where emotions such as anxiety, frustration, perhaps even anger, compelled me to engage at a practical level (see Case Studies B and C). Making the researcher's emotionality or affectivity transparent is, however, not only relevant because emotions often constitute the driving force behind practical engagement in the field (cf. Smith and Kleinman 2010), but also because this engagement can be of epistemological relevance, inasmuch as it provides a deeper understanding, or rather situated knowledge, of what is at stake for people involved in particular situations, events, or processes, such as long-term HIV therapy.

My intense involvement in the treatment trajectory of Zeinabu, a woman who had interrupted her ART as the consequence of a prolonged period of psychological impairment (see Case Study C), illustrates, for instance, the intimate causal connections between involvement, trust, and access to new avenues of gaining knowledge. I contend that it was my practical and emotional involvement in her ART reinitiation that opened doors that had been closed before. It was only after I had demonstrated that I cared about Zeinabu's well being in a practical way that she and her family started to talk openly about spirits, evil powers, witchcraft, and local healing practices, themes that they had not addressed before. Zeinabu even took me to a healer in her neighborhood whom she had consulted after repeated experiences of what I considered psychological dissociation, but that she interpreted as a sign of being "possessed." In this way, I was granted a more thorough insight not only into the detrimental syndemic effects of mental ill-health and HIV, but also into the complex superimpositions of various understandings of illness causalities and how they are discursively and practically managed in patients' social environments.

Through my involvement in Zeinabu's case, I also experienced in a particularly intense way how difficult it could be for patients to navigate through the hospital's intricate routine procedures, to keep up with endlessly occurring structural obstacles, and to deal with health professionals' arbitrariness, time constraints, and lack of expertise. My own deep frustrations and depletions that I felt accompanying Zeinabu during the lengthy process of ART reinitiation, in turn, rendered it comprehensible to me that after such deterring time, money, and energy-consuming experiences, some potential ART patients would simply cease to make further efforts and would rather resort to more accessible traditional health practitioners.

My practical involvement in Zeinabu's and other patients' cases also evoked the question of being biased, of opposing authority that *I* deemed unjust, of emotionally being driven to take the side of patients who epitomized vulnerable, poor, seemingly oppressed "victims." Roy D'Andrade (1995) has hinted at the problematic identification of what is "good" and "bad" inherent to such moralizing models as the "militant anthropology" proposed by Nancy Scheper-Hughes (1995), which challenged anthropologists to be politically engaged, to be involved witnesses rather than dispassionate observers. Although I disagree with D'Andrade on several points in his reproduction of Scheper-Hughes' appeal, I *do* agree that "badness and goodness are not simple properties of things but complex interactions between events and human intentions and welfare. ... Almost always what happens is the result not *just* of a knowing intentional act but of a complex web of causes" (D'Andrade 1995, 405f—emphasis in original). Thus, too hastily putting blame on particular actors in a particular field certainly is a risky attitude. Nevertheless, I hold the opinion that in the case of seriously ill people unable to negotiate access to life-saving ARVs by themselves, being the dispassionate, detached observer *or* the involved witness was not a choice at my disposal. While I deem my involvement to have been the only ethically justifiable decision in these situations, I still made constant efforts to reread emotionally challenging episodes, such as Zeinabu's ART reinitiation, which involved myself as an actor, during my analysis in order to question my own bias and appreciate, for instance, a psychiatrist's fragmentary training and pressing time constraints instead of solely focusing on his seemingly chilling indifference toward his patient's well being, or a clinician's anxiety and self-doubts rather than her disdainful reproaches alone.

Notes

1. Unless further specified, whenever I speak of Tanga, I refer to the city rather than the district or region.
2. At the beginning of my first field stay (September 2008), 1,000 TSH equaled ca. 60 US Cent. At the beginning of my second field stay (May 2011), 1,000 TSH equaled ca. 45 US Cent.
3. It is important to note here that these ethnic groups have to be viewed as social constructs that were reinforced during the period of colonial rule. Historian John Iliffe thus argues: "In precolonial Tanganyika each individual had belonged to several social groups: nuclear family and extended family, lineage and chiefdom, and perhaps clan and tribe. Circumstances had led some to emphasize one identity. . . . Yet groups and identities had remained so amorphous that to write of them is to oversimplify them" (Iliffe 1979, 318). Nonetheless, ethnic affiliation constitutes an important marker of identity for many Tanzanians. Each person I asked about his/her ethnic group (*kabila*) quickly came up with a decisive response, and on several occasions, respondents ascribed particular aspects of others' behavior explicitly to their ethnic affiliation.
4. Individuals' religious affiliation with Christianity or Islam, for instance, does not preclude their concurrent adherence to vernacular religious practices. In Chapter 8, I will provide examples of such "religious parallelism."
5. Health care delivery in Tanzania is ordered in a six-tier pyramidal pattern as follows: (1) Village health posts, consisting of one to two village health workers who have received three to six months of training, and who provide mostly preventive health services and care of minor ailments in homes. (2) Dispensaries that cater to between six thousand and ten thousand people, which are ideally run by a clinical assistant with two years of basic medical training, and "provide maternal and child health care, treat simple medical problems during pregnancy such as anemia, assist with normal deliveries, and offer basic outpatient curative care" (Kwesigabo et al. 2012, S37). (3) Health Centers that cater to fifty thousand persons, which are supposed to be run by "Clinical Officers (secondary school graduates with 3 years of basic medical training) . . . have 10-20 beds and provide reproductive health services and minor surgery" (Kwesigabo et al. 2012, S37). (4) District Hospitals, which are run by Assistant Medical Officers, that is "clinical officers with a further 2 years clinical training . . . supported by clinical officers and enrolled and registered nurses" (Kwesigabo et al. 2012, S37), and which provide "outpatient and inpatient services . . . including laboratory and x-ray diagnostic services and surgical services, including emergency obstetric care" (Kwesigabo et al. 2012, S37).

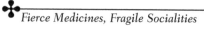

. (5) Regional Hospitals, which offer specialist services and whose staff include specialized medical officers in addition to Clinical and Assistant Medical Officers. (6) Referral/Consultant Hospitals, finally, which provide tertiary care "requiring advanced technology and highly skilled personnel" (Kwesigabo et al. 2012, S37).

6. Other Swahili terms for spirits are *mashetani* and *mapepo*. A clear distinction between these is difficult to establish and varies from one place or person to another. As Linda Giles states: "There is a great deal of variation in how these terms are used and some informants use them interchangeably. Many point out that, in fact, they are simultaneously general terms and specific types. For example, one can talk about any spirit as a jini or one may refer to a certain type of spirit—a 'jini proper.' Part of the problem in usage derives from the fact that jini and shetani are Arabic terms which are found in Middle Eastern and Islamic manuscripts. Thus their local interpretation has been coloured by Islamic interpretation and Middle Eastern concepts, which have been adopted to varying degrees by the local coastal people, depending on their literacy, Islamic training or religious tolerance of the spirit world" (Giles 1987, 240).

7. For further explications on this term, see Bruchhausen (2006, 286).

8. For a more detailed discussion of locally used Swahili terms for "traditional healer," and their users' respective underlying intentions in terms of positioning in relation to the discourse of "tradition" vs. "modernity" through the use of these terms, see Bruchhausen (2010) and Marsland (2007).

9. The topic of pediatric ART will not be covered in detail in this book due to matters of space. For a detailed exploration of its specificities, see Mattes (2014a).

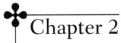

Chapter 2
Antiretroviral Treatment as a Global Mobile Force

Treatment for the Privileged and the Neglect of a Global Threat

After "the 'Dark Ages' of a world ravaged by a disease without any antiretroviral drugs" (Zuniga et al. 2008, 4), the advent of highly active antiretroviral combination therapy (HAART)[1] in the mid-1990s constituted a landmark in the fight against HIV/AIDS. The new combinations of multiple antiretroviral drugs in single compounds prevented the virus from replicating and quickly becoming drug resistant. Consequently, they could decrease patients' virus loads (ideally to a nondetectable level) and allow their damaged immune systems to recover. The introduction of the medicines thus initiated the transition of HIV/AIDS from a (usually) lethal disease to a more or less chronic infection (Whyte 2012), and, with the years, the conceptual framework of HIV/AIDS-related global health policy and management changed from crisis and exceptionality to long-term management, control, and normalcy (Beaudin and Chambre 1996; Kenworthy, Thomann, and Parker 2017; Rosenbrock et al. 2000).

Nevertheless, even though highly effective ARVs were introduced in the mid-1990s, the scope of these life-prolonging technologies remained restricted to the Global North for several years, while millions of untreated people continued to die of AIDS in less privileged areas of the world, such as sub-Saharan Africa. To a certain degree, this delay constituted an old indifference in a new disguise. Before the dawn of the treatment era, the mass proliferation of HIV/AIDS in many parts of the world had first remained undetected and was then later neglected (cf. Smith and Whiteside 2010, 3). But even when the dramatic scope of the HIV/AIDS epidemic, particularly in Africa (but also in other "underdeveloped" regions of the world), became ever more obvious, the international donor community made no serious efforts to increase access to ARVs beyond the boundaries of Europe and North America. Most African health systems were considered to be too underfunded to provide the expensive drugs through a public sector program, their infrastructure too deficient to secure a steady supply of ARVs and reliably monitor treatment progress over long periods of time for thousands of potential patients (cf. Schwartländer, Grubb, and Perriëns 2006). Such arguments were often built on broad sweeping generalizations about the alleged failures and deficiencies of African states (cf. Crane 2013). In addition, culturalist arguments were brought forward in an effort to legitimize the prioritization of HIV-prevention interventions over treatment in Africa. Africans were assumed to be incapable of complying to the rule of regularly taking ARVs at a certain time of the day (Messac and Prabhu 2013, 119), which raised the specter of rapid and wide-scale development of drug resistant virus strains that would eventually spill over to the "developed world" (Garrett 2007, 18; Jones 2004, 397). While such a discourse resonated with deeply historically rooted stereotypes about African difference (cf. Comaroff 1993), the ultimate reason for opposing a global ART rollout was economically motivated. In 1996, the costs for providing a patient with ARVs for one year ranged between ten and twenty thousand USD. Facing such prohibitively high costs, so the argument went, the international community's hands were tied. Even in 2002, when generic drug manufacturers had already begun to offer ARVs at a fraction of the first brand-name pharmaceuticals' costs, the authors of an influential cost-effectiveness analysis advocated against spending larger parts of the limited available resources for the HIV/AIDS response in sub-Saharan Africa on ART provision, since "prevention is at least 28 times more cost effective than HAART [and] funding HAART at the expense of prevention means greater loss of life" (Marseille, Hofmann, and Kahn 2002, 1851). Starting at around the turn of the millennium, the predominant focus on cost–benefit calculations, however, became increasingly contested. The study by Marseille and colleagues was strongly criticized for its narrowly economistic, utilitarian line of argumentation, and its implicit lack of attention to the international community's insufficient financial investments in global HIV treatment (Boelaert et al. 2002). Critics reframed the problem of the inaccessibility of ART in large parts of the world as an ethical issue, one that needs to be addressed *in spite* of concerns regarding cost-effectiveness.

These sentiments reverberate with the argumentation of the global activist movement that emerged in the late 1990s, which reformulated access to HIV treatment as a human right and successfully pressured governments and multinational pharmaceutical corporations to initiate processes that would eventually lead to significant ARV price reductions. Before taking a look at this activist coalition, however, it is necessary to explore why ARVs were so prohibitively expensive in the first place.

Intellectual Property Law and the Activist Response to the Treatment Gap in the Global South

In 1994, the WTO completed the Trade-Related Intellectual Property Rights (TRIPS) agreement, a multilateral agreement that came into force on 1 January 1995 and "revolutionized global patent law by requiring the standardization of [intellectual property] law among all [WTO] members" (Westerhaus and Castro 2006, 1230). This agreement required intellectual property in all fields of technology to be protected by patents on respective development processes and end products. Pharmaceutical companies were one of the major profiteers of this international covenant, as they were allowed to patent newly developed drugs and other health products, and thus to set monopolistic prices and prevent generic manufacturers from copying them for a period of twenty years. This was intended to enable the companies to amortize the investments they had made in the research and development of their products and to maintain the incentive for constant innovation within the drug industry as a whole.

The resulting long-lasting high price levels of the patented ARVs newly placed on the market from 1996 onward constituted an insurmountable barrier to low- and middle-income countries with underfunded health sectors and no domestic drug industry to finance public sector HIV treatment. Consequently, at the beginning of the twenty-first century, only some fifty thousand people in sub-Saharan

Africa had access to ARVs (WHO 2002a, 1), mostly through pilot initiatives and international research projects (cf., e.g., MSF et al. 2011; Nguyen et al. 2007), personal ties with charitable individuals or nongovernmental organizations in the Global North (cf. Nguyen 2010), or by purchasing them on the private market.

Susan Whyte and colleagues (Whyte et al. 2006) have compellingly described the dilemmas people faced in the era prior to public mass treatment programs in Uganda, when only newborn babies but not their HIV-positive mothers who were participating in PMTCT programs were treated with ARVs, and the inclusion criteria for research projects that included ARV provision were only met by a lucky few. Health workers felt obliged to not even mention the existence of HIV drugs to patients whom they deemed too poor to afford them, and families had to make painful decisions about which of their HIV-positive members was most in need of collective support to buy the medicines, a situation that often meant the withdrawal of support for the life projects—such as schooling—of other family members.

In order to at least partially mitigate the drastic consequences of the TRIPS agreement for public health care provision across the globe, in November 2001, the Fourth WTO Ministerial Conference in Doha, Qatar, issued the Doha Declaration on TRIPS and Public Health, which "affirmed the right of governments to take measures to protect public health" (Hoen 2009, xv) against the interests of profit-oriented transnational pharmaceutical corporations in the case of national emergencies. The first of these measures, compulsory licensing, "enables a competent government authority to license the use of a patented invention to a third-party or government agency without the consent of the patent-holder against a payment of 'adequate remuneration'" (Hoen 2009, xv). The second measure, parallel importation, applies to "cross-border trade in a patented product without the permission of the manufacturer or publisher. Parallel imports take place when there are significant price differences for the same good in different markets" (Hoen 2009, xv).

The applicability criteria for these so-called "TRIPS flexibilities" were, however, not so easy to fulfill, even though the generalized HIV epidemics in many countries indisputably constituted a national health emergency. Indeed, "multinational pharmaceutical companies and their home governments fiercely opposed [their] practical implementation" (Hoen 2009, 3). They threatened national governments who made or intended to make use of them with sanctions on the basis of bilateral free trade agreements that "limited the circumstances under which compulsory licenses may be issued or extend the life of patents beyond 20 years—a practice known as TRIPS plus" (IRIN News 2014). Moreover, effectively applying the TRIPS flexibilities required the successful iteration of a highly complex and administratively burdensome legal procedure, which constituted an enormous challenge for many low-income countries lacking the necessary expertise (Hein 2007, 43).

The Doha Declaration therefore did not per se contribute decisively to the scale-up of ART access across the globe that started in the early 2000s. Rather, the turning point came with the Indian pharmaceutical company Cipla's announcement in 2001 that it would sell a generic version of a triple-therapy antiretroviral compound for 350 USD per person per year.[2] The resulting drastic price reduction in ARVs—including of the branded products—due to increasing competition on the pharmaceutical market enabled many low- and middle-income countries (and their external donors) to finally initiate public sector treatment programs (AVERT 2014).

Since the onset of generic ARV production by Cipla and other companies that followed suit, treatment programs in the Global South have predominantly relied on the supply of low-priced pharmaceuticals from generic manufacturers in India, "the pharmacy of the developing world" (Hoen 2009, xvii). In 2005, however, India was obliged to amend its patent law to the regulations laid down in the TRIPS agreement, which "severely constrain[ed] generic competition and supply, particularly for newer medicines" (Waning, Diedrichsen, and Moon 2010, 2).

Until today, the TRIPS agreement, plus related subsequent trade restrictions imposed on governments in the Global South through bilateral free trade agreements with the home countries of large transnational pharmaceutical corporations, continue to negatively affect global access to HIV treatment, particularly to second- and third-line ARVs. Even though throughout the recent years the price for second-line medications has decreased, new regimens that can be used as third-line options remain exceedingly expensive, which is "extremely problematic as more and more treatment programs need access to these drugs for people who have exhausted all other treatment options" (MSF 2013, 5).

Countering this impasse continues to be a central concern of a globally connected treatment activist coalition, which had already played a crucial role in bringing down the prices of the first- and second-line ARVs most widely used in resource-limited settings. This "new" movement was fueled by experienced AIDS activists in the US and Europe who felt a moral obligation to turn their attention to the treatment gap in resource-poor settings once they had gained access to effective combination therapies and recovered their health themselves (Smith and Siplon 2006). These activists increasingly connected with their counterparts in the Global South, where newly emerging grassroots organizations had started to fight for HIV treatment and boldly protest against the profit seeking of multinational pharmaceutical companies protected by international trade regulations. Domestic activist groups increasingly linked up and, in collaboration with well-established international NGOs, formed a globally operating AIDS treatment access coalition that advocated for access to ART as a human right, strongly opposed the subjection of pharmaceutical production under global intellectual property rules, and significantly contributed to building up the political pressure that would eventually result in the adoption of the Doha Declaration in 2001.

The South African Treatment Action Campaign (TAC), cofounded by former anti-Apartheid activist Zackie Achmath in late 1998, came to be one of the largest and most recognized grassroots organizations involved in treatment activism in the world (Geffen 2010). While in some of its battles against multinational pharmaceutical manufacturers (see Hoen 2009; Messac and Prabhu 2013; Robins 2004; Smith and Siplon 2006) the TAC allied with the South African government, at other times, the government was the organization's target and antagonist. This was especially the case during the years when president Thabo Mbeki and other high level members of the country's administration had adopted a stance of "AIDS denialism," refuting HIV as the cause of AIDS and decidedly resisting activists' call for delivering ART within the public health system (Fassin 2007; Nattrass 2007; Robins 2004). The activists' persistent confrontational activities significantly contributed to the fact that in 2003, the government finally reversed its policy and established a national treatment program.

Another important player in this context has been Brazil, whose progressive AIDS politics have served as a role model for the global treatment access movement. Even during the early years of the Brazilian AIDS epidemic, "grassroots and regional states' interventions were not antithetical to each other" (Biehl 2004, 107), and the fruitful collaboration of activist and governmental actors continued after the advent of ART. As early as 1997, Brazil started to offer free HIV treatment through the public health system,[3] setting an important example of how ART could successfully be provided in the context of a low- and middle-income country. The vital difference between Brazil and many other low- and middle-income countries, however, was that it had a well-performing domestic pharmaceutical industry. Even though Brazil had introduced pharmaceutical drug patents in 1997, a large proportion of the antiretroviral medications provided during the first years of its national treatment program were nationally produced drugs that had been previously developed (Hoen 2009, 46), a situation that largely precluded the need to import expensive brand-name drugs from abroad. When, later on, the need to provide newer brand-name drugs increased (Biehl 2010, 176), notwithstanding the pressure of the US government and pharmaceutical multinationals (Alcorn 2007; Smith and Siplon 2006), the Brazilian government issued compulsory licenses and produced generic copies of patented medicines in order to force the patent holders to significantly reduce prices.

The actions of what anthropologist João Biehl (2004) has referred to as "the activist state" Brazil had a significant bearing on further developments with regard to access to HIV treatment across the globe. On the one hand, it strengthened the global treatment access movement by making clear "that a framing of issues that pits human rights against the right to reap profits, and that privileges the former over the latter, has strong resonance in the court of public opinion" (Smith and Siplon 2006, 102). This was acknowledged by a passage in the Doha Declaration, which explicitly affirmed that the TRIPS agreement "can and should be interpreted and implemented in a manner supportive of WTO members' right to protect public health and, in particular, to promote access to medicines for all" (WTO 2001, 1).

On the other hand, Brazil's domestic ARV production created "a market for generic drug components" and simultaneously "raised international competition that led to an overall decrease in drug prices" (Biehl 2004, 117). The dropping prices of the raw materials for ARVs as an outcome of this was a crucial element in enabling Cipla to make its 2001 offer, which in turn initiated a further spiral of price reductions in ARVs on the global market. This facilitated MSF, in collaboration with TAC, to set up a large pilot initiative that proved ART provision in a resource-poor setting to be feasible (MSF, Department of Public Health at the University of Cape Town, and the Provincial Administration of the Western Cape 2003; Robins 2004), and fueled a nascent shift in the attitude of the international donor community that increasingly came to see global ART provision as financeable and morally imperative (Messac and Prabhu 2013).

By uniting forces, the domestic protest groups and grassroots initiatives across the world that formed the treatment advocacy coalition accomplished a great deal of their aims. First, after unmasking the relatively low actual cost of ARV production and putting significant pressure on pharmaceutical manufacturers through raising the awareness of the global public, prices of brand name ARVs dwindled. Second, in supporting the governments of low- and middle-income countries to pass or hold on to legislation that allowed for the implementation of compulsory licensing, the movement contributed to wider competition in the international generics market, which translated into further decreasing ARV prices. Third, "it encountered the prevalent market- and charity-based approaches with a compelling rights-based narrative that had tremendous resonance with many target audiences" (Smith and Siplon 2006, 156).

The contribution of Tanzanian activists in bringing about these transformations has been marginal. Nadine Beckmann and Janet Bujra have analyzed the political dynamics within NGOs and (self-) support groups of people living with HIV/AIDS, pursuing the question of why, in comparison to South Africa, "non-governmental public action by [Tanzanians living with HIV/AIDS] had little impact on national policy formulation, legislation or strategic planning" (Beckmann and Bujra 2010, 1044). They attribute the nonformation of a significant activist collective to the "limited 'political opportunity structures' for contentious politics in Tanzania" in the late 1990s (Beckmann and Bujra 2010, 1044). Contrary to South

Africa, where the founders and many members of the TAC could look back on long-term political activism and resistance against the Apartheid regime, in Tanzania, there was no "'repertoire of contention'—politically conscious subjects, ways of organizing and building alliances, political space for unrest" (Beckmann and Bujra 2010, 1044). Instead, the authors contend that the groups into which Tanzanian people living with HIV/AIDS organized themselves "exhibit a patron-client mode of politics rather than one based on the solidarity of common interests or organizational capacity developed through past struggles" (Beckmann and Bujra 2010, 1045). This configuration of patron–client relationships between NGOs and transnational donors led to "factionalism and infighting within the [people living with HIV/AIDS] community" (Beckmann and Bujra 2010, 1046) for the continuous support of donors, who had no interest in inciting political unrest among their beneficiaries. "Rather than building a movement," Beckmann and Bujra found that "collective action [of people living with HIV/AIDS] more often feeds into compliance with state and donor agendas" (2010, 1052).

Beckmann and Bujra's conclusions to a large extent concur with the findings of Hansjörg Dilger, who specified four main reasons for the nonformation of "publicly articulated challenges to the state or the international community in relation to their alleged responsibility for people living with HIV/AIDS" (Dilger 2013a, 186) in Tanzania since the 1990s (in comparison to the situation in the US). First, there had been a "lack of a unifying identity and common goal" (Dilger 2013a, 187) among the members of the existing NGOs/(self-)support groups, which were to a large extent made up of young and middle-aged, low-educated women from rural areas, whose most pressing concern was to alleviate their immediate economic hardship by receiving small loans. Second, the members did not have sufficient social and cultural capital in the form of "knowledge, political experience or educational background" that would have enabled them to "establish an activist agenda or to organize publicly visible events such as the Treatment Action Campaign in South Africa" (Dilger 2013a, 188). Third, there was a specific relationship between NGOs and the state in Tanzania during the 1990s, which Dilger labels as "maintaining the political status quo" (Dilger 2013a, 189). The fact that the "NGOs' existence depended ultimately on government permission and they were only allowed to engage in political activities if they were registered as political parties" had the consequence that "it was almost exclusively on the premises of the NGOs (and rarely in public) that members of HIV/AIDS support groups expressed their critique of governmental authorities" (Dilger 2013a, 189).

Finally, Dilger also pays particular attention to forms of collective action within the domain of religion. On the one hand, Dilger points to the specific relationship between Tanzanian NGO members and organized religion. He found that most NGO members were practicing Christians and Muslims for whom "belief and a moral life as defined by Islam or Christianity were crucial for the ways in which people with HIV/AIDS perceived themselves in relation to their illness" (Dilger 2013a, 190). Furthermore, religious congregations often served as a source of psychological and material support. One of the effects of this was that (often conservative) religious moral norms did not ignite and constitute a principal target of activists' protests, unlike in the US, where "'the Church's' moral stance had been one of the driving forces of AIDS activism" (Dilger 2013a, 190). Furthermore, political lobbying for the needs of people living with HIV/AIDS—for instance, in the form of publicly demanding expanded availability of and access to HIV treatment—was evidently not on the agenda of religious nongovernmental actors. Instead, Dilger concludes that "in the NGOs in Dar es Salaam faith and belief have . . . become primarily a source of individual level comfort and hope for people living with HIV/AIDS" (Dilger 2013a, 190f).

Access for All and the Emergence of the Transnational Treatment Apparatus

The conceptualization of AIDS as a threat to global security, increasing pressure from globally connected activists, decreasing drug prices, and mounting scientific evidence of the feasibility of ART in low-income countries (Kasper et al. 2003; Moatti et al. 2003) all came together and finally induced international political commitment to set the global ART rollout in motion. In 2002, the WHO strategically issued the first guidelines on the scaling-up of ART in resource-limited settings (WHO 2002b), driven by the hope of reproducing a transition of HIV in low- and middle-income countries just like "in the [world's] richest countries" where ARVs "have dramatically improved mortality and morbidity, prolonged lives, improved the quality of life, revitalized communities and transformed perceptions of HIV/AIDS from a plague to a manageable, chronic illness" (WHO 2002b, 8). Putting millions on ART evoked positive expectations of decreased mortality rates (Tawfik, Kinoti, and Chad Blain 2002), curbed HIV incidence through treated patients' lower infectivity (Blower and Farmer 2003), the dilution of the dynamics of stigmatization, and a boost in readiness to undergo HIV testing within target populations.

Underpinned by the conviction that the exceptionally large endeavor of global HIV/AIDS treatment must be sustained by equally exceptional financial means, the Global Fund (GF) was established and became operational in 2002. This public–private partnership receives the largest part of its funding from the governments of the US, Japan, and several European countries, and smaller parts from foundations like the Bill and Melinda Gates Foundation and other private sector actors. As a mere financing mechanism with a strong emphasis on "country ownership,"

> the GF does not have its own programs or projects, but finances proposals that are developed by the countries themselves. The aim of this principle is to encourage bottom-up processes and Southern participation, and it represents a shift away from conventional development approaches as followed by other financing institutions in health like the World Bank or PEPFAR, where countries have to apply within much narrower strategic frameworks than in the case of the GF. (Bartsch 2007, 161)

In just over a decade, the Global Fund has become one of the most important providers of financial resources in global health, financing a wide array of HIV/AIDS interventions across the globe. In order to be eligible for funds, countries have to actively apply and meet a number of specified criteria. One of these is the creation of so-called Country Coordinating Mechanisms (i.e., a team that coordinates the national Global Fund supported activities and is comprised of representatives from the government, civil society organizations, and people living with HIV/AIDS). Once an applicant country's proposal has been approved, "principle recipients" in the receiving countries administer the Global Fund grants. These may be governmental institutions or nongovernmental organizations who in turn contract local organizations as "subrecipients" for the implementation of HIV interventions on the ground. Frequent recipients of large amounts of funding from the Global Fund (and PEPFAR, see below) are FBOs with close relations to specific churches; and in some cases, this funding has enabled these organizations to significantly enhance their power position in relation to the state (Patterson 2010).

Only one year after the establishment of the Global Fund, another major program was initiated. Then US president George W. Bush launched the bilateral PEPFAR initiative with an initial commitment of 15 billion USD (for the first five years), which, at least up to the point of writing this, still finances AIDS interventions, predominantly in Tanzania and fourteen other focus countries. In contrast to the Global Fund, PEPFAR provides not only financial resources for the purchase of ARVs and other medical equipment, but also technical assistance in the form of training for medical professionals or the construction of medical infrastructure. A further difference between the Global Fund and PEPFAR at the time of my research was that the activities of the latter were exclusively led by transnationally operating US-based organizations, which may (or may not) collaborate with local NGOs. In the endeavor to fulfill its obligation of accountability to the US Congress, PEPFAR places strong emphasis on obtaining regular reports on the number of patients treated at the health facilities it supports, in order to provide quantitatively measurable evidence of the continuous progress of the program and thus keep the resources flowing. As the total number of patients enrolled in ART through PEPFAR support is considered to be the strongest indicator of the program's efficacy, the rapidity of treatment scale-up is its first priority, often at the cost of the quality of care it provides (cf. Eibl 2010).

The assemblage of HIV policies, guidelines, and strategies issued by the WHO and UNAIDS, multinational financing mechanisms like the Global Fund, and large-scale initiatives like PEPFAR with its myriad of subcontracted implementing organizations "represent an unprecedented intervention on entire populations by NGOs and foreign powers" (Nguyen 2009a, 198). By determining the form, extent, enrollment criteria, involved actors, and underlying morals of national HIV treatment programs across the globe, they constitute a salient example of the workings of transnational governmentality "in places where the State does not reliably carry out biopolitical functions associated with ensuring population health" (Nguyen 2009a, 202).

Through the interventions of this global HIV/AIDS treatment apparatus, the promise of pushing the process of normalizing HIV/AIDS beyond the boundaries of the Western world increasingly seemed to come true. While the initial targets of providing treatment to three million people in need by the end of 2005 (known as "3x5") (WHO 2003) and providing "universal access"[4] to ARVs by 2010 (WHO 2006) were not met on time, the goal of putting 15 million people on treatment by 2015 was indeed achieved (UNAIDS 2015, 109). To this day, the number of people who initiated ART each year has steadily increased from one year to the next, and in June 2017, 20.9 million people were accessing treatment globally (UNAIDS 2017b, 1). In view of the rapid treatment scale-up, over the recent years, the rhetoric of organizations such as WHO, UNAIDS, PEPFAR, and the Global Fund became ever more optimistic. In 2012, UNAIDS envisioned "the beginning of the end of AIDS" and the "start of an AIDS free generation" (UNAIDS 2012, 9). Two years later, it claimed that, building on past achievements, by 2030 "the AIDS epidemic can be ended as a global threat to health" (UNAIDS 2014, 6). In 2016, the United Nations General Assembly issued a political declaration committing to this ambitious aim (United Nations General Assembly 2016).

Simultaneous to the impressive global scale-up of ART delivery, the WHO kept updating its treatment guidelines. Whereas in the revised version of 2013, the CD4 level indicating ART initiation of patients without any clinical signs of disease progression was elevated to 350 cells/µl (WHO 2013, 92), the version of 2015 finally recommended that "ART should be initiated among all adults with HIV regardless of WHO clinical stage and at any CD4 cell count" (WHO 2015, 24). With each revision of the guidelines, the number of people eligible for ART across the globe increased, which implicated that accomplishing the aim of universal access to HIV treatment receded further into the distance.

At the end of 2016, 47 percent of the adults and 57 percent of the children below the age of fourteen living with HIV worldwide had no access to ART (UNAIDS 2017b, 1), and by November 2017, only half of the least- and middle-income countries among the WHO member states had implemented the Treat All Policy (WHO 2017,

1). In Eastern and Southern Africa, 60 percent of all people living with HIV were accessing treatment in 2016 (UNAIDS 2017b, 2). Notwithstanding the enormous progress that has been made since the beginning of this millennium, these numbers raise the pressing questions of how to generate the immense resources needed in the years to come for the continuous exponential treatment scale-up, globally achieving satisfactory retention rates, countering emerging drug resistances of long-term ARV users, and providing reasonable care for people living with HIV over their life time.

HIV/AIDS and the Introduction of ART in Tanzania

The introduction of ART as a national public health intervention can be viewed as a major element of the process of transnationalization and projectification of health care provision in Tanzania. It not only constitutes an excellent example of the increasing shift of state responsibilities onto the international development apparatus, however. It also illustrates the implicit challenges of incorporating a supposedly universalistic health intervention into the administration of a national health system, of providing the necessary financial resources and infrastructure, of technically implementing such an intervention within health institutions, and of effectively shaping the individual interactions between health professionals and patients through which the social meaning of the intervention is produced and transported on the ground. The following overview of the development of the HIV/AIDS epidemic and the governmental response in Tanzania shows how the above-described shift in global health politics from prevention to treatment initiated a corresponding change of direction at the national level. This prepares the ground for a subsequent detailed exploration of the translation process of ART as a global mobile force into local social realities at the community level (i.e., at particular HIV clinics in Tanga's neighborhoods) (Chapters 3 and 4).

In 2016, an estimated 1.4 million HIV-positive people was living in mainland Tanzania (UNAIDS 2017c, 44), 110,000 of whom were children below fifteen years of age (UNAIDS 2017a, 1). Whereas the national prevalence rate among adults aged fifteen to forty-nine years decreased from 7 to 4.7 percent between 2005 and 2016

(TACAIDS 2014, iv; UNAIDS 2017a, 1), geographic variation in 2016 ranged from 11.4 percent in Njombe region to 0.3 percent in Lindi region (The United Republic of Tanzania 2017, 2). Moreover, while across all age groups, HIV prevalence among women was twice as high as among men, in the age segment of twenty to twenty-four years, the chances for women of being HIV-positive were almost four times higher than for men (The United Republic of Tanzania 2017, 2). Finally, according to the latest available national report, particularly high rates of HIV infection were also found among certain urban "key populations," such as people who inject drugs (50 percent), sex workers (31.4 percent), and men who have sex with men (23.3 percent) (TACAIDS 2014, ix). Addressing the "concentrated epidemics" among these populations has only recently become an additional focus of Tanzanian HIV interventions (Moen et al. 2013).

The first three AIDS cases in Tanzania were registered in the Kagera region in the very northwest of the country in 1983. By 1986, HIV infections were reported from all twenty-five regions of the country (TACAIDS 2013a, 1). The onset of the AIDS epidemic struck Tanzania at a particularly inopportune moment. A severe economic decline in the wake of the 1979 oil crisis, the resulting global economic depression, and the war against Uganda that Tanzania had fought in 1978–1979 all combined to leave the country in a state of crisis. In 1986, after previous unsuccessful attempts, Tanzania managed to get a loan from the IMF and the World Bank. Arguably, these institutions were only ready to grant the loan after Julius Nyerere, the "Father of the Nation" who had led Tanzania into independence and a period of socialist *Ujamaa*[5] politics, had stepped down in 1985 (cf. Sullivan 2011b, 103), and "the chief obstacle to liberalization of the mainland economy" (Iliffe 1998, 217) had thus been removed. The loan was granted, subject to the implementation of a multitude of SAPs that were expected to result in decreased state spending and economic stabilization. As indicated above, these policies had numerous detrimental effects on service provision in the public sector, particularly with regard to health care provision.

Even though a National AIDS Task Force (which later became the National AIDS Control Program), a national institution in charge of HIV control and the development of respective intervention strategies, was established as early as 1985, the critical state of the national health care system in the late 1980s and early 1990s, in combination with the Tanzanian population's increasingly precarious living conditions, offered fertile ground for the HIV epidemic to thrive and reach its peak at an estimated national prevalence rate of 8.4 percent in the mid-1990s (NACP 2013, 16).

During the first years of the national epidemic, the response to HIV/AIDS was predominantly driven by the Ministry of Health. In 1992, a multisectoral approach was set down in the "Medium Term Plan II," a policy document guiding HIV interventions from 1992 to 1996, and through which "projects and activities [were] started in sectors like education, labor, agriculture, in the private sector, and among the youth" (TACAIDS 2002, 8). But the progress that was made over the following years, also with regard to the decentralization of the national HIV/AIDS response that was called for in the Medium Term Plan II, was limited (cf. Dilger 2005, 20). Only in the aftermath of President Benjamin Mkapa's New Year address of 1999, in which he declared HIV/AIDS "a 'national disaster' and called on the entire nation, including the Government, political, religious, and civil leaders and nongovernmental organizations, on the importance of taking new measures to put the nation on a war-footing with HIV/AIDS" (TACAIDS 2002, 1), were more concrete advances discernible.

In 2001, after ten years of negotiations in numerous decision-making committees, a National Policy on HIV/AIDS was finally approved (The United Republic of Tanzania 2001), which for the first time explicitly defined the provision of ART as a right for every Tanzanian living with HIV/AIDS (WHO 2005, 2). In the same year, the Tanzania Commission for AIDS (TACAIDS) was established and put in charge of directing the multisectoral national HIV/AIDS response, including "advocating, mobilizing, and distribution of funds" (TACAIDS 2013b, 61). Until today, TACAIDS and the National AIDS Control Program (NACP) within the Ministry of Health are the most important governmental bodies entrusted with the guidance and coordination of the Tanzanian response to HIV/AIDS.

During the first two decades since the documentation of its first AIDS cases, Tanzania's efforts to counter the disease have predominantly focused on impact mitigation, providing care to people living with HIV/AIDS, and preventing new HIV infections by increasing knowledge about HIV/AIDS in the general population, promoting the use of condoms and the reduction of sexual partners, increasing the regular use of HIV counseling and testing (VCT) services, and striving for universal screening of donated blood for HIV infection. The success of these efforts, however, has remained limited. An analysis of the first sixteen years of Tanzania's response to HIV/AIDS assessed that "despite substantial efforts by the Government of Tanzania and its Development Partners since 1986 . . . HIV prevalence rates continue to rise in nearly all parts of the country" (TACAIDS 2002, v). TACAIDS ascribed this to a variety of reasons, such as the "lack of human and financial resources; inadequate capacity of the implementing institutions; excessive bureaucracy and centralization; insufficient coordination; and limited integration of development partner activities" (TACAIDS 2002, vi).

The Establishment of the National Treatment Program

The situation of HIV treatment at the turn of the millennium was similarly disillusioning. In the absence of concrete numbers of patients taking ARVs in the early 2000s, the "Health Sector Strategy on HIV/AIDS 2003–2006" that was issued by the NACP in February 2003 stated that

> the use of [ARVs] is limited only to a small proportion of patients who would . . . need it. Drugs are being prescribed by any medical practitioner, most of them untrained in the management of HIV/AIDS using ARVs. Drugs are mostly dispensed by untrained medical personnel [who] do not give adequate information to patients who use them. There is no adequate counseling for patients on the use of ARVs and hence adherence is often very erratic. In short, the current use of ARVs in Tanzania although limited can only be described as uncontrolled and chaotic. (NACP 2003a, 161)

Two years after the commitment to provide ART was fixed in the national AIDS policy, in resonance with the above-described policy shift toward a global treatment rollout, the turn toward a more systematic inclusion of treatment in Tanzania's efforts to fight HIV/AIDS finally took shape. Fulfilling the human right to treatment was not the only decisive factor behind this development. Financial calculations were just as important: "Despite the current low prices of drugs the provision of ARVs can potentially cripple the financial health services in terms of funding and resources," warned the Health Sector Strategy (NACP 2003a, 161). Yet it continued by arguing, "These costs are expected to offset with the benefits of the health services by other means, such as decreased burden of disease, [and] reduced morbidity and mortality from HIV/AIDS" (NACP 2003a, 161).

In close cooperation with the William J. Clinton Foundation, the Harvard AIDS Institute, and the WHO, the Tanzanian Ministry of Health developed the "HIV/AIDS Care and Treatment Plan 2003–2008," which set the aim to provide ART to more than four hundred thousand people and to monitor and track the disease progression of an additional 1.2 million people who were not yet clinically eligible for ART initiation by the end of 2008. In October 2004, public ART provision began in the country's four referral hospitals and selected regional hospitals—including the one in Tanga—and district hospitals, with the aim of expanding treatment to all district hospitals within three years (NACP 2003b, 11).

The launch of the national treatment program was supported by a wide array of bi- and multilateral donors. The Global Fund; the Norwegian, Canadian, Swedish, German, and Danish Governments; the William J. Clinton Foundation; the World Bank; and PEPFAR all contributed to meeting the costs of expanding ARV provision, which were estimated at 539 million USD for the first five years (WHO 2005, 2). Since the initiation of ART rollout, Tanzania has experienced a massive influx of external resources for implementation. Between 2006 and 2011, approximately 2.2 billion TSH of externally funded money was spent on the fight against HIV/AIDS in the country (TACAIDS 2012b, 19). Roughly two thirds of this amount went to treatment (TACAIDS 2012b, II). These and subsequent enormous financial flows enabled an impressive scale-up of ART provision. In 2016, 850,000 people (i.e., 62 percent of all people living with HIV) were on treatment (UNAIDS 2017a, 2).

One of the most crucial problems, however, centers on retaining the large number of ART patients on treatment in the long term. Cohort studies that have been conducted from 2005 onward have shown that only 72 percent of children and 63 percent of adults were still on ART thirty-six months after their treatment initiation (NACP 2011a, 17). Between 2005 and 2009, the dropout rate of patients during the first year of therapy even increased, from 28.6 to 39.8 percent (NACP 2011b, 57). As at the time of my research, there was no functioning centralized patient tracking system in place—the possibilities of cross-checking patient data in different health facilities across the country were very limited. It therefore remained unknown whether the patients registered as "no longer on treatment" had died, continued treatment at another facility, or had really interrupted their therapy. These challenges speak for the necessity to increase—and better understand the obstacles to achieving—the *quality* of the national treatment rollout, rather than simply putting as many people as possible on ARVs in the shortest possible period of time.

Notes

1. The first antiretroviral drug for the treatment of HIV, Azidothymidine (AZT, brand name Retrovir), was approved in 1987 (Molotsky 1987). However, treatment with AZT alone or in combination with other drugs of the same class (nucleoside reverse transcriptase inhibitors) only proved effective for a limited period before the HI-virus grew resistant against the regimens. The crucial novelty in HAART was the combination of usually three different drug classes that intervened at different stages of virus replication, which significantly delayed the development of drug resistance (Messac and Prabhu 2013, 116f). In this book, the acronym ART refers to these combination therapies (i.e., to HAART).

2. The sale of generic ARVs was legally possible on the basis of transitory implementation periods provided in the TRIPS agreement: "While, in general, the TRIPS agreement only grants a one-year period to adjust national legislation to TRIPS provisions, developing countries were entitled to delay the date of application for a further period of four years (until 1 January 2000). In cases where a developing country already had a system of patent protection in place, but is obliged 'to extend product patent protection to areas of technology not so protectable in its territory on the general date of application of this Agreement for that Member' (TRIPS article 65.4) there would be an additional transitional period of five years until 2005. This was the case in India, which had introduced a Patent Act in 1972 protecting only production *processes* but not products as such. Least developed countries (LDCs) also have a transitional period of ten years (in 2002 this was extended until 2016 with respect to patents for pharmaceutical products)" (Hein 2007, 41).

3. The creation of this national treatment program was based on a law that referred to Brazilian citizens' right to access health care and medicines as laid down in the Brazilian constitution. It was signed in 1996, in large

part as a result of well-organized pressure from civil society groups and people living with HIV/AIDS who successfully sued state and municipal governments in order to be provided with the necessary treatment (Galvão 2005, 1112).

4. Defined at the time as treatment coverage of at least 80 percent of the population in need (WHO 2010b, 5).

5. *Ujamaa* (Swahili for family ties, village community, community spirit) was the term for Nyerere's model for a self-reliant socialist society, which became a central tenet of his vision for Tanzania's development, as laid down in the Arusha Declaration of 1967.

Chapter 3
Translating Global Technology into Local Health Care Practice

The introduction of HIV treatment in Tanzania actuated thorough transformations in countless involved health institutions, which had to find a way to meet the multiple exigencies that the provision of this complex biomedical technology implies. These institutions not only had to handle the sophisticated matter of prescribing and delivering the pharmaceuticals, they also had to accommodate the "baggage" with which these medicines arrived, namely the

> protocols and guidelines on how to manage the supply of medicines, and who to treat and why; resources for training and additional benefits for salaried health workers; . . . strict guidelines on how to ensure adherence (to prevent drug resistance from emerging); and new notions of responsible and therapeutic citizens who "live positively," disclose their status, and refrain from drinking alcohol or taking traditional medicines. (Hardon and Dilger 2011, 149)

This chapter takes a look at how health institutions in Tanga have grappled with this arduous task under particular structural and material circumstances. Furthermore, it explores how this assemblage has impinged upon—and been shaped by—the clinicians, nurses, pharmacists, and other health professionals who constitute the social foundation of these institutions and are the crucial actors in realizing ART provision on the ground.

These health professionals play an eminently important role as intermediaries between global health policy and local health care practice (Richey 2012). It is they who predominantly implement the supposedly "neutral" and "universal" scientific biomedicine under specific, often constrained local conditions, and who must translate international and national standards into everyday practice. "From day to day, African health personnel provide biomedical care, engage donor and state policies and programs, and interact with members of the same communities in which they live," writes anthropologist Noelle Sullivan (2011b, 43). "Thus, their position at the interstices of state, global, local, and biomedical domains allows for the consideration of how these multiple scales intersect, in practice" (Sullivan 2011b, 43f). Biomedical professionals have nevertheless gained relatively little attention from social science scholars interested in the complex interrelations between global and local spheres with regard to health interventions, and in the formation of what could be called "local biomedicines." This is regrettable, because

> without empirical examination of how contemporary African biomedicine is learned, lived, and practiced, we will describe medicine only in relation to its own theory of itself (as found, for instance, in textbooks) rather than in all the richly contextualized historical and cultural complexity of its actual local instantiations. (Wendland 2010, 23)

In light of this research gap, some researchers *have* paid particular attention to the role and experiences of African health workers in the "actual local instantiations" of such interventions, as well as their contribution to the scientific understanding of HIV/AIDS. In his account of the formation, trajectory, education, and role of African doctors in Uganda, Kenya, and Tanzania, historian John Iliffe emphasizes the role of East African doctors in demarcating and responding to the emerging AIDS epidemic in the 1980s and 1990s.

> It was they who first recognized AIDS in the region and, with expatriate collaborators, chiefly uncovered the epidemiology of the disease when transmitted by heterosexual contact, as it was to be in most of the world. . . . Further, East Africa's doctors were largely responsible for devising national AIDS control programs which became the models for other regions of heterosexual transmission. (Iliffe 1998, 220)

While Iliffe points to extrapolations from the local to the global that made an important contribution to the scientific understanding of AIDS in the early days of the epidemic, Karen Booth directs her attention to processes unfolding in the opposite direction. On the basis of her research on the everyday practices of nurses entrusted with HIV care and prevention in Nairobi in the early 1990s, she argues:

> Nurses daily produce policy by brokering and selectively translating relationship[s] among biomedicine and development; donors and the state; past and present economic, political, and sexual relations; and experts and patients. In this process, nurses actively interpret, challenge, and reframe "expert" knowledge about HIV. . . . On the local level, therefore, policy in the form of everyday institutional practices reflects . . . tensions and accommodations between the national and the international. (Booth 2004, 20)

Susan Whyte and colleagues made similar observations in their examination of how Ugandan health professionals managed the "contradictions between the declared commitment to [patient] confidentiality on the one hand, and on the other, the need to certify people as HIV positive and therefore entitled to support and treatment" (Whyte, Whyte, and Kyaddondo 2010, 82). The authors show that the health workers were not morally bound solely to the ethical protocols underlying the care and support programs that they worked in and which are deemed universally applicable. As members of social networks and local communities, they also had other moral obligations. At times, these required actions that would be regarded as unethical in terms of the programs' ethical protocols, for instance deliberately disregarding patient confidentiality and doing favors for people they knew in order to provide the most effective health care (Whyte et al. 2010, 96).

While the abovementioned studies refer to the era prior to HIV mass treatment, two recent anthropological studies stand out in providing valuable insights into African health workers' everyday experiences in times of large-scale public ART scale-up. Conducting fieldwork in a district hospital in northern Tanzania, Noelle Sullivan pursued the question of how "reconfigurations in health sector governance, donor-sponsored health programs, and local norms and values [are] converging in the hospital, and how . . . they impact the possibilities and limitations of interactions on the ground" (Sullivan 2011b, 36). One conclusion of her work is that the unprecedented magnitude of foreign donors' financial support and technical assistance in ART provision in Tanzania created discrepancies in the landscape of health facilities, where HIV treatment centers became "enclaves of abundance" in contrast to other hospital departments that struggled with a continuous lack of personnel and economic scarcity. In describing the conflicts among health workers over the allocation of financially lucrative opportunities to participate in trainings facilitated by transnational NGOs, Sullivan reveals the ambiguity of these enclaves. While they did provide urgently needed highly specialized health care, they simultaneously "eroded the staff's relationships . . . with each other as the economy of scarcity put them in competition with each other" (Sullivan 2011a, 218). Thus, while the massive influx of money, materials, and social technologies undeniably enhanced local health care infrastructure and the career opportunities of some medical professionals in an invaluable manner, it also produced unforeseen tensions among health workers.

Margaret Kyakuwa's doctoral dissertation on caregiving among nurses in Uganda is equally instructive. Kyakuwa took the nurses of one public and one NGO-run HIV clinic as "a practical example of how global technologies and ideas, when exported to different contexts, are reworked at the local level and thus experienced differently" (Kyakuwa 2011, 43f). Similar to the work of Whyte and colleagues, albeit with a particular emphasis on the experiences of HIV-positive nurses taking ARVs themselves, Kyakuwa demonstrates how these professionals adapted global treatment standards to local circumstances and needs. Based on her detailed observations of situations in which nurses "creatively (re)designed therapy and care practices in ways that went against national and international guidelines," Kyakuwa concludes that "these nurses were not passive victims of the challenges they faced, but acted with agency to counteract the negativity they encountered" (Kyakuwa 2011, 214).

This chapter attempts to add to these works by illuminating the constraints that health care providers perceived with regard to their daily work routines at HIV treatment centers in Tanga, which ranged from structural and managerial shortcomings to intrainstitutional power relations, physically straining workloads, and psychologically and emotionally challenging everyday encounters. I propose that taking a close look at these experiences is of particular importance, because the manifold social factors that have an influence on the working conditions at HIV treatment centers are largely overlooked in the measurement of program effectiveness, according to the logic of the major funding bodies of global HIV treatment (cf. Seckinelgin 2012). As described in the previous chapter, Tanzania's national HIV treatment program is strongly shaped by and predominantly dependent on PEPFAR and the Global Fund, which not only provide enormous amounts of money, but also determine the program's underlying policies and targets. The program is thus obliged to meet the reporting requirements of these major initiatives, for whom success, effectiveness, and efficiency are predominantly measured by numeric indicators: the number of patients tested for HIV or put on treatment, the number of lives or life years saved through treatment, the number of health professionals provided with professional trainings, or the number of people reached through a prevention intervention. Based on the logic of "performance-based funding," and in consideration of PEPFAR's accountability to the US Congress and taxpayers and the Global Fund's accountability to its donor shareholders, reporting on the accomplishment of predetermined quantitative targets is an essential precondition for the continuous replenishment of the program's resources. Quantitative indicators of the "progress" of HIV treatment in a specific location, however, often do not provide any information on the *quality* of the intervention in that place. Instead, they erase from the picture exactly those experiences of the "frontline" health workers that might provide explanations of *why* certain problems like poor treatment retention rates occur and how they can be tackled, and whose better understanding might provide hints about how global health policy can be translated into more effective health care provision on the ground.

In order to appropriately appraise health professionals' everyday struggles in Tanga's treatment centers, I will first take a look at what was expected of them according to official guidelines that meticulously determined the "social design" of ART provision in these institutions. The ensuing exemplary description of the introduction of ART services in one specific health center and a detailed exploration of health professionals' views on their work in this and other insufficiently equipped and overcrowded government health care facilities will then illustrate the challenges that stood in the way of meeting the standards and requirements laid down in the national guidelines.

Simultaneous to the geographic expansion of ART provision in Tanga, the involved implementing organizations and medical institutions have made increased efforts to tighten the nets of patient surveillance. This will become clear in the subsequent elaborations on a skills workshop for health professionals and volunteer community care workers that constituted an essential component of these efforts. This workshop could be viewed as an example of an attempt to counter local recalcitrance to a therapeutic regime that was deemed by its initiators to be universally applicable. It also constitutes a vivid example of transnationally exerted biopower trickling down from the arena of global health politics to the very personal everyday interactions in local health facilities and communities.

Finally, the chapter turns to the financial instability of ART delivery that has increased both on the global and national scale in the wake of the global financial crisis of 2008. The subtle effects that this instability had on the working conditions of health professionals on the ground point to a *temporal*—in addition to the *spatial*—particularity as another factor impinging on the concrete articulation of global ART in specific localities.

Localizing Global Health Policy: The National Guidelines for the Management of HIV/AIDS

In April 2002, the Tanzanian Ministry of Health and Social Welfare (MoH) issued the first edition of the National Guidelines for the Clinical Management of HIV and AIDS in order to provide guidance to the few health care workers who were involved in ART provision at the time. A second edition was released exactly three years later, when the national treatment program had already been running for a few months, and ever more health workers were being confronted with the need to quickly learn as much as they could about this newly available therapy. A third edition of the guidelines was released in 2008. Although a fourth edition of the guidelines was released in April 2012, in the following, I will refer to the third edition, since it was this version that I saw lying around on the shelves and desks in health centers and being flipped through by the hands of busy clinicians.

The direct link between global and national HIV policy becomes clear on one of the guideline's first pages, explaining, "Current developments and knowledge in the field of HIV and AIDS has necessitated the review of the [second] edition and formulation of this document" (NACP 2008, 5). The explanation refers particularly to the revised WHO guidelines on ART provision in resource limited settings (WHO 2006), which set the global standards for HIV treatment and whose integration into national treatment programs across the world was highly recommended. In fact, the WHO itself—in partnership with the US-based NGOs Family Health International and the William J. Clinton Foundation—functioned as a consultant partner in revising Tanzania's national guidelines.

While the guidelines cover a wide range of topics, their largest part elaborates on how to provide ART within treatment centers. This includes extensive details on available pharmaceutical regimens, the management of their side effects, and recommended treatment combinations. But it also contains passages that in a detailed manner prescribe the "social circumstances" of the service set-up with regard to treatment enrollment, patient monitoring, and adherence counseling. As these passages provide an excellent insight into the social complexity and challenges of ART provision, they shall partly be quoted in detail.

Let me begin with a section entitled "Scope of Activities to Provide Care and Treatment," which features an extensive list of "core elements of HIV services that need to be provided at CTC level" (NACP 2008, 26):

- Education about behavior change and condom use for infected people (prevention for positives)
- Orientation to the care and treatment program
- Education and regular counseling on life-long disease management, in particular on treatment adherence
- Education and counseling about actions that may delay disease progression and reduce co-morbidities by addressing issues regarding nutrition, food safety, clean water and use of insecticide treated bed-nets
- Routine clinical care and nutritional assistance to malnourished patients
- Proactive exclusion of co-morbidities such as TB and effective referral to TB clinics
- Prophylaxis for [opportunistic infections] as indicated by these guidelines . . .

- Assessing eligibility for ART (clinical staging, social eligibility and CD4 counts . . .)
- Effective referrals to essential hospital services such as antenatal clinics for [P]MTCT; family planning advice before and while on ART; [sexually transmitted infection] or other specialized clinics
- Recording and reporting according to the established electronic and paper system
- Registration and appointment systems for effective treatment continuation
- Referral to community services such as HBC, social welfare, and legal support

While this detailed script demonstrates the challenging diversity of CTC staff's tasks, the subsequent section on the "Staffing and Team Approach" is particularly instructive with respect to the expected quality of the relationship between patients and professionals as well as among professionals themselves.

> For a CTC to function well, adequate and trained staff need to have clearly outlined roles and responsibilities. Since HIV and AIDS are now manageable chronic diseases, the principles of chronic disease management need to be followed. Team approaches involving a patient and a family carer and a healthcare team consisting of at least a triage nurse, a doctor and a treatment/adherence nurse, will ensure the building of an ongoing relationship between patient and the health care team for lifelong care. . . . Weekly CTC team meetings to discuss bottlenecks and case studies will help to build the team spirit, while quarterly staff meetings between heads of relevant units involved in HIV care . . . will help to build better internal cooperation and patient referrals. (NACP 2008, 28)

Due to the immense importance of patients' consistent drug intake to the success of ART, the guidelines place particular emphasis on the correct management of nonadherent patients. Aside from "regimen-related strategies" to enhance adherence, such as simplifying regimens and reducing patients' daily pill burdens, they list "patient-related strategies" that include enhancing patients' understanding "that the first ART regimen has the best chance of long-term success" and thus better establishes their "'readiness' to be on life-long treatment." The "clinician and health team-related strategies" once more turn to how patients are to be treated. They include "building a trusting relationship with patients" and "adopting provider attitudes and behaviors that are supportive and non-judgmental to encourage patients to be honest about their adherence and about problems they have with adherence" (NACP 2008, 146). While this already points to the social skills that counselors are required to have at their disposal, a later passage elaborates on these needs much more explicitly:

> Relationship building skills are essential for building rapport and "joining in" with clients. [They] include common courtesy (greetings and introductions appropriate to culture and context), emotional presence, and appropriate vocal tone and speech rate. The relationship building process requires counseling staff to show empathy by putting themselves in their clients' shoes in order to better understand the client's perspective and communicate this understanding to the client. Empathy is the ability to tune into the client's feelings and respond in a way that the client knows that he/she has been heard. Empathy is not the same as sympathy, which is feeling sorry for another. The ability to demonstrate empathy is a key skill in promoting rapport between a counsellor and client such that the client opens up, even to the extent of disclosing very personal information.
>
> Empathy is evidenced when one:
>
> - Listens to all the feelings and not selectively
> - Responds with understanding without trying to minimize or change the client's feelings
> - Does not try to judge, solve, advise, tell or question. (NACP 2008, 217f)

The subsequent subsection on "information gathering skills" complements these explanations and delineates in detail the body postures and gestures that will signal the health professionals' empathy and thus allow patients to feel at ease:

> Listening . . . involves knowing what to listen for, suspending judgment, recalling expressions, looking for themes, resisting distractions and reflecting on what is being said. Effective listening also involves complete focus on the client and not doing other tasks while listening to him/her, encouraging the client to speak out and acknowledging their feelings. . . . Listening also involves asking questions if you do not understand. Attending skills are a very important aspect of listening skills and involve:
> - Establishing good eye contact
> - Having a relaxed body posture

- Ensuring good body language
- Listening to feelings
- Eliciting concerns

To apply attending skills one needs to face the client squarely in the face by adopting a posture that indicates involvement with the client, and adopt an open posture such as leaning towards the client with a slight inclination towards him or her which says "I am interested in what you are saying." The counsellor should maintain good eye contact but not stare at the client as this may be seen as threatening and the client may feel they are under scrutiny. Eye contact must be used in moderation, the counsellor needs to be relaxed and should not be fidgeting or nervously engaging in distractive facial expressions. (NACP 2008, 219)

It was difficult to discern the extent to which health professionals involved in ART provision, and particularly adherence counseling, were familiar with these instructions. I could neither verify how large the print run of the national guidelines had been nor how many books had been delivered to Tanga's treatment centers. Even though a nurse at the Bombo Regional Hospital pointed out how lucky I had been to get one of the rare hardcopies of the guidelines, I had the impression that at least every clinician prescribing ARVs owned a copy too. In fact, it was predominantly the clinicians who consulted the guidelines, for instance when they needed to verify which ARV regimen would best fit a specific patient's needs. Even if the guidelines had been widely available, however, it is questionable how useful they would have been to the many nurses with very limited knowledge of the English language. Only the extracts of the guidelines that specifically concerned the treatment prepara-tion of patients and the content of respective "adherence classes" (see Chapter 4) were available in Swahili—though according to my observations, even these translated versions were hardly utilized in practice.

No clinician or nurse ever explicitly alluded to the national guidelines' sections on the social arrangement of ARV provision and adherence counseling over the course of my fieldwork. Nevertheless, many of the professionals whom I specifically asked had a similar imagination of a health worker's appropriate demeanor and pro-ductive relationship with patients. As will be shown below, in many cases, it was the working conditions at the treatment centers them-selves that hindered health workers in building up favorable social circumstances for ART provision, which they held to be just as important for their patients' well-being as the provision of effective pharmaceuticals.

The Structural Context of Tanga's Care and Treatment Centers

The Bombo Regional Hospital's CTC

In July 2005, the first doses of ARVs were administered at the Bombo Regional Hospital, the largest health facility in the region, which is situated on the cliff coast at the brink of the Raskazone peninsula. This commencement of ART provision in Tanga was realized in collaboration with the TAWG, whose HBC network provided the hospital staff with access to a large number of patients in need of treatment. While the drugs were initially provided at the TAWG headquarters, in 2006, the treatment center relocated to the second floor of a newly renovated hospital wing at the very edge of the compound (Figure 3.1). Only a small conference hall and the morgue

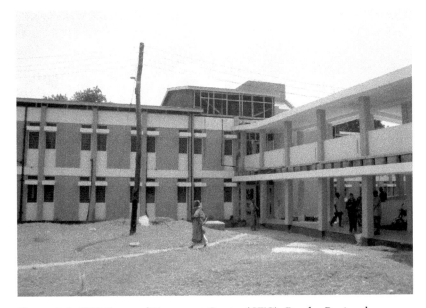

Figure 3.1. HIV Care and Treatment Center (CTC), Bombo Regional Hospital © Dominik Mattes 2009.

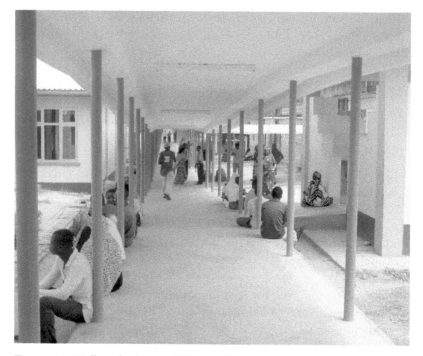

Figure 3.2. Hallway leading to CTC, Bombo Regional Hospital © Dominik Mattes 2009.

sat even further off and closer to the sea. Due to the somewhat peripheral location of the CTC, patients had to cross the entire hospital area and pass through a long roofed hallway that was usually lined with crowds of people seeking shelter from the blistering sun while waiting to be treated at one of the adjacent departments (Figure 3.2).

The establishment of ART services at the Bombo Regional Hospital had been shaped by a high degree of provisionality. The financial support stemming from the MoH and the Global Fund were limited, and only two clinicians and two nurses were initially delegated the difficult task of ARV provision, without having received extensive prior training. They had to learn by doing, trying to solve their uncertainties by calling more experienced colleagues from the MoH and consulting the Internet and professional literature. In November 2006, PEPFAR began providing financial and technical support through AIDSRelief, a consortium[1] that funded health care infrastructure, hired medical staff on short-term contracts, provided trainings in specialized HIV care, and supported the implementation of facilities in compliance with international treatment standards and long-term patient surveillance. With this support, ART service provision at the Bombo Regional Hospital improved significantly. More nurses, a pharmacist, and laboratory technicians were hired, trainings were offered, and the center was equipped with furniture and medical equipment. During my fieldwork, the center's work-force, although always fluctuating slightly, more or less constantly comprised four clinicians (one medical officer, two assistant medical officers, one clinical officer),[2] eight nurses, two nurse attendants, two pharmacists, one receptionist, three data clerks, and one lab technician. The latter was located at the hospital's central laboratory, which had a CD4 testing machine and provided the CTC with other lab services required for enrolling patients on ART and monitoring their progress.

In addition to the professionals, so-called volunteer peer educators played an important role in the clinic routine. HIV-positive and living with ARVs themselves, they often assisted the nurses as "positive examples" when preparing new patients for treatment, provided their peers with continuous education about HIV and ART, and, most importantly, constituted a link between health facilities and the community, since many of them were simultaneously community care providers and leaders of (self-)support groups that they had founded in their neighborhoods. This type of "task shifting," as it is called in WHO policy, to nonprofessionals with sporadic if any training was and is widely practiced in East Africa and beyond (see, e.g., Kyakuwa 2009; Kyakuwa, Hardon, and Goldstein 2012) in order to decrease the work burden on overwhelmed health workers.

As of July 2011, an impressive cumulative number of 9,475 patients had enrolled in HIV care at the Bombo Regional Hospital (Figure 3.3). Reflecting the uneven ratio at the national level (TACAIDS 2014, 16), female patients over the age of fifteen ever enrolled in HIV care outnumbered males in the same age cohort by almost 100 percent. Between 1 April and 1 July 2011, 138 patients had been initiated on ART, and a total of 3,475 patients had received care.

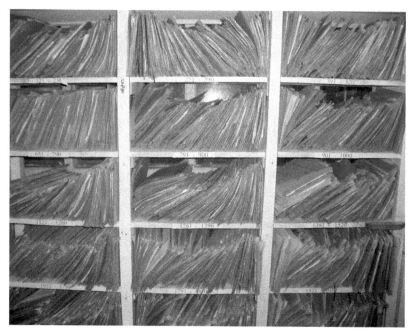

Figure 3.3. Patient files at CTC, Bombo Regional Hospital © Dominik Mattes 2009.

CTCs at Health Center Level

Until January 2009, the Bombo Regional Hospital was the only public facility providing ARVs for a catchment area of about 40 km in diameter. From February 2009 onward, the decentralization of public sector ART delivery was pushed further as the treatment apparatus expanded to two health centers within the city boundaries and a third one situated 15 km away in the countryside. By then, some 7,100 patients had been enrolled in HIV care at the Bombo Regional Hospital, whose CTC staff hoped for a significantly reduced workload once the new centers became operational.

The *Tumaini* Health Center[3] was located in a densely populated residential area at the junction of a busy commercial street and a larger circular road that circumscribes what could be called Tanga's inner city. Its CTC was housed in four tiny rooms, right behind a large waiting area at the entrance to the health center, in the first building facing the commercial street. Inside this waiting area, one could at times hardly hear oneself talk due to the street noise.

During the first eight months, until the refurbishment of these rooms was completed, ART services were offered in provisionally arranged rooms in a corner of the gallery surrounding the health center's neatly planted patio. During that time, patients had to wait in the open, where, to the obvious discontent of some, peer educators loudly counseled them about living with HIV within earshot of the crowds of patients waiting for their consultations in the adjacent departments. The space of the newly renovated rooms was in turn so limited, and the wooden walls dividing the consultation rooms from the waiting area so thin, that it was hardly possible to observe any discretion, since the conversations between individual patients and the consulting clinician could easily be overheard by others.

The situation at *Maendeleo* Health Center, located close to one of Tanga's main arterial roads and a large and populated market for secondhand clothing, was similar to that at *Tumaini*. During the first seven months that it was in operation, the space of the provisional CTC was insufficient and did not provide a waiting area protected from the sight of passersby, which raised such vexation among some patients that they threatened the staff to continue their therapy back at the Bombo Regional Hospital if they did not address the problem. Unfortunately, the new building that finally housed the HIV clinic also turned out to be too small. While it was the only facility where I regularly encountered two practicing clinicians, they had to share the only available consultation room, which precluded even the attempt at preserving their patients' confidentiality and conducting proper physical examinations when—as was often the case—intimate body areas were affected.

The CTC at *Uhuru* Health Center, which was located 15 km from Tanga's center on the very edge of a small village on the southbound highway, was a bit more spacious. Even though the number of patients who had been referred there from the Bombo Regional Hospital, as well as those newly enrolled at the clinic, increased roughly at the same pace as at *Maendeleo*,[4] the atmosphere at *Uhuru* CTC was considerably more relaxed, mostly due to the fact that the health center was built in the open rather than a densely developed neighborhood and was therefore generally less crowded. Nonetheless, efforts to maintain patient confidentiality at the clinic were not significantly greater than at the other health centers. Often, several patients were present in the consultation room at the same time, the door remained open, and other patients, nurses, or administrators dropped in during consultations.

The staffing of the health centers differed only slightly from one to the other. While at all facilities, two clinicians were supposed to be in charge of prescribing drugs and examining patients, usually only one was present, either because the second had not (yet) been hired, was attending training, had been summoned to work at another ward, or was simply absent for unknown reasons. Apart from the clinicians, the personnel included usually two to three nurses, a pharmacist or assistant pharmacist, and a data clerk. In the face of a general lack of medical workforce, some of the staff had been called back from retirement.

Installing the new HIV clinics within already existing health centers turned out to be a challenging and tense process. Once the three health centers had been selected by the NACP, based on an evaluation of their financial, spatial, and human resources, a lot of preparations had to be made. Waiting, consulting, storage, dispensary, and data entry rooms had to be arranged in already crowded facilities, staff had to be trained, and drugs and other equipment had to be stocked. The first months of managing the new patients encompassed a lot of improvisation and learning by doing. Theoretically, all of the clinicians and nurses in the new centers had to attend a two-week national training on ARV management and assist in the enrollment procedure at the Bombo Regional Hospital for one week prior to beginning their work. Several nurses and clinicians complained that they had not received any special training beforehand.

Just as at the Bombo Regional Hospital's CTC, at the *Tumaini*, *Maendeleo*, and *Uhuru* Health Centers, health policy had to materialize into clinical practice. Material technologies (laboratory equipment, registry books, databases, report forms) and social technologies (HIV disclosure, trustful professional–patient relationships, patient empowerment) had to be applied, enacted, and promoted (see Chapter 4). The application of medical protocols was intended to facilitate standardized forms of decision making. These facilities thus constituted ideal sites in which to observe in situ how medical technologies, standards, and policies, as global forms, were being grounded in the particularities of the local. In order to illustrate this grounding process, let me first describe the structural context of the treatment rollout from the Bombo Regional Hospital to the health centers, before examining the personal experiences of the involved clinicians, nurses, and pharmacists who functioned as brokers "between the global assemblage of therapy and the life world of the ARV clients" (Richey 2012, 834) in often highly strained working environments.

Medical Professionals' Perspectives on the Management of HIV Mass Treatment

The Intricacies of ART Expansion

The expansion of HIV treatment delivery to the health center level began with two "outreach days," held one month apart. On these days, a team of ART-experienced clinicians, nurses, and pharmacists from the Bombo Regional Hospital travelled to the new facilities in order to teach the staff correct patient management routines in situ. All patients who had previously agreed to continue their therapy at the new treatment centers and whose appointments for drug refills coincided with these dates were asked to turn up early in the morning.

In order to better understand the difficulties of ART provision in new target institutions, let me provide an exemplary outline of the first outreach day at *Uhuru* Health Center. At eight o'clock in the morning on that day, around eighty patients and the local staff were awaiting the Bombo Regional Hospital's outreach team in the center's packed meeting hall. Stacks of patient files piled up on a large reception desk in the front, which was decorated with flower arrangements. After the team had arrived and exchanged lengthy polite greetings with the waiting crowd, one nurse from the Bombo Regional Hospital team began to explain the precise procedure for obtaining drug refills on that day. She instructed the patients on how to be correctly transferred from the Bombo Regional Hospital to the new facility and provided them with details about the range of services that would be provided at *Uhuru*. Her voice was regularly drowned out by enervated and angry patients who had apparently been wrongly informed about the purpose of the outreach day. Others had not understood the numerous details of the nurse's explanations, or were indignant over the necessity to go back to the Bombo Regional Hospital and ask for an official transfer letter.

Irrespective of the resulting strident discussions, the staff began to process the patients who were scheduled for control visits and drug refills. The patients had to go through the same "stations" as at the Bombo Regional Hospital (which will be covered in detail in Chapter 4). First, their weight, temperature, and blood pressure were measured at the reception desk before they were referred to a small consultation room where they received their prescription for their next supply of ARVs and—if deemed necessary—a physical examination. Patients then proceeded to the drug storage room where they received their medicines. Finally, they were given their new appointment date at the exit desk, where for a final time they had to answer questions about the exact procedure for taking the drugs.

When I joined a nurse and a volunteer from the outreach team and two local nurses at the exit desk in order to see what other topics emerged in the conversations with the patients, it turned out that many other "proper" forms of conduct set out for treatment were being negotiated. Caretakers of children on ART, for instance, were instructed to explain to the children why they had to take the medicines, in order to spur their treatment adherence; married couples were advised not to have sexual intercourse more often than twice a month in order to "stay strong" and to always use condoms.

Arranging sufficient space for patient waiting areas, offices for patient consultations, data entry rooms, and drug dispensaries in the face of limited spatial capacity constituted a significant challenge at not only the *Uhuru* Health Center. All of the renovated and newly constructed facilities ultimately turned out to be too small to accommodate the high patient numbers. In addition to doctors having to share consultation rooms, measures could not be taken in any of the centers to separate patients with highly contagious infectious diseases such as tuberculosis from others in the congested, badly ventilated waiting rooms. Furthermore, patients' treatment preparation was hardly ever organized into separated classes according to the patients' level of knowledge, as suggested in the national guidelines (see Chapter 4)—to name just a few.

Another challenge lay in equipping the new treatment centers with properly trained staff. In this regard, AIDSRelief and the NACP's efforts to provide ART specializations seemed insufficient. Several nurses and clinicians working in the new treatment centers lamented that they had to provide HIV treatment without ever having completed the relevant training. "I haven't attended any [training] about ARVs," explained one clinician, six months after she had started prescribing ARVs to patients. "To be honest, it was really difficult. All these abbreviations of the medicines were really troubling me but . . . I took the guideline for the very beginners and started writing in my notebook" (Dr. Viola, 21 August 2009). A nurse who had come back from retirement to work at another health center and had only attended the one-week "internship" at the Bombo Regional Hospital's CTC before taking up her work pointed to similar difficulties:

> When we applied for this post which I'm having now, [the people from AIDSRelief] didn't care whether somebody has any knowledge about ARV drugs. They told us you are . . . going to the seminars to study about that. So it will depend on my [initiative] how much do I want to know, even if they haven't sent me to school. . . . So I am just learning from Dr. Irene [her superior], and since I came here, I have had two seminars. . . . You must not pretend that you know while you don't know. You have to ask so much! But I think as I am doing [my daily work], I'm catching [up] a lot and they are promising us that there will be more and more seminars. (Nurse Latifa, 14 August 2009)

The problem concerning skilled workforce did not only consist of equipping the health centers with adequately prepared personnel but also of *retaining* them in the long run. AIDSRelief only provided nonpensionable short-term contracts that did not meet the staff's desire for sustainability and social security. Furthermore, it was reported that a certain percentage of specialized staff had returned to other hospital departments due to the increased risk of occupational acquisition of HIV and tuberculosis and the excessive documentation and reporting requirements involved in ART provision. As the visibly annoyed clinician in-charge of one CTC explained:

> They don't have that spirit to come to work at the CTC. Because at the CTC there is too much work, too much documentation. Whenever you take a ball pen, only in two days it is finished, compared to the outpatient department where they can be with a pen for a week or two weeks! (Dr. Irene, 18 August 2011)

Finally, the medical technology and the supply of health care consumables for routine procedures were rather unreliable. The regular periods wherein the Bombo Regional Hospital's CD4 machine was out of order due to permanent excessive demand[5] not only led to immense processing delays but also to additional, sometimes unbearable, transportation costs for patients who were consistently told to come back on another day after their laboratory results turned out to be invalid. Reagents for lab examinations such as liver and kidney function tests were occasionally unavailable, in one case for several weeks in a row. The supply of no-cost pharmaceuticals for opportunistic infections, which fell within the scope of governmental responsibility, was often interrupted, which obliged patients to resort to the private market and cover the costs themselves. Even the simple breakdown of a copy machine in one instance prevented nurses from implementing routine tuberculosis screenings for several days, since they were missing the respective protocol forms.

The lack of staff and the unstable supply of medical equipment and working materials substantially compromised health workers' ability and willingness to apply standardized protocols in their daily working routine. In interviews, however, it became apparent that the obstacles to the workflow at the treatment centers were not only exacerbated by unsteady material supplies and insufficient human resources, but also by unsatisfactory management. In addition, the CTC staff had to cope with, at times, severe emotional challenges.

The "Human Substrate" of ART Expansion: Grappling with the Workload

The sheer number of patients visiting the treatment centers on a daily basis posed one of the greatest challenges to the health workers and had a large impact on their working procedures. In mid-2009, a few months after the initiation of ART provision at the additional three health centers, the CTC staff at the Bombo Regional Hospital reported decreased workloads as they had managed to transfer a considerable number of patients to these facilities. This situation would not last long, however. Patient numbers kept rising rapidly at all treatment centers and quickly brought the providers back to the limits of their capacities. In August 2011, a doctor at the Bombo Regional Hospital explained:

> We now have nearly 10,000 patients, so the clinic is congested. It can happen that [the clinicians] see an average of 120 patients in one day.

> There are . . . five clinicians here, but due to their additional responsi-
> bilities, they are not always at work. . . . Often, you find three clinicians
> to deal with 100–120 patients. It's a lot of work. . . . For one to see forty
> patients per day is impossible! You cannot take a thorough patient history
> or conduct a thorough clinical examination because there is this long
> queue of patients waiting for you. So you find that the quality of care is
> going down. (Dr. Rashidi, 18 August, 2011)

Many nurses felt equally overburdened and were well aware of
the discrepancies between the actual daily practices of processing
the patient masses and the expected standard of care as laid down
in the national guidelines. Referring to the almost unmanageable
number of daily patients, one nurse emphasized her inability to
provide the "emotional care" that patients need:

> It gets to the point that you're simply exhausted. You don't manage any
> more to sit down with patients and explain them anything. You serve
> 120, 150 people; that's not the same as dealing with ten! If it was ten
> people, you'd have the time to listen to them, to talk to them, but 150 at
> a time?! You just want them to be finished with everything soon, so that
> they can go and relax. Some get exhausted, others complain, so it's really
> difficult. It would really be good to take care of less patients . . . because
> the patients here need consolation more than anything. Medicine is
> what they get, but what they really need is love and consolation. (Nurse
> Halima, 16 February 2009)

The insufficient number of staff and the resulting time pressure
experienced by health professionals not only compromised the provision of emotional support to patients but also adequate medical
treatment through the staff's deviance from standardized working
protocols:

> Patients are served here, but the service is not good. Because . . . if we
> take the "triage"[6] over there: you can't sit there alone and manage all
> [the patients]. So it will happen that you sometimes miss things. For
> example you miss [taking the] vital signs and you only take them from
> those who you suspect to [really] need them taken. (Nurse Asiya, 25
> May 2009)

At times, the staff shortage at the CTCs resulted in extreme situations. Dr. Irene told me that when she herself was away participating
in a training or on sick leave, for instance, patients sometimes had to
be sent away because there was no other clinician available:

To me it's a torture, because when I'm not there for one or two weeks, the clients are treated by nurses. The serious cases are taken to this one doctor at the outpatient department. That doctor doesn't have any knowledge of ART. So even [in the case of] opportunistic infections, sometimes he doesn't know if this drug is not supposed to be taken with this kind of ART. Maybe the patient is on antituberculosis [medication] and ARVs and he is sick. [The doctor] can see the patient has an oral thrush and just prescribes Fluconazole—but Fluconazole is not recommended. . . . When I come back . . . I just keep quiet because it's not the fault of the patient, it's not the fault of that doctor. . . . When you go, there's nobody there. The nurses just take their phone: "Please, doctor, there is a patient, how can we help?" You just question the nurse, then you tell her, "Prescribe this and this and this," so it is kind of disturbing. . . . Sometimes I think, why don't I just change the job because I am too much worked and . . . there is no support. (Dr. Irene, 17 August 2011)

Many nurses who in similar situations were obliged to transgress their field of responsibility and prescribe ARVs themselves did not give it serious consideration. Some, however, were quite aware of the consequences that it could have should something go wrong. Yet in the face of the patients' urgent concerns, they could not help but continue the practice.

In addition to the lack of human resources and the high number of patients, the CTC staff's manifold concurrent responsibilities contributed to their hardly manageable work burdens and, on many occasions, obstructed the daily workflow. Clinicians had to reconcile their duties at the CTCs with their tasks in other wards or different health centers; they had to make house calls and fulfill their teaching obligations at the local school for assistant medical officers; they were involved in international research projects and public health interventions; they had to assess potential new treatment centers and supervise ART rollout to other health facilities, as well as HBC activities in Tanga; they had to produce reports for multiple transnational organizations involved in HIV care; they sat on scientific panels and governmental advisory boards; they were on-call a few nights a month and sometimes on the weekend; and in some cases, they ran private practices or pharmacies in their neighborhoods after their working hours at the hospital.

Aside from having simply too many tasks to accomplish, some health care providers felt that their patients' incessant need for immediate medical attention was the primary reason why their work was particularly demanding: "You can work and work, but you cannot say, 'I'm not gonna see this patient until tomorrow.' An accountant or engineer can say, 'Today is enough. I will continue tomorrow,' but for us, we must work," said a clinician, who added that he had not taken a vacation for the past two years (Dr. Ndovu, 13 September 2009).

Toward the end of my research in fall 2011, it was clear that the tense situation of the medical professionals working at the public treatment centers could not be expected to change for the better any time soon. On the contrary, the US government's endeavor "to phase out investments in infrastructure [for ART provision] concomitant with increased URT [United Republic of Tanzania] responsibility for this area" (TACAIDS 2012a, 42), which had been agreed upon in a bilateral agreement, seemed to be having its first concrete consequences on the ground. Dr. Irene, for example, elaborated on the daily impediments to her work due to decreasing PEPFAR (and Global Fund) funding:

> We can see there is no training; no cars to go to clients or to visit other sites to [provide] clinical mentoring or to [provide] supportive supervision; sometimes the cars have no fuel, sometimes [there is not even] support to buy a bus fare for those who are supposed to go there; no refreshment training, so some staff just forget what is supposed to be done; and even to maybe buy furniture or laboratory reagents and equipment . . . I heard they said there's no money to buy this, no money, no money. (Interview, 17 August 2011)

Workflow Management and Intrainstitutional Communication

Not all of the difficulties emerging in the CTCs' daily working routines could be ascribed to structural shortcomings, a general lack of human resources, and overburdening workloads. There were also organizational issues at play. Several nurses, pharmacists, and clinicians critically commented on their superiors' lack of ability or insistence on efficiently organizing the staff and workflow in their health facilities. One nurse, for instance, ascribed the lack of systematic organization of patients' treatment preparation at her treatment center to one of her superiors' incompetence, rather than to the insufficient number of available nurses:

I don't see any staff shortage. . . . There are many staff; but when it comes to self-organization, I think the [clinician] in charge has not ordered his things properly. You go talk to him, but he does not have [the necessary] perseverance. Sometimes people don't come to work, I don't know which seminar they're at or what's going on, and he doesn't know either. He doesn't even know what's going on here and sometimes people stay away for a whole week! (Nurse Frances, 18 June 2009)

Frances also mentioned another problem related to her superiors' managerial shortcomings: the frequent occurrence of missing patient files not only added another burden to the nurses' already arduous workdays, but also raised significant discontent among the affected patients, who may have already waited for several hours but could not proceed to their consultation with the doctor without the file. One reason for this, Frances observed, were deficiencies in the rotation of patient files from one station of the patient-processing itinerary to the next:

The filing system is not good. Over there at the data [entry], those people don't enter the [data] in the computer fast enough, so the client comes here and you have found his/her laboratory results, but you notice that the file at that shelf [at the reception] is gone. You look for it all over the place. It can take a long time before you find the file. (Nurse Frances, 18 June 2009)

On the very day I conducted the interview with Frances, the problem of missing patient files was particularly salient. Frances attributed this to the absence of some of the data entry clerks, who were attending a three-day training. The remaining staff was unable to compensate for their colleagues' absence, which resulted in patient files piling up in the data entry room rather than being transferred back to the nurses who needed them in order to attach laboratory results and process the waiting patients.

Frances's colleague Mariamu raised another cause for dissatisfaction. She perceived the lack of clarity of the entire processing routine of patients as in great need of improvement, and, in addition to the lack of good staff organization, identified her colleagues' low work morale as an underlying problem. When I asked her whether she would change anything in the CTC's working routine if she had the chance to, she replied:

Maybe the thing to be improved is the self-organization. . . . You know, sometimes there are [staff] who come here in the morning and they only wear their [uniforms], but don't do their work. So you can find someone who . . . works a lot but someone else doesn't do a thing. . . . The problem here at the CTC is that the staff have not organized themselves well. . . . It happens that someone comes in and [shortly after] leaves again. They say, "I'm leaving," and you don't know where they are going, what they are doing, if they leave in order to take care of their own private business or if they have to leave on official business. (Nurse Mariamu, 17 June 2009)

While the frequent absenteeism of staff, the related inadequate management of the available personnel, and colleagues' low work morale were mentioned by several nurses and clinicians, others hinted to further negligence on the part of their superiors with regard to the consistent documentation of ART provision and surveillance. One pharmacist pointed to significant gaps in the correct entry of data in the patient database concerning patients' current pharmaceutical regimen, transfers to other CTCs, those lost-to-follow-up, and deaths, which was crucial for the long-term monitoring of individual patients' treatment response and the overall progress of ART provision at the facility.

I can tell you one thing: we have a database here, and it has a lot of things, very, very important things, but nobody cares about this [here]. If we call the [clinician] in charge and ask or explain anything about the database, he does not care. Only AIDSRelief cares about this when they come. When they came the last time, we talked a lot about the database and the loss to follow-up, but [here] nobody cares. . . . Maybe [the superiors] don't know the importance of the database. (Pharmacist Joy, 16 July 2009)

Joy explained that she was the only one at her treatment center who was able to input information into the database properly. Not only did her superiors show little interest in the matter, but her colleagues were not very fond of the time consuming and painstaking documentation work either. When she was not present at the treatment center, Joy concluded, it could happen that large amounts of crucial data on the patients visiting the facility on that day were simply lost.

A further problem consisted of the lack of platforms for regular exchange among staff. Some health workers at the Bombo Regional

Hospital, for instance, questioned why, over the course of several years, there had been few occasions for systematic exchange within the team about the challenges they perceived in their work and where they saw need for improvement. One professional explained that within three years, there had been only three staff meetings. Mariamu, who at the time of our interview had been employed at the CTC for only two months, also expressed her discontent about the lack of communication or assignment of clear responsibilities to certain work areas:

> There are no staff meetings here. If there were staff meetings, we our-
> selves could teach each other that maybe when we come in the morning,
> we do this or maybe when a certain person enters there, there's a certain
> thing that has to be done like this and this. . . . But because there is no
> staff meeting, people just do whatever they want. (Nurse Mariamu, 17
> June 2009)

While Mariamu suggested that regular meetings could result in a higher level of clarity and standardization of certain work steps at the clinic, a colleague of hers pointed to a further positive effect that a more institutionalized form of exchange within the CTC team could have on the staff's working morale:

> In other departments, you find that every morning they have a morning
> meeting. They present the cases they have seen yesterday. . . . The people
> sit down and talk . . . "Yesterday we had this issue and that one, how are
> we going to solve that one?" . . . Maybe every end of the week we should sit
> down [too] and talk about the things that have happened throughout the
> week. I believe this would help and it would also increase the motivation
> to work (*ule moyo pia wa kufanya kazi*). (Nurse Asali, 11 February 2009)

At the same time, however, Asali pointed out how difficult it would be to get all of the staff together for a meeting, because everyone was already so exhausted by their daily work. "If you tell them, 'People, there is a meeting tomorrow,' everyone simply disappears," she complained.

Complicating the matter further, communication about organizational problems across hierarchies among the staff was a sensitive issue. Some health workers simply did not feel entitled to express any critique vis-à-vis their superiors or their colleagues who had been employed for longer periods of time. One clinician who had more work experience than her colleagues, but had only been hired on a short-term contract a few months before I interviewed her, for instance, did not address the pressing problem of her colleagues' permanently unstable and incalculable presence during their shifts because "although I am sneering at the service, here at the CTC, I am the most 'junior' one" (Dr. Eliza, 20 August 2009). Other health workers simply stated that they had stopped sharing their ideas about how to improve the working routines at their facilities. Too often they had observed that nothing would change after they had put forward their suggestions.

Social Recognition and Supervision

A further issue concerning recognition of the health workers' commitment was the inadequate remuneration of overtime hours. Several clinicians and nurses complained that they were only partially compensated for regularly occurring overtime and that, at times, they had to go without any extra duty allowance for several months. One nurse interpreted this as a consequence of the management's disinterest in their employees' often precarious economic situations and related her own low occupational incentive to this indifference:

> There is no motivation in terms of the workers being cared for by their leaders (*viongozi*). For example, I have worked here from the morning until 4 p.m., and I don't have money in my pocket. . . . I'll be hungry at this time of the day, I haven't eaten anything since the morning . . . the money I get is not enough. . . . If you depend on that salary only and you get out late here, you can't do any other activity that brings you [additional] income. So . . . if those executives up here motivated [their employees] a little bit, maybe the work performance would be better; the people would be more engaged rather than just wait for their salary. (Nurse Sanura, 9 June 2009)

Adequate payment was, however, only one among several factors shaping the health workers' motivation levels. Receiving feedback on their achievements constituted an equally important but mostly unattended concern. Joy was particularly disappointed in this regard. She proclaimed that a former colleague of hers had even quit his job due to the management's failure to display appreciation for their staff. "What can I say?" she asked. "Motivation is very important for workers, [but] most of the workers don't have [any]. Even if they perform well, nobody cares. Nobody cares; that is very bad"

(Pharmacist Joy, 16 July 2009). It was not only the recognition of *good* performance, however, that seemed to be missing. "To get feedback that today I have done a good job or I have failed in a certain instance? There is no one to tell you that," stated Mariamu, whose remark resonated with other health workers' laments that there were basically no consequences for bad work performance. In their eyes, this contributed to some colleagues' problematic stance of indifference with regard to their own engagement.

Health workers' sensations of being unsatisfactorily supervised were intensified by their feelings that superiors displayed inconsistent and preferential treatment of the staff. Some claimed that superiors allocated training opportunities to specific employees on the basis of personal preferences rather than their need for qualification (cf. Sullivan 2011a). One nurse even suspected her supposedly privileged colleagues of not even participating in the full trainings, but only going at the beginning in order to receive the allowance. These allegedly discriminatory practices stood in stark contrast to the perceived resentment of the CTC staff's colleagues from other wards, who assumed that all CTC staff not only had much higher basic salaries[7] but also benefitted from several additional allowances. Several nurses explained that occasionally this encumbered the practical collaboration between the CTC and other departments.

In sum, insufficient mitigation of high workloads through targeted managerial and organizational interventions, superiors' poor routine of providing feedback and guidance, unequal allocation of training opportunities, and tensions with envious colleagues produced a considerable amount of frustration among many CTC staff, who were additionally struggling with the emotional challenges they faced in their daily work.

Emotional Exigencies: Fear, Despair, Mental Overload, and Frustration

In addition to the many challenges posed by the working conditions within the CTCs that made it difficult to motivate existing staff, the potential danger of acquiring HIV at the workplace constituted a significant barrier to further recruitment. For some of the nurses and clinicians I spoke to, the constant risk of pricking one's finger with an infected syringe posed a serious concern:

> Of course you are very worried because the gloves we use for taking blood . . . are those [thin] disposable ones. I wear two pairs, but sometimes they are big and slip off my small hands and you take the blood without wearing them. . . . You don't have tranquility then, so this is one thing that makes me be worried about contamination. (Dr. Viola, 21 August 2009)

For some, this potential, fearful risk had already become a painful reality. Asali reported that she had once hurt herself with a contaminated syringe. Fortunately, she had been quickly provided with postexposure prophylaxis, and three months later, she had tested HIV-negative. Half a year after Asali told me this, I learned of another nurse who had pricked herself and at the time was still waiting for the test results that would provide her with certitude about her status. Yet another nurse told me that she knew several colleagues who claimed with certainty that they had acquired HIV at their workplace. They could not prove it, however, which is why none of them had received any compensation from the government.

In the face of the often-occurring co-infection of HIV-positive persons with tuberculosis, many health workers perceived the risk of acquiring TB in the overcrowded and poorly ventilated treatment centers as an even greater threat than accidental HIV infection. In fact, during my fieldwork, I encountered two cases of medical staff who had contracted TB at their workplace.

In spite of the comparably high exposure to serious and/or incurable infectious diseases in HIV clinics, however, the main source of psychological distress perceived by CTC staff consisted of coming to terms with their own limited capacity to alleviate patients' multilayered "social suffering" (Kleinman, Das, and Lock 1997), which not least endangered their adherence to the treatment regime:

> Maybe the patient misses his/her next appointment. . . . Maybe you call him/her and he/she tells you, "Sister Christina, I have failed to take your medicines. It's not like I don't like them, but I don't have food. When I take these medicines, they make me feel bad." So you find that the patient stops taking the drugs because of his life circumstances. . . . Such situations also make you yourself as a nurse feel bad; you get a *burnout* [English expression in original Swahili quote]. (Nurse Christina, 16 June 2009)

In addition to patients' poverty, health staff had to cope with narratives that were often fraught with appalling depictions of stigmatization and discrimination. To some, these narratives caused considerable emotional turmoil:

> It's really something that touches me, something that bothers me. You meet small children . . . who are orphans, whose relatives have not helped them, who [are] finally stranded at an orphanage. When you really listen to their stories about their itinerary until they arrived at the orphanage—these stories make you sad. Honestly, this profoundly touches me as a human being (*katika hali ya ubinadamu inanigusa sana*). They have gone through enormous misery. I think here at the CTC, the [staff's] psychological distress is bigger than at these other wards . . . because the [patients] have gone through great suffering. . . . *Here* they mostly have the stories that make you hurt. (Dr. Rashidi, 18 August 2011)

While some health workers reacted to the suffering they encountered on a daily basis with a blend of resignation and fatality, stating simply that they could not help but continue with their daily routine, others were seriously struggling. Dr. Viola, for instance, was profoundly upset and desperate when she reflected on a young patient of hers who had died a few days earlier:

> Honestly, it affects me very, very much. I'm even thinking about staying home for two or three days. . . . You don't get used to that, never! If you look at [these patients], their life is miserable. They are in bed and cannot [move] anymore, because their legs hurt. What will they eat?! . . . Or you have prescribed them medicines, but they even had to beg others for the fare to the hospital, so where are they supposed to get the money from for the medicines? And [you know that] if they don't buy the medicines, their illness will finish them off! It affects me a lot. But I can't do anything, because I don't have the means to help everyone. (Dr. Viola, 21 August 2009)

The frustration caused by the discrepancy between patients' needs and health workers' own limited means to provide care and support may explain why time and again, the nurses and clinicians made extraordinary efforts to help patients in particularly difficult situations (cf. Kyakuwa 2011). Many regularly covered patients' transport costs or contributed to the payment of their medicines out of their own pocket. Several also tried their best to provide particularly destitute patients with emotional support. Moreover, the nurses' and clinicians' engagement did not stop at the end of the workday. Patients in their neighborhood who needed medicines or other kinds of support often consulted them privately—at all times of the day and also on the weekends. "Even if [this] overwhelms you, if someone is already bedridden, you must see it as an appeal to your humanity (*lazima uchukue na utu*) and ask yourself, 'What if it was me?!'" Nurse Sanura commented (Interview, 9 June 2009).

Unsurprisingly, some professionals told me that this permanent demand for their services, in addition to insurmountable structural impediments to their work and their own inability to alleviate patients' physical and social suffering, caused situations of physical and emotional overload. A salient strategy to cope with what occasionally was labeled as "burnout" consisted of temporary social withdrawal and technological disconnection. Several clinicians told me that when they felt too overwhelmed, they switched off their mobile phones after working hours so that they would not be reachable by desperate patients during their time off. Christina went even further:

> When I experience [a situation of emotional breakdown], I get home and close my door. . . . I even lock it with the key, and I hide underneath my blanket. . . . When I have stress like that, I close my door, and I sleep and sleep. (Nurse Christina, 16 June 2009)

None of the nurses or clinicians who revealed such experiences of feeling overwhelmed to me indicated that they had shared these with their colleagues as a way of mitigating their pain, which once more underlines the necessity of regular team meetings. Such meetings might not only serve as a platform to collectively find strategies to deal with particularly challenging patients, but also for the mutual exchange of recognition, emotional support, and moral encouragement.

In sum, medical professionals working at HIV clinics in Tanga had to accomplish the demanding task of striking a balance between two rather distinct forms of caregiving. On the one hand, they were expected to allocate enough time for patients, treat them with compassion, gain their trust, and establish equitable relations with them. On the other hand, they had to prepare them for their treatment in the best possible manner and make all reasonable efforts to enhance their chances of enjoying a sustainable positive treatment response, even if this occasionally involved rather vehement disciplinary measures to support treatment adherence. Both forms of caregiving were postulated in the national guidelines. As demonstrated above, however, diverse factors, ranging from structural hardships to emotional distress, had a negative influence on the staff's ability and willingness to achieve this balance in accordance to international standards. The large number of patients alone prevented health workers from paying sufficient attention to patients' social and emotional concerns, and from establishing the level of mutual trust that was expected to contribute to higher patient retention rates. While many of these issues remained unaddressed by the administrations of the Bombo Regional Hospital and the health centers themselves, AIDSRelief did attempt to take measures against patient attrition and insufficient adherence rates, predominantly by building up a comprehensive and reliable system of follow-up for the countless ART patients dispersed across the city. It is to these attempts that I turn next.

How to Get Ahold of an ART Patient? The Tightening of Patient Surveillance

In May 2009, I had the opportunity to participate in a three-day workshop that AIDSRelief offered for local HIV/AIDS service providers (i.e., health workers, volunteer community care providers [most of whom were also peer educators at one of Tanga's CTCs], and health officials). When Edna and I arrived at the Bombo Regional Hospital's conference hall where the workshop was held, a short and sturdy man welcomed us with a wide, sympathetic smile. He introduced himself as Jerry, one of the workshop leaders whose office was located at the AIDSRelief headquarters in Dar es Salaam. In a high pitched voice, he explained to us that the workshop was part of the pilot initiative called the "Community Based Treatment Support Services Program," which was to be conducted in four selected pilot sites in the Tanga region. The concept, Jerry continued, was simple: as patients spend only a few hours per month in the HIV clinics and the rest of their time in their communities, it was only logical, particularly with regard to the lack of medical professionals, to entrust the peer educators of the CTCs with the additional task of upholding steady contact between patients and clinics and supporting them in adhering to their therapy. At the Bombo Regional Hospital, Jerry appraised, this system was already well established in comparison to other health facilities under AIDSRelief supervision.

While we were chatting with Jerry, the conference hall slowly filled up with some twenty participants. The opening consisted of a collective prayer led by one of the workshop participants. "Retention of people living with HIV/AIDS in ART treatment and HIV prevention: A call for a community response for treatment support and care for people living with HIV/AIDS," read the title of the handout that was then distributed, to inform everyone about the agenda for the following three days. As Jerry had mentioned, the workshop aimed first and foremost to improve patient follow-up through the establishment of a tight care and control continuum that would extend from the health facilities deep into Tanga's communities. Every ward of Tanga was to have at least one self-organized group of ART patients, which was to be closely linked to the nearest CTC through its HIV-positive chairperson, who would simultaneously function as a community care provider and peer educator at the clinic. The groups were supposed to officially register at the office of the Council HIV and AIDS Control Coordinator (CHAC) so that they could claim support from local government authorities; the authorities, in turn, would be able to keep better track of the number of people receiving ART in their jurisdiction. Additionally, the workshop was meant to foster the setting up of an umbrella network that would comprise all existent and prospective (self-)support groups in Tanga, centralize their interests vis-à-vis the local government, and establish ties with the organizations providing treatment, care, and support for people living with HIV/AIDS in the city.

Finally, the workshop also pursued the more subtle aim of shaping health care providers' and volunteers' individual manner when interacting with patients in a way that would result in trustful professional–patient relationships. It thus serves as an example of how transnational governmentality in relation to ART provision played out, not only on the institutional level, but also on the individual level. In the following, I will provide a thick description of this multilevel, biopolitical intervention.

The Formation of a Surveillance and Support Network

The first day of the training was dedicated to enhancing the links among Tanga's organizations and institutions working in the field of HIV/AIDS. Aside from nurses from each of the city's HIV treatment centers, the participants included representatives of PASADIT, TAWG, TRC, a local orphanage for HIV-positive children, the CHAC and District AIDS Control Coordinator (DACC), and the chairpersons of four (self-)support groups, each of whom was associated as a peer educator to one of Tanga's public CTCs. Once all of the participants had received their per diem,[8] they provided one another with a short report on their institution's work. The report of the nurse from the Bombo Regional Hospital's CTC was particularly instructive with respect to the strategies for dealing with patients who, without any notice, had stopped picking up their drug refills on the scheduled dates and no longer showed up for their control visits. Every Friday, the nurse explained, the CTC forwarded a list of these "defaulters" to the HBC providers at TRC and TAWG, who would then try to locate the patients under their supervision.[9] If the reason for the patient's disappearance could not be established within the following three months, they were registered in the database as lost-to-follow-up (LTFU).[10] The number of these cases at the Bombo Regional Hospital had increased from 162 in 2007 to 297 in 2008–2009. Due to the continuing stigma associated with HIV, the nurse continued, many patients felt ashamed and enrolled in ART using false names and addresses, which significantly complicated the location of patients who dropped out of therapy.

At this point, Jerry intervened, insisting that not a single patient should start ART without agreeing to participate in a (self-)support group or an HBC program, so that they could be visited in case of an emergency. Patients who refused to be visited by health professionals, he suggested, were to indicate the names of fellow patients who could be informed instead. In order to make this a more binding requirement, patients should not only be invited to join a (self-) support group and an HBC program at the CTCs, as was the current routine, but they should sign an agreement during treatment preparation. This would also save professionals from increasingly occurring allegations of having breached patient confidentiality and guarantee that the practice of tracing patients in their homes was ethically justifiable and legally safeguarded against potential objections. As a few of the workshop participants had at least once been alleged as having illegitimately disclosed a patient's HIV status—in fact, shortly before the workshop, one such case had even made it into the national newspapers—Jerry's idea was met with approval.

Up until the end of my fieldwork, however, it had not yet been implemented in any of Tanga's treatment centers.

Subsequently, the topic shifted to the creation of the umbrella network of local (self-)support groups. There were disagreements among the participants about whether such a network was necessary and who should be in charge. While an NGO representative generally criticized the local government authorities for their lack of initiative in creating a supportive environment for people living with HIV/ AIDS, a leading CTC clinician more concretely attacked the current CHAC for not meeting her responsibility of registering (self-)support groups and keeping track of the current number of groups within the city. Apart from this, she suggested strengthening and supporting the already existing groups themselves, rather than investing too much time and energy in the creation of a new network. Too often, such endeavors had ended unsuccessfully. Even the NACOPHA was not functioning effectively, three years after its establishment. Despite this skeptical appraisal, the group stuck to the idea of forming the network, not least because of Jerry's insistence on the immense benefit that would result from it for all involved.

After coming under pressure from the clinician's above-stated allegations, the somewhat puzzled and defenseless CHAC consulted with her counterpart at the district level and pledged to come up with a list of all (self-)support groups in Tanga, including the names of their chairs and their contact details, by June. Decisions on possible funding options for the precise further proceedings were postponed to another stakeholder meeting in the near future. During the entire discussion about building the network, the four present (self-)support group chairpersons remained largely silent. Apparently, in this context, the concept of "stakeholders" referred to the higher-ranking medical professionals, NGO representatives, and local government authorities, rather than people living with HIV/AIDS themselves.

"We Want the Science"

The following days of the workshop addressed health professionals' and volunteers' practice of dealing with patients at the clinic and in their communities. In the NGO and local government representatives' stead, more peer educators and (self-)support group leaders, nurses in charge of adherence counseling, and HBC providers were in attendance. During the morning of the second day, the participants were to gain a detailed understanding of the microbiological workings of HIV and ART in order to be able to provide their patients with accurate information. In small groups, they were asked to discuss questions like, "What exactly happens within the body after HIV infection?" and "How do ARVs decrease viral load?" In their discussions, the participants resorted to the same metaphoric language that was commonly used to explain the workings of ARVs to patients at the treatment centers: ARVs, they said, were "HIV's birth control" and they "put HIV to sleep."

When the results were finally discussed in the plenary, Jerry and his equally eloquent cofacilitator Margaret often intervened, corrected, and complemented the presented responses. Jerry emphasized that patients needed much more detailed information on how ARVs work inside their bodies in order to become convinced of the medicines' power and thus adhere to treatment. Once more, he asked the participants to explain exactly how ARVs intervene in HIV replication. With a canny smile, he jokingly offered 5,000 TSH to the person who could produce the correct explanation. "This is the CD4," a nurse began to explain while drawing on a flip chart.

> This is the virus, that came in here. The way these medicines work is they put a coat around the CD4 so that this virus cannot get out any more and multiply itself. So this virus stays right here. This coat of the medicine is out there. [The virus] cannot come outside and produce more children, so it dies right here inside.

Not quite content with this explanation, Jerry asked one of the present HBC providers to step in.

> Well, so this virus, let's say it is *dormant*. If the patient takes the medicine, the virus remains *dormant*, so it cannot continue to reproduce itself [*kuzaana*]. It will reproduce itself again when the patient takes the medicine today, tomorrow he/she doesn't take it, and the day after tomorrow he stops taking it. But if he/she takes the medicine well, at the right time, the virus remains *dormant*.

Jerry was still not satisfied. "We want the *science*," he insisted, "which explains why the amount of the virus decreases. We have said that if someone starts taking medicines, the viral load is reduced. How is it reduced?" A clinician finally made another attempt. Her response was far more detailed and included scientific jargon like "RNA," "DNA," "reverse transcriptase," and "cell receptors." This pleased

Jerry much more, but, thanking the clinician, he finally decided to answer the question himself. Building on the clinician's response, he made great efforts to provide every microbiological detail involved in HIV replication and its prevention through ARVs, and subsequently translated these into the metaphoric language that many of the participants were used to in order to make them more comprehensible. Nonetheless, he insisted that the participants needed to understand the science behind these metaphors.

He then showed a computer-animated educational video on HIV replication by the German pharmaceutical company Boehringer-Ingelheim.[11] As the film was in English, which most of the participants could not understand, he turned off the sound and provided ad hoc comments and explanations in Swahili. Despite this, it is questionable whether the video's highly technical terminology (e.g., CD4 receptors, RNA replication, extracellular glycoproteins, etc.) had increased the participants' understanding—particularly of those who had no medical training, such as the community care volunteers and volunteer peer educators—to such an extent that they would be able to provide their future patients or peers with significantly better information than before. When the film had ended, most of the participants' questions, in fact, concerned Jerry's side note about rarely occurring genetic defects that resulted in HIV immunity, rather than the actual subject of the video.

Upon my own question about how this detailed and complicated information was to be transferred to patients within the limited time dedicated to the transfer of biomedical knowledge during treatment preparation and in consideration of most patients' rather limited educational background, Jerry replied:

> There are people who [believe] that ARVs are the [Tanzanian] president's plans to kill everybody having HIV; so when you start to distribute the drug, [they believe] you want to kill them. . . . If you bring that patient to the adherence class . . . he/she is not listening, because what he/she believes about HIV is not what you are talking about. [Therefore,] the patient should know exactly [how] HIV enters [the body], how HIV destroys the cells, how the body defends itself, and how . . . the ARVs act against the virus . . . just to encourage the patient to be able to accept the issue of being adherent to that drug, [to make him/her understand] that these drugs help me.

Jerry did, however, acknowledge that the transfer of comprehensive knowledge to patients was hampered by the lack of staff and the deviance from official guidelines on treatment preparation due to time constraints. In order to tackle this problem, he continued, AIDSRelief was conducting a pilot study in Mwanza on alternative treatment preparation set-ups. In the study sites, treatment preparation had been outsourced to "training centers" run by the Catholic Church, where more time could be invested in educating patients than in overcrowded treatment centers. The outcome of this intervention in comparison to a control group was yet to be seen.

"Where Do We Get Them?" Surveillance and Support in the Community

The afternoon session started with the question of why patients interrupt their therapy. The participants came up with several reasons: patients' assumption that they have been cured, often in relation to experiences of religious healing practices; their lack of education and knowledge; their lack of proper nutrition; their preoccupations with confidentiality; and the distance to the treatment centers. Margaret asserted that patient participation in (self-)support groups was one of the most effective solutions to many of the major obstacles to treatment adherence, and invited the participants to simulate through role play situations of creating and productively utilizing such groups. First, she asked for a volunteer to come to the front and show the audience his/her skills in convincing a community member to join a (self-)support group. Tumaini, a woman in her midthirties who chaired a (self-)support group in her ward, stood up and had a try:

> I have come from the CTC up there [she said to her imagined neighbor]. I'd like to be your friend. What do you think about it, me being your friend? I've been living with HIV for five years now, and I'd like to share the secret of my success with you. How does that sound to you? You'll be happy when we'll be together, when I give you the secret of my success. If you want to be my friend, I'd like you to join my group, which will meet every Saturday. Are you ready? . . . I'd like to give you courage, hope, happiness. . . . We meet each other and share our thoughts. What do you think?

After another participant's similar performance, different recruitment approaches were discussed with the audience. Then, in the next role play scene, the communication chain, from the CTC via a (self-)support group leader and his fellow group members to a patient who had interrupted her therapy, was simulated.

The lengthy discussions that evolved among the participants after these role plays provided insight into the wide array of problematic issues that nurses, HBC providers, and the volunteer group leaders faced in their daily interactions with ART patients. Patients' "traditional" medical beliefs and "erroneous customs" (*mila potofu*), the risk of involuntary disclosure of patients' HIV status, wives' concealment of their HIV infection from their husbands and vice versa, and the problem of providing the right advice to serodiscordant couples who would like to have a child were only some examples. The participants tried to come up with practical solutions and counseling strategies for each of these issues. One such solution involved making an effort to continuously provide patients and community members with correct information about HIV, a strategy that was passionately supported by Margaret, who repeatedly encouraged the participants to fulfill their role as "community teachers" (*walimu wa jamii*). Moreover, she suggested that they should also approach their ward leaders and try to involve them as powerful allies in the endeavor of "community sensitizing." After these discussions, the day ended with a collective prayer.

On the following morning, Margaret resumed the topic of systematically recruiting people into (self-)support groups. "Where do we get them?" (*Tuwapate wapi?*), she wrote on a flipchart, and collected the participants' answers: in their neighborhoods, in the churches, in the CTCs. The participants then developed "action plans" that specified who of the volunteers would be assigned to the respective CTCs, how many patients would be recruited within a certain time period, and when and where their group meetings would take place.

While they were busy writing down the agenda for their (self-)support groups, the issue of payment for the volunteers came up. With very few exceptions, neither the community care workers providing HBC nor the (self-)support groups' chairpersons received any payment for their work. In a somewhat accusatory tone, one volunteer emphasized that "every single day of God" (*kila siku ya mungu*), they invested several hours to their work, implying that they should receive at least some sort of compensation. Another volunteer posed the question of what AIDSRelief's selection criteria were for

admitting participants to workshops and trainings whose per diems
for many constituted the sole irregular compensation for their extensive engagement. In response, Jerry delivered a long, flattering monologue in which he explained the "assessments" that preceded each
training, and during which the targeted health facilities were asked
to provide a list of extraordinarily committed and reliable volunteers
whose continuing education promised the greatest effect. Thereby
implicitly revealing to the participants that they had been chosen
on the basis of their previous merits, he apparently managed to ease
some of their discontent. Jerry also stressed how much expertise they
could gain through the seminars they were invited to, and how much
they would benefit from this in the future. Furthermore, he passionately pointed to the moral value of their involvement, appealed to
their continuous aspiration to help their fellow community members,
and assured them that society gave them plenty of credit for their
invaluable work. Margaret backed up his passionate plea, affirming
that the worth of voluntary commitment could not be weighed in
gold. "This is work for God," she said. "The salary comes from God;
it doesn't come from this world (*malipo ni kwa mungu, malipo siyo
kwa duniani*)." While some participants clapped their hands in agreement, others seemed to be less convinced by such appeals to their
religious humility. Even though they remained silent, I felt that the
new care arrangements that have been increasingly introduced with
the scale-up of ART (i.e., the delegation of large parts of the responsibility for educating, monitoring, and taking care of patients to lay
community members) were indeed worthy of more critical inquiry. Yet
Jerry and Margaret obviously deemed a more profound discussion of
this issue unnecessary, perhaps even pointless, given that there would
never be enough resources available to adequately pay the myriad of
volunteers involved in ART provision and surveillance.

In the afternoon of the third day, more strategies for improving
patient follow-up were discussed. Every group leader was asked to
hang up large posters with the name, meeting place, and dates of
their group meetings in their wards' churches, mosques, CTC, and
ward office, in order to reach the largest number of potential group
members possible. Jerry then introduced a report form for systematically informing CTC staff and HBC supervisors about the number
of LTFUs and death cases, as well as group members' current health
condition and work situation.

Toward the end of the day, the participants finally engaged in long and heated discussions about who should be in charge of the "Network of people living with HIV/AIDS in Tanga." After they had finally come to an agreement, they elected two leaders who were mandated to convene twice a month and see to it that every ward in Tanga had an officially registered (self-)support group and team of supervisors. The latter were expected to make every effort to increase motivation within the community to undergo an HIV test; provide HIV-positive community members with relevant information; support people living with ARVs to adjust their lifestyle, keep their clinic appointments, and regularly take their medicines; and urge influential persons like religious leaders to address the needs of their HIV-positive community members.

Jerry further reminded the present (self-)support group leaders to motivate their groups to build up their own income-generating projects in order to stand on their own feet rather than become trapped in an endless cycle of donor dependency:

> Let us try to encourage the people to stop begging around (*waache kuom-baomba*). Our groups are not there to *be helped*. Let us say this together: "Our groups are not there to *be helped!*" [Audience repeats] . . . Once you have allowed yourself to get to that level [of begging], you have degraded yourself and people will despise. . . . Have we understood each other, eh?! . . . The crucial thing about being helped is *us*! *We* help *ourselves*!

It was not without a certain irony that Jerry's mantra of self-reliance was not accompanied by any suggestions of how to accomplish this, considering the massive difficulties that many of Tanga's (self-)support groups had already encountered in their attempts to set up small-scale stockbreeding, farming, or whatever other income generating projects that would help increase their individual members' income (see Chapter 7).

"Talking to Them in a Nice Manner": Establishing Trust in the Clinic

The next topic concerned the trustful relationship with patients. Recounting stories of patients who had been treated impolitely by CTC staff in another city, Jerry emphasized how detrimental medical professionals' rudeness was for patient morale and treatment adherence. He vividly simulated negative examples of nurses who did not establish eye contact with their patients, talked to them in an uncaring manner, ordered them around, and scolded them—much to the amusement of the participants, who knew very well that Jerry's parody was not too far removed from the reality. Subsequently, he pleaded with the participants to pay close attention to the way in which they interacted with their patients, and to abandon disrespectful conduct. While it was indeed difficult to deal with patients' manifold problems, he insisted that, as mentioned in the national guidelines, respectful treatment was a crucial element of providing professional support and significantly contributed to positive therapy outcomes.

> There is no bigger help than to talk to them in a nice manner (*hakuna msaada zaidi ya kuongea nao vizuri*). . . . To look someone in the face when talking to him/her gives him/her confidence that he/she is alive and worth something. Have you understood? . . . Let us exert ourselves very much to make sure that we approach [patients] with the pledge to show them that they live, that their blood is circulating! They are agonized by pain, [from] which they need to be alleviated. Let us not increase their pain!

Aware of the overwhelming number of patients that the health workers had to handle at the CTCs, Jerry preempted the question of how this desirable professional–patient relationship could be achieved in spite of the professionals' consistently high stress levels. He strongly urged the participants to always share their problems with one another and support each other in every possible way so that difficult situations could be solved in a collective effort. Everyone simply agreed with this suggestion, without any remarks on potential hindrances to such collegial exchange and team spirit. Particularly with the above-quoted health workers' complaints about the detrimental lack of communication at their treatment center in mind, the absence of any discussion about how the cohesion and solidarity within a CTC team could concretely be improved made Jerry's appeals appear more like a somewhat utopian vision than a realistic strategy for stress reduction. Nevertheless, among the workshop participants themselves, his plea seemed to have the desired effect. Several delivered emotionally laden declarations of their unconditional will to provide the best possible support to people living with HIV, in close collaboration with the representatives of the other institutions present. After these mutual attestations of goodwill, the workshop finally ended with another collective prayer, and the visibly exhausted participants were released into the golden light of the late afternoon.

Between Empathic and Disciplinary Care: The Tribulations of ART Surveillance

As the discussions among the participants during these three intense workshop days show, the improvement of ART provision and the creation of an effective continuum of patient surveillance from health facilities to patients' homes exacted great commitment from all involved actors. Medical professionals and peer educators were expected to render the messages they transferred to patients during treatment preparation more scientific; ways had to be found to talk patients into participating in (self-)support groups and to prevent them from interrupting their treatment; logistical tasks had to be accomplished, such as the assignment of "territories" to individual (self-)support group leaders so that the entire city could be covered; systematic ways of reporting to health facilities and government authorities had to be introduced; and government authorities had to be pressured to correctly register the (self-) support groups, keep track of their development, and provide them with material and social support using whatever (mostly meager) means they had on hand. Aside from all this, micropolitical tensions between hospital staff and local government representatives had to be overcome, and the volunteers' commitment and work morale had to be invigorated in the absence of any substantial financial compensation.

The workshop also made clear that the volunteers, who were entrusted with the great responsibility of keeping their fellow patients (and community members) "on track," were confronted with the demanding task of reconciling empathic and disciplinary caregiving, similar to the professionals working at the CTCs. On the one hand, they were expected to "lure" new patients into joining a (self-)support group, and establish close social ties with them in order to continuously provide them with correct scientific information about HIV and ART, assist them in adjusting their lifestyle, help them to manage the adverse effects of ART (see Chapter 4), and—if possible—contribute to mitigating their economic hardships by including them in their groups' initiatives. On the other hand, they were expected to watch over their conduct and regularly report their current health state and social situation to the CTCs. This included reporting treatment "defaulters," who could then be subjected to disciplinary actions at their next visit to the treatment center (see Chapter 4). In this sense, the volunteers acted as an extension of biomedical patient surveillance, which aimed to reach deeply into Tanga's communities as well as individual patients' domestic and private lives.

Similar to the observations in the treatment centers, the workshop further elucidated the fact that effective ART delivery and surveillance within a public mass treatment program is a highly complex endeavor that demands enormous investments, in terms of not only making the necessary infrastructure available, but also reshaping social configurations, both at the level of institutional management and at the micro level of everyday interactions between individual patients and medical professionals or involved volunteers. Many professionals and volunteers went out of their way to instantiate these transformations and provide high quality care, as laid out in the national treatment guidelines; but, as discussed above, their efforts were often compromised by structural shortcomings and unfavorable social dynamics.

Dr. Irene's complaints about decreasing financial support from AIDSRelief pointed to another factor that complicated ART service provision and substantially endangered the delivery of HIV treatment far beyond Tanga: the decrease in donor funding for the scale-up of HIV treatment in the aftermath of the 2008 global financial crisis. Aside from Dr. Irene, only one further clinician explained that AIDSRelief had reneged on an earlier announced rise in medical staff's salaries due to the nearing phase-out of its support in 2015. All of the other health professionals whom I consulted on this issue either had no insight into the national treatment program's financial arrangements, or simply referred me to "those up there at the national level" if I wished to obtain further information. Following their advice, I tried to find out more about the program's financial status quo at NACP and TACAIDS in Dar es Salaam. The results of these efforts are presented in the following section.

The Temporal Particularity of a Treatment Regime

The Global Financial Crisis and the Fragileness of Global ART

The extension of HIV/AIDS treatment across Africa (and other resource-limited areas of the world) has been accompanied by doubts about its sustainability from the beginning (cf., e.g., Garrett 2007). But in the wake of the global financial crisis of 2008–2009, these concerns became particularly relevant. In 2010, phasing out, flat lining, and funding shortages of PEPFAR, the Global Fund, and other major financiers meant that "for the first time in the history of the response, international investments for AIDS [in Africa] decreased by 13 percent from 2009 to 2010, from US$ 8.7 billion to US$ 7.6 billion" (UNAIDS 2012, 9). Significantly, this pullback occurred just after the WHO had revised its HIV treatment guidelines and lowered the threshold for ART initiation (WHO 2010a). The estimated global number of people in need of ART had thus risen by almost 50 percent, to 14.6 million people (WHO 2010b, 10).

In November 2011, another weighty incident followed. Due to scaled back pledges and insufficient financial replenishment from its contributors, the Global Fund fell 1.3 billion USD short of the 13 billion USD budget, which even according to modest estimations was needed in order to finance the continuation of already running HIV/AIDS programs at their current pace (McNeil 2011). This prompted the cancellation of funding round eleven[12] and the announcement that no new grants could be signed before 2014. The Transitional Funding Mechanism (TFM) designed as an emergency cushion for the treatment and prevention programs whose funding would come to a halt before then precluded funding for any program scale-ups. "This means that in countries with grants coming to an end, many people already waiting for life-saving HIV treatment, will not benefit from Global Fund resources for at least two years. Unless the situation changes, millions of people will die waiting for access to treatment," warned the International HIV/AIDS Alliance (2012, 6f), pointing out that fifty-five countries had been in the process of preparing round eleven applications in order to sustain their national AIDS response over the coming five years (see also MSF 2012a).

The cancellation of funding round eleven, the restricted access to the Global Fund's TFM, and the simultaneous phasing out of several large-scale public and private donors who had invested in ART provision for years, including PEPFAR, significantly endangered the continuation of national treatment programs in several African countries (MSF 2012a, 2012b). In April 2014, PEPFAR "was at its lowest funding level since 2007" (Collins 2013). The Global AIDS Coordinator (and head of PEPFAR) at the time, Eric Goosby, justified this with the claim that the program was "'getting better and smarter' in service delivery," and pointed to PEPFAR's agenda to increasingly transfer the financial responsibility for HIV treatment to the respective receiving countries' governments (IRIN News 2014). However, "after several years of mostly flat funding" and recent decreases in a wide range of multi- and bilateral donors' financial support to the global HIV/AIDS response "against a backdrop of constrained aid budgets" (Kates et al. 2017, 3), the prospects of global HIV/AIDS treatment continue to be disconcertingly uncertain, and not only in Africa. The following section will specify how this uncertainty played out in the national context of Tanzania and how it was perceived by experts from NACP and TACAIDS.

From Emergency to Sustainability: The Dilemma of Donor Dependency

Since 2006, the proportion of foreign donor funds covering the expenditures for Tanzania's national HIV/AIDS interventions has been above 90 percent, with a peak of 97.8 percent in 2009–2010 (TACAIDS 2012b, 19). In 2010–2011, PEPFAR contributed 67 percent and the Global Fund 19 percent of this large share of external sources (TACAIDS 2012b, 9). "This high dependency on two external financiers puts the whole program under risk if any unanticipated fall-out of funding happens," warned the authors of a financial gap analysis of Tanzania's response to HIV/AIDS in 2011 (Maina and Ngowi 2011, 64).

Regarding the procurement of ARVs and diagnostic consumables, the reliance on external sources was particularly striking. Global Fund rounds four and eight covered the majority of these costs; round four came to an end in October 2010; the first phase of round eight—for which Tanzania was only granted 24 percent of the requested 500 million USD—ended in May 2012 (TACAIDS 2012b,

13). The HIV-related components of Tanzania's proposals for Global Fund rounds nine and ten were rejected, among other reasons, for being too unfocussed, which was explained as the result of the multitude of stakeholders pressing for their interests to be included in the proposal (Interview with a high ranking TACAIDS official, 23 August 2011). Hence, renewed efforts had been made to submit a sound proposal for round eleven. In light of the increased number of people eligible for ART initiation in alignment with the 2010 WHO guidelines, the desired grant was to fill a financial gap of 281 million USD in the provision of ART, which amounted to 27 percent of the projected costs until 2017 (Maina and Ngowi 2011, 68). "It's like we're looking in the cinema, and we're trying to see what will be next," commented a high-ranking NACP staff member in mid-2011.

> Funding really is a big challenge. We were hoping that the Global Fund will be our main supporter. But of course, the Global Fund is funded mainly by the Americans, the very same Americans whose interest has changed. If it's true that the Global Fund [round eleven] will not be approved, we will suffer. Surely we will suffer.[13] (Interview, 14 July 2011)

Only a few months later, the Global Fund officially announced the cancellation of funding round eleven, and the financing gap beyond 2012–2013 was estimated to be over 90 percent. As TACAIDS warned,

> Now, all hopes of entering a new phase of the HIV response are effectively put on hold until at least 2014, and progress on many fronts may actually be reversed due to shortage of funding. The effects on individuals and communities will be devastating. (TACAIDS 2012b, 14)

The capping of PEPFAR funding from 2010 onward and the uncertainty about the form and scope of the US government's support for Tanzania's treatment program after 2013 exacerbated concerns about the program's sustainability. Since the beginning of PEPFAR's involvement in Tanzania up to 2013, Tanzania had received 1.9 billion USD from the program (GFATM 2013, 5), which made it the principal donor funding the national treatment rollout. PEPFAR's direct contribution to the Tanzanian ARV stock through the procurement of second-line and pediatric compounds was minor. Instead, it focused mainly on services and system strengthening (PEPFAR 2013, 2), for instance, the improvement of patient monitoring, building and renovating health facilities, and providing trainings for health professionals. In 2010, the US and Tanzanian governments signed the Five-Year Partnership Framework in Support of the Tanzanian National Response to HIV and AIDS, covering the period of 2009–2013, known as PEPFAR II. The agreement included the objective to "maintain care, treatment and support services existing at initiation of [the] framework," as well as to "expand prioritized care, treatment and support services, dependent on available resources" (PEPFAR 2010, 13). However, a footnote on the same page read: "While funding for existing services is expected to remain stable, the channels for implementing these services are expected to change over time. In particular, the [US government] hopes to transition some service delivery to indigenous partners" (PEPFAR 2010, 13). This corresponded to the overarching aim of PEPFAR II of "transitioning from an emergency response to promoting sustainable country programs," whereby the partner countries are supported "in taking leadership of the responses to their epidemics" (PEPFAR 2009). According to the TACAIDS Country Progress Report of 2012, the

> transition of responsibility from U.S. Government to URT [United Republic of Tanzania] is expected in the areas of procurement, blood and injection safety, and management of centralized data. . . . The U.S. Government also plans to phase out investments in infrastructure concomitant with increased URT responsibility for this area. (TACAIDS 2012a, 42)

The somber outlook for Tanzania's treatment program in 2011–2012 was not only the result of the uncertain future of Global Fund and PEPFAR assistance. Since the beginning of the global financial crisis, other donors had also phased out their support (TACAIDS 2012b, 17f) or, like the Canadian International Development Agency (cf. Lamtey 2012), shifted their focus away from treatment. This reflected an ongoing paradigm shift of global health policy from vertical disease-specific health interventions driven by a logic of exceptionalism to more horizontal approaches of health system strengthening (Smith and Whiteside 2010).

One means to at least partially counter Tanzania's donor dependency consisted in the government's efforts to establish the so-called Tanzania AIDS Trust Fund (ATF), which was to be fed by domestic revenues, public fundraising activities, contributions from the private sector, short-term investments, and the remaining external donors. This, however, was expected to only "reduce donor dependency by 34 per cent" (Lamtey 2012), and by no means to carry the immense financial weight of the interventions when it comes to the worst. "If at all that scenario comes in," foresaw a high ranking TACAIDS official in the summer of 2011, "we don't have the Global Fund money, we don't have PEPFAR money [referring to the time after the closure of PEPFAR II], then the Trust Fund by almost 95 percent will finance treatment, because that is something we cannot afford to continue without. . . . But even with that the money will not be enough" (Interview, 23 August 2011).

In December 2012, this worst case scenario was averted as Global Fund round eight for the national treatment program was extended to a second phase, covering the period until 2015 (GFATM 2013). The uncertainty concerning the program's sustainability beyond that point, however, remained. In August 2013, Fatma Mrisho, the Executive Chairperson of TACAIDS at the time, reported that the Canadian and Danish governments would no longer contribute to Tanzania's fight against HIV/AIDS, and that PEPFAR was also going to reduce funding based on the premise that "HIV/AIDS in the country is no longer an emergency case, hence local efforts could easily handle the pandemic in a sustainable way as the infrastructure was already there" (Daily News, 22 August 2013).

Since then, Tanzania has fortunately managed to repeatedly avoid imminent treatment funding gaps by securing more funding from the Global Fund (Buguzi and Namkwahe 2016).[14] Yet in light of the government's nation-wide adoption of the Test and Start approach[15] in October 2016 (PEPFAR 2017a, 39), a move that significantly increased the number of treatment-eligible people in Tanzania, independent observers prospected that even with Global Fund investment, a gap will remain in the country's resources to fight HIV, TB, and malaria over the following three years.[16]

As far as PEPFAR is concerned, in early December 2013, the program was extended by another five years. Within the framework of PEPFAR III, handing over ownership of HIV treatment programs to the Government of Tanzania—a strategy that had already posed significant challenges to local health care provision during the preceding years (Marten 2014)—remains a priority (PEPFAR 2017a).

Aside from this, however, Tanzania was fortunate enough to be included in the recent PEPFAR Epidemic Control Strategy's list of thirteen "priority high-burdened countries" for which the strategy "sets a bold course for achieving control of the HIV/AIDS epidemic . . . by the end of 2020" (PEPFAR 2017b, 1). At first sight, this implies a secure continuation of treatment-relevant funding for the years to come by one of Tanzania's largest donors. In light of US president Trump's propositions of drastic budget cuts for the fiscal year 2018—including a cut of 850 million USD from PEPFAR and another 250 million USD from the Global Fund (Lavers 2017)—however, the sustainability of this commitment seems to be anything but certain. And even though Tanzania's AIDS Trust Fund was finally launched in December 2016 (Msikula 2017), it seems unlikely that the country will be able to significantly reduce, let alone avoid its dependency on external funders in the near future.

Chapter Conclusion

The challenges that professionals and volunteers involved in ART provision and surveillance in Tanga faced on a daily basis point to the "messiness" of grounding global health policies and standards in a specific locality and the need to pay close attention to the particular institutional, social, and material contexts shaping HIV treatment on the ground. Four points, it seems to me, are particularly important in this regard.

The first relates to the (infra)structural limitations of ART implementation at the treatment centers. Although a certain material affluence of Tanga's HIV clinics was certainly discernible in comparison to other hospital departments that were less endowed with international donor funding, I would not necessarily conceptualize the CTCs as "enclaves of abundance" (Sullivan 2011a), as their affluence was still rather limited in relation to the actual material and human resources that effective management of the rapidly growing patient masses required. Furthermore, the (infra)structural insufficiencies indicated that the decentralization of ART services and the exponential increase in ART patients in Tanga came at the cost of a compromised quality of service provision and patient care, which necessarily deviated from internationally formulated standards.

This deviation—and this leads to the second point—was caused not only by (infra)structural deficits, but to a significant extent also by problematic "micro-social undercurrents" in the treatment centers in the form of inhibitive organizational deficits, communicational barriers, and emotionally overburdened health workers. This illuminates the limitations of the Tanzanian government's practice of focusing on the transnational apparatus of HIV treatment, with its "prioritization of certain quantitative indicators, often purely numerical or financial, in the measurement of social, economic or institutional well-being" (Malpas 2003, 2343f) and its "emphasis on the uniform, the calculable, and the formal" (Malpas 2003, 2345). The universally applicable metrics that this apparatus applied to measure the success of its own operations, in order to legitimize its constantly growing financial demands, were far from taking local health workers' psychosocial concerns into account, and thus implicitly disregarded aspects that were detrimental to the provision of high quality care (cf. Pfeiffer 2013, 181). Yet as the ethnographic exploration of the manifold challenges facing ARV provision in Tanga's health facilities has made clear, reinforced efforts must be made not only to sustain the financial and technological support for ART rollout, but also to address the social and psychological dynamics within health facilities. Strengthening staff supervision or personnel management capacities may be just as important for the success of long-term ART provision as delivering drugs to the largest number of patients possible.

Third, my observations during the process of incorporating standardized ARV provision into local health centers illuminated not only the difficulties of complying with (inter)national standards when putting people on treatment in overburdened and understaffed treatment centers, but also some of the challenges of monitoring and maintaining these people on treatment in the long run. The description of the AIDSRelief training sheds light on how transnational NGOs commissioned with the implementation of ART provision intended to counteract these challenges by tightening patient surveillance; engendering trustful professional-patient relationships; and fostering a philanthropic attitude among volunteers who were essential in the endeavor to extend into the communities the reach of biomedical control over the increasing patient masses. Building on extensive observations of the working routines and power dynamics

in Tanga's treatment centers and the struggles for a socially meaningful and economically secure life of both individual patients and the
(self-)support groups whose formation was so insistently promoted
by AIDSRelief, the subsequent chapters will elaborate in depth on
how effectively these strategies were applied in practice.

Fourth and finally, this chapter points to the critical dependence of Tanzania's national treatment program on the fluctuations
of the global economy and closely correlated interest shifts within
the arena of global health politics. While the massive external
resources that had been channeled into ART in Tanzania during
the first years of its treatment program held out the prospect
of survival and the resumption of a meaningful life for many
thousands of people living with HIV, the increasingly insecure
sustainability of the program obfuscated this positive scenario.
External donors' efforts to foster national ownership of the program
in light of their own reduced resources began late, and to this day,
the respective demands on the Tanzanian government are largely
unaccomplishable. The resulting uncertain outcome of the current
transitory situation of ART rollout in the country (as well as across
the globe) adds a critical temporal dimension to the spatial particularity of HIV treatment (cf. Marten 2014, 259ff) that needs to be
taken into account when assessing its challenges and achievements
in Tanga and other localities.

Notes

1. The consortium was constituted by the US-based NGOs Catholic Relief
   Services and Interchurch Medical Assistance, the US-based consulting
   firm Futures Group (formerly Constella Futures), and the University of
   Maryland's Institute of Human Virology.
2. There are various types of biomedical practitioners working in Tanzanian
   CTCs (and at other health facilities), to whom I collectively refer in this
   work as "clinicians." The following is an outline of the function and training trajectory of these different types of clinicians, as provided by Sullivan
   (2011b, 24):

   "*Clinical Officer* (CO): The vast majority of biomedical care provided
   within clinics and hospitals in Tanzania is done by clinical officers, who
   receive approximately three years of medical training in clinical medicine,
   community health, and some training in sutures, bone setting, and minor
   surgical procedures.

Assistant Medical Officer (AMO): An Assistant Medical Officer receives an additional two years training after the CO training at a university or college of medicine, and can perform routine surgeries such as caesarian sections, appendectomies and laparotomies. They also have more specialized training in diagnosing more complex ailments compared to COs. Within the district hospital structure, they normally serve as the head of each ward or department, and complex cases are most often referred to them.

Medical Officer (MO): A physician, holding a Degree in Medicine. The majority of physicians in Tanzania do not practice medicine below the regional hospital level. Many work as administrators within the Tanzanian Ministry of Health and Social Welfare, within specialized hospitals, within regional hospitals, or in the private or NGO sector."

3. The names of the health centers are pseudonyms. In the section on the health staff's experiences further below, I omit or have changed descriptive details that might reveal the identity of the quoted individual health workers to those familiar with the CTCs in question.

4. It has to be noted, however, that obtaining such statistics from the health centers was a difficult endeavor. The DAC in charge of collecting these reports constantly put me off from one month to the next, data clerks at the health centers were unavailable or lamented that their computers were broken. As a result, I can only provide snapshots of the patient numbers at the three centers at different moments (*Tumaini*, 15 July 2009: 320 patients; *Maendeleo*, 2 July 2009: 110 patients; *Uhuru*, 19 September 2009: 208 patients), and even the validity of these numbers is questionable, since different persons reported different numbers at the same health center for a given point in time.

5. Due to the limited daily processing capacity of the CD4 machine at the Bombo Regional Hospital, each CTC at the health center level was assigned a maximum of fifteen blood specimens that could be sent to the laboratory per week.

6. Every time patients returned to a CTC for their ARV drug refill, nurses were first supposed to measure their "vital signs" (blood pressure, pulse rate, temperature), conduct a tuberculosis screening, and note their current weight in their files at the triage desk, before they either referred the patient to one of the doctors (in case of further complications) or filled in a prescription form themselves (which was officially not allowed) and sent them directly to the pharmacy to receive their drug refills.

7. During the first years of PEPFAR involvement in Tanzania, the salaries that AIDSRelief paid to CTC workers specifically hired through the consortium were indeed reported to have been slightly higher than those paid by the government. By the time of my research, however, this practice had apparently been abandoned. Several nurses and clinicians told me that it made no difference in terms of the basic salary if one was hired by AIDSRelief or directly by the government. The following figures may provide an approximate point of reference: while an assistant medical officer told me that he

had a gross income of 645,000 TSH, of which 513,000 TSH remained after tax deduction, several nurses explained that their gross income amounted to 450,000 TSH (net 350,000 TSH).

8. Tanga locals were given 32,000 TSH and participants from outside of Tanga 65,000 TSH—considerable amounts of money bearing in mind that the latter sum equaled the official Tanzanian minimum wage per month as of 2009.

9. Shortly before the nurse's report, the TRC representative had mentioned that out of the 605 patients that had been reported to the Red Cross's HBC section as lost-to-follow-up during the previous year, 400 had been located, which leaves 33 percent whose whereabouts and health situation remained unknown.

10. Pharmacist Joy's abovementioned explanation about the consistency of this follow-up practice suggests that this "ideal" routine was prone to frequent irregularities.

11. See http://www.youtube.com/watch?v=RO8MP3wMvqg. (Last accessed 8 February 2016.)

12. Until 2011, the Global Fund periodically issued calls for proposals under its "rounds-based channel." The grants provided in each of these funding rounds ran for five years. After the first two years (phase one), grants were only extended for another three years (phase two) subject to satisfactory performance during the first phase.

13. In recent years, the tendency of the US (and other international donors) to predominantly finance "vertical," disease-specific global health interventions has been balanced by increased attention to broader global health issues such as health system strengthening, capacity building, and the improvement of maternal and child health services (Marten 2014, 58). This has implicitly resulted in the decreasing allocation of resources for the global fight against HIV/AIDS (Reddi 2010).

14. See, e.g., http://www.aidspan.org/gfo_article/global-fund-has-provided-bri dge-funding-378-million-11-shortened-grants. (Last accessed 22 January 2018.)

15. In accordance with the WHO guidelines from 2015 (WHO 2015) this entails that every person found to be HIV-positive should be put on ART immediately regardless of CD4 count and clinical condition.

16. http://www.aidspan.org/gfo_article/tanzania-requests-700-million-hiv-tb-and-malaria-global-fund. (Last accessed 22 January 2018.)

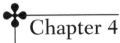

Chapter 4
Generating Treatment Adherence
Neoliberal Patient Subjectivities, Biomedical Truth Claims, and Institutional Micropolitics

In the mid-1970s, a shift took place in the logic, discourse, and practice of public health. Albeit restricted to a particular field of social interaction, this shift can be viewed as a late reflection of the transition from sovereign governance to governmentality. Whereas during the first half of the twentieth century, public health practitioners largely imposed their interventions on individuals and populations in a rather authoritative manner, from the mid-1970s on, they increasingly conceived of their task as assisting people in the "process of self-governance through advice they offer and through seeking to promote social institutions that facilitate 'healthy' choices" (Petersen and Lupton 1996, xiii).

Profoundly influenced by the neoliberal rationalities that gained momentum in the "Western world" at that time, what would come to be known as "the new public health" relied "upon the model of the rational, unified self, consciously making decisions about one's conduct in everyday life in the quest for self-improvement and social success" (Lupton 1995, 8f). Public health experts and medical professionals, in turn, had to provide people with sufficient information about potential health risks in order for them to make adequate decisions and adjust their lifestyle in favor of their health on their own accord. In short, the neoliberal notions of empowerment, self-responsibility, and rational choice became central tenets of health care provision and public health interventionism (Miller and Rose 2008, 18).

Closely related to this was a particular imagination of the ideal relationship between health care providers and patients. Medical professionals should avoid approaching their patients in a paternalistic and authoritative way; instead, the relationship between them and those seeking their help should take on the form of reciprocally felt obligations between equal parties (Mol 2008, 33f). The idea of "non-directive counseling," focusing on "clients' self-determination, autonomy, and self-reliance" (Rasmussen 2013, S542), also emerged in the 1970s in the context of social work theory in the US (Richey 2012, 835). It perfectly blended in with the idea of an equitable professional–patient relationship and the "logic of choice" (cf. also Miller and Rose 2008; Mol 2008) underpinning the new public health.

During the pre-ART era, these credos of the new public health found entrance into HIV counseling (UNAIDS 1997). Some years later, they also informed the way in which HIV/AIDS activists and public health experts came to envision the successful set-up of ART provision in resource-poor settings. Shortly before the implementation of a national HIV treatment program in South Africa, for instance, the South African public health practitioners David Coetzee and Helen Schneider suggested that, in view of the five million people infected with HIV in their country at the time,

> Alternative approaches to the traditional management of chronic diseases ... are needed if the stringent adherence requirements of ART are to be achieved. The evidence from pilot projects is that high levels of adherence stem from a new kind of contract between providers and clients. This contract is premised on very high levels of understanding, treatment literacy and preparation on the part of users, the establishment of explicit support systems around users, and community advocacy processes that promote the rights of people living with HIV/AIDS. The responsibility for adherence is given to the client within a clear framework of empowerment and support. This is very different to the traditional paternalistic and passive relationship between health care workers and patients—changing this represents the key innovation challenge of an ART program. (Coetzee and Schneider 2003, 772)

As Steven Robins argues, this call for a fundamental change of power relationships partly resulted from South Africa's previously failed attempts to tackle the problem of expanding treatment-resistant tuberculosis. Aside from the fact that "directly observed therapy" (DOT)[1]—the paternalistic principal control strategy of this endeavor—had not produced the desired effects (Robins 2006, 321), it was also not practicable to apply this strategy in the context of HIV treatment, considering the far larger number of expected patients. Instead,

> clients would be entitled to free government health care, including ARV drugs, but they would also need to demonstrate that they were "responsibilized citizens"—specifically through treatment adherence, disclosing their HIV status, using condoms, abstaining from alcohol abuse, and having healthy diets and lifestyles. (Robins 2006, 321)

Robins indeed saw such forms of empowering and "responsibilizing" of ART patients realized at the pioneering sites of ART provision in South Africa that were run by Médecins Sans Frontières (MSF) in collaboration with the Treatment Action Campaign (TAC). He did concede, however, that aside from the provision of education and information to patients, the activists' success in fostering the desired new form of "health citizenship" (Robins 2004) also had to be ascribed to patients' "personal empowerment that comes from having survived the passage from 'near death' to recovery" (Robins 2006, 317).

Several factors thus played a role in animating patients to commit to their therapy and adopt a "positive identity" and "healthy lifestyle." These included achieving biomedical treatment literacy, the deeply transformational experience of physical resurrection after ART initiation, and gaining a new sense of belonging and recognition achieved through activist collectives of peer AIDS survivors. In many cases, Robins argues, these experiences were so compelling as to transform the patients into "foot soldiers of global health" who became engaged in activist work and "educated" other patients with the aim of "recruiting new members into their biopolitical projects and epistemic communities" (Robins 2009, 81).

Conducting research on community organization, HIV activism, and ART in West Africa during the years immediately preceding the global ART rollout, Vinh-Kim Nguyen observed a similar convergence of externally induced self-fashioning and novel forms of claims making, which he subsumed under the concept of "therapeutic citizenship—a form of stateless citizenship whereby claims are made on a global order on the basis of one's biomedical condition" (Nguyen 2005). He described how, since the mid-1990s, people living with HIV/AIDS in Burkina Faso and Ivory Coast have been directed to transform themselves through an outright "onslaught of empowerment workshops, role-plays, [and] self-esteem exercises," in which they were trained "to 'live positively' and to 'come out into the open' in order to 'break the silence' and 'overcome the stigma' surrounding life with HIV in Africa" (Nguyen 2005, 125). During the pretreatment era, people's adoption of these technologies of the self was first and foremost to facilitate the formation of patient communities and self-help groups as a resource of mutual psychosocial support.

When the first rations of privately donated ARVs were then finding their way into these patient collectives, the ability to apply confessional technologies, in the sense of producing compelling testimonials about one's seropositivity (and stimulating others to open up and talk about themselves), became a matter of survival. In a situation where the demand for the life-prolonging pharmaceuticals always outstripped the available supply, the ARVs were preferably given to those who were expected to be most useful in pushing HIV prevention by contributing to a destigmatization of the disease (cf. Nguyen 2010, 98ff).

In the era of institutionalized treatment programs, in turn, the term "therapeutic citizenship" "describes the way in which individuals living with HIV appropriate ART as a set of rights and responsibilities" (Nguyen et al. 2007, S34). On the one hand, therapeutic citizenship is "a political claim to belonging to a global community that offers access to treatment for the ill," while on the other hand, it is also "a personal engagement that requires self-transformation" (Nguyen et al. 2007, S34). The technologies of self that patients are taught to apply in the context of treatment programs have extended significantly beyond the focus on confessional technologies of the pretreatment era. Now, "these more intimate technologies target the way we care for our bodies, constitute our families, talk to our lovers, raise our children, as well as our sexuality" (Nguyen 2009a, 205). Patients are expected to apply these technologies not only in order to contribute to a decrease in new infections by being open, but also to create the ideal environment for faultless treatment adherence and for the pharmaceuticals to achieve the greatest possible effect.

This chapter explores to what degree the concepts of "health" and "therapeutic citizenship" lend themselves to an analysis of the processes of treatment enrollment and patient surveillance in Tanga.[2] As will be shown, the tenets of equitable professional–patient relationships, patient empowerment, and self-responsibility that are implicit in these novel understandings of citizenship resonated in Tanzania's National Guidelines for the Treatment of HIV and AIDS (NACP 2008). However, the extent to which this ideal social set-up of ART provision was realizable—and even desirable—in settings of HIV mass treatment differed from the settings of the pilot treatment programs observed by Robins and Nguyen, and is a matter of ethnographic inquiry. As delineated in the previous chapter, nurses, clinicians, and other health care providers involved in ART provision in Tanga were exposed to the enormous pressure of enrolling as many patients as possible on ART in the shortest amount of time. While this already posed a great challenge in itself, unsatisfactory personnel management and substantial infrastructural insufficiencies frequently hampered their work.

Producing the Adherent Patient: Treatment Enrollment and Surveillance in Practice

The dispensing of life-prolonging medicines through Tanzania's national treatment program provided HIV infected persons with the long awaited opportunity to reengage in their social roles, resume economic activities, and regain a sense of agency with regard to their future. ARVs thus became a substantial element in HIV-positive persons' biological and social lives. However, this "redemption" did not come without significant prerequisites. An adherence rate to the strict treatment regime of at least 95 percent had to be maintained permanently in order to prevent virus strains from becoming resistant to the medications (Laing and Hodgkin 2006, 25f). Achieving this high rate is all the more important in resource-poor countries like Tanzania, where second- and third-line medications were only available to a limited extent and—not least due to the often unavailable technology for conclusively verifying treatment resistance—clinicians were often hesitant to move patients on to the next treatment line in case of an unsatisfactory immune response. In stating that "the loss of effectiveness of the first line regimen . . . will have wide public health implications for the entire country," the National Guidelines for the Management of HIV and AIDS (NACP 2008, 217) confirm that the development of drug resistance among ART patients is not only viewed as a danger to individual persons' health. It is also considered a significant threat to the health of the body politic.

Ensuring that as many patients as possible fully adhered to the therapeutic preconditions of ART thus constituted doctors', counselors', nurses', and peer educators' foremost priority. How important it was for patients to regularly take their medications at the right time of day and to adhere to a lifestyle that would support the medicines in doing their work was thus communicated over and over again during the procedure of treatment enrollment, as well as patients' routine control visits. Before exploring these procedures in more detail, however, a short reflection on the notion of "adherence" as opposed to "compliance" will be instructive.

Nearly thirty years ago, James Trostle (1988, 1299) problematized compliance "as an ideology that assumes and justifies physician authority" in reference to the predominant self-understanding of medical professionals throughout the decades following the development of antibiotics in the 1950s. The respective "assumptions about patient-doctor relationships," he argued, "can be summarized as follows: The physician is the proper ultimate authority over the actions of his or her patients, in exchange for a physician's services a patient owes fees, cooperation, and compliance, non-compliance is usually the patient's fault" (Trostle 1988, 1305).

Whereas compliance thus implies patients to be passive and obedient recipients of medical services and advice, adherence is "defined as the active, voluntary, and collaborative involvement of the patient and provider to produce desired preventive and therapeutic results . . . and acknowledges the vital role of the patient as partner in the goals and outcomes of treatment" (Ssewaya 2011, 6). The notion thus inherently reflects the neoliberal conception of the self-responsible patient citizen who complies with medical prescriptions on the basis of his or her own well-informed decisions rather than mere subordination to medical authority.

Consequently, both in Tanzania's policy documents as well as in the discourse of medical and other professionals working in the field of global ART, adherence is the term of choice when referring to patients' desired behavior, as it implies their agency with regard to therapy-related decision making as well as a balanced relationship between patients and health workers. Accordingly, Tanzania's National Guidelines for the Management of HIV and AIDS outlined how CTC staff were expected to build rapport, be empathic, and thus establish a trusting relationship with their patients. The guidelines' section on adherence counseling opened with the instruction: "When a client accesses the CTC for the first time it is important that information be provided that will encourage a life-long partnership between the client and CTC staff" (NACP 2008, 222); and an important way of facilitating such a partnership was to ensure a high level of transparency of the procedures at the CTC for the patients.

With these instructions in mind, let me proceed to how treatment enrollment and monitoring was practically organized in Tanga. In the detailed description of the involved procedures, I draw on my observations at the four public CTCs introduced previously. While individual ethnographic examples (for instance of provider–patient interactions during treatment preparation) thus stem from varying sites, together, they represent the entirety of the system of patient enrollment and surveillance, whose structure was virtually identical at all four facilities.

Reception and Laboratory

The majority of people who sought ART at one of Tanga's CTCs had either been referred from one of the city's VCT centers or from the Bombo Regional Hospital's inpatient departments. In the first step, they had to be registered at the respective CTC's reception. At the Bombo Regional Hospital, the reception constituted a large counter table behind which thousands of patient files occupied several meters of filing shelves, while at the health centers, it merely consisted of a desk located in a small extra room or set behind a screen in the waiting area.

In order to have a CTC file opened, patients had to indicate their full name, address, date of birth, and phone number; the name and address of their treatment assistant (a relative, friend, or neighbor who had to be familiar with their living situation and was supposed to support their daily drug intake after ART initiation); and the names of their head of household, ten-cell leader, and chairman of the district. Oftentimes, patients had to provide these details in the immediate presence of other people waiting to be registered, who could overhear every word they were saying. Visibly uneasy with this situation, some patients spoke in a very low voice, only to be admonished by the receptionist or nurse to speak up. Furthermore, printouts of lists of patients who had been referred to the health centers' CTCs were hung on the wall in the Bombo Regional Hospital's reception area and included patients' full names, ages, and addresses—yet another signal for an institutionalized disinterest in maintaining patient confidentiality.

Once patients had registered and a file had been opened, they received a "CTC 1 Identity Card," a blue piece of cardboard containing their personal details, on which at every drug refill and control visit, nurses should note the progression of their CD4 count and the medications they had received. Subsequently, they were sent to the CTC laboratory to have their blood taken, but only if it was one of the three days per week that were assigned for taking patients' blood; if this was not the case, patients had to return another day. The blood samples from all of Tanga's CTCs were then sent to the central laboratory at the Bombo Regional Hospital, where a complete blood count, CD4 count, and chemistry profile of the liver functions were conducted. Patients were then scheduled to return to the CTC a few days later in order to receive their lab results and, if ART initiation was indicated, to attend the so-called adherence classes. These constituted the core device used to transfer the therapy's central biomedical concepts and to instruct patients on how to realize a "responsible" lifestyle.

"The Doctor Is the One Who Decides!" The Adherence Class

Every prospective ART patient was obliged to attend three consecutive adherence classes within a period of two weeks in the company of a "treatment assistant." The crowded classes with twenty to thirty predominantly female participants[3] took place in a usually dimly lit room.[4] The door leading to the equally crowded hallway mostly remained open, and the piercing crying of the children whose blood was being drawn on the opposite side of the hallway made it difficult to follow the nurse's instructions. Other patients often crossed the room to talk to another nurse in the adjacent room, whose creaking door easily competed with the children's screaming.

During the lectures, that lasted up to two hours—and sometimes induced severely weakened patients to fall asleep on the rear benches—the nurses applied manifold didactic techniques, such as multiple repetition, direct probing, the coercion of inattentive attendees in the presence of the others, and the creation of anxiety by issuing warnings about the "exam" that they would have to pass following the classes. It is little wonder, then, that the nurses were often addressed as "teachers" (*walimu*), for teachers were also generally conceived of as figures with nearly unrestrained authority.

The National Guidelines for the Management of HIV and AIDS meticulously prescribed the content of adherence counseling during a patient's first three visits to the CTC (NACP 2008, 226–32). However, another set of guidelines, prepared by AIDSRelief in Swahili and English, simultaneously circulated in the CTCs and was more often referred to by the nurses involved in adherence counseling than the national guidelines. The AIDSRelief guidelines were formulated in somewhat simpler language and, in a clearer manner, distinguished the topics of each of the three adherence classes. The first class should focus on explaining the differences between HIV and AIDS, ways of transmitting the virus and preventing transmission, and the meaning of CD4. The second class was to explain what ARVs are, who should be put on treatment, what were the conditions for patients to be initiated on treatment, the benefits and side effects of the medications, the meaning of "perfect" adherence, and how to prevent the development of drug resistance. During the third class, finally, the content of the first two classes should be reviewed, the importance of good treatment adherence once more emphasized, and more thorough information provided on resistance and the risks of transmitting resistant virus strains to others. "Partial adherence, no matter how good, will put you at risk of developing resistance," read the final section of the instructions for the third class, and in bold letters it continued: "You should take 'all' your ARVs or 'none' at all. All or none!!!!!!!" (punctuation in original).

In practice, this clear division of topics according to the classes was hardly ever realized. Almost all of the approximately thirty adherence classes that I attended basically included the same array of topics. Often, the patients did not stick to their schedule and simply attended whatever class was convenient for them, with the effect that the audience was usually made up of people with different levels of knowledge. This, in turn, prompted the nurses to simply cover and repeat the topics they held to be most relevant in each class. Aside from slight variations, they usually addressed the distinction between HIV and AIDS, forms of transmission and protection against the virus, forms of opportunistic infections, and finally the functioning of ART, the correct way of taking and storing the drugs, the range of side effects they could evoke, the danger of drug resistance, and dietary requirements.

In the following, I will take a look at how exactly so-called adherence nurses "injected" their audience with the relevant biomedical knowledge about HIV/ART and what strategies they used to instill the particular patient subjectivities that were expected to translate into what was considered an ART patient's "proper" behavior throughout her or his lifelong therapy.

Establishing Medical Authority and the Rules of Treatment

The first thing that the nurses explained to prospective ART recipients was that ARVs were not "emergency medication" that had to be administered immediately. Rather, they emphasized thorough preparation, inner preparedness, and strong-mindedness as essential for the treatment's success. The concept of *kukubali(ana)* (Swahili: "to accept," "to agree") featured centrally in this context. If patients had any doubts about their ability to accept their disease and respective medicines, they should postpone ART initiation until they felt ready to do so.

In order to facilitate patients' readiness to adhere to the rules of HIV treatment and to set the conditions for it to become a routine-like part of their everyday lives, some nurses vividly emphasized the drugs' transformative power and evoked the "normalcy" that would consequently find its way back into their lives.

> Once you've started the medicines, it's you and them forever! ... The medicines are your life. If you take them well, we will not see you being sick every single day, we will not see your children having problems, you won't leave orphans behind, you will build your house well, if you are studying you will continue studying. However, he/she who takes the medicines deficiently will place a troublesome burden (*mzigo kwa kuhangaika*) on his/her children, because you will not have the strength to help them. Have we understood each other, *jamani* (Swahili term for addressing a crowd of people)?! (Nurse Katherine, 15 May 2009)

The only way for patients to reach this promising state was through strict, lifelong adherence to the treatment regimen. The nurses mostly described the HI-virus in terms of "small bugs" incessantly "attacking the body's soldiers" until the ARVs "put them to sleep." Should the bugs "awake again," in the case of a treatment interruption, they would feel "well rested" and therefore "attack with even more fervor." The detrimental consequences of such a reawakening were often depicted just as vividly as the positive outcome of successful treatment. The development of drug resistances was explained metaphorically. "ARVs have a certain habit," Nurse Ruth, for instance, began her explanations during the adherence class on Christmas Eve 2008.

> Nurse Ruth: They "read" the viruses inside your body, all right? Once they have "read" the virus as having the shape of a circle, they will continue keeping it dormant, okay? . . . Now, if you take [your medicines] arbitrarily—one time you take it at a quarter past eight, another time you don't take it at all—the virus changes. Instead of having the shape of a circle, it will have three or four corners. Do we understand each other here?!
>
> Audience: Yes.
>
> Nurse Ruth: Now, tell me, will the ARVs you take every day that usually read circles be able to recognize these squares?
>
> Audience: It's not possible; they won't recognize it.
>
> Nurse Ruth: It is not recognized. It will multiply into many copies of itself. . . . *Pa-pa-pa-pa* [imitating the sound of a machine gun], millions within one minute. . . . The next morning, you take your ARVs again at half past eight, but they help no more. You will wonder, you take the medicines, but opportunistic infections haunt you. TB comes back, herpes zoster, repeated bouts of fever, PCP [pneumocystis-carinii-pneumonia—a lung infection often occurring as a consequence of a suppressed immune system]. You are admitted to the hospital. . . . It is this [messy] use of ARVs . . . that will bring us bad things. So, I repeat it again, people, if there's anyone who knows that he/she will mess around with taking ARVs in one way or the other, I want you to not start it altogether and to first wait until you are really ready for it. Okay? Have we understood each other here?!
>
> Audience: Yes.

Occasionally, the specter of treatment failure was interrelated to national economic interests and global economic inequalities, with the latter given as the cause for the limited availability of second- and third-line medications in Tanzania.

Once you have caused the virus to become resistant against the medicines, I don't know what we should do. Because we don't have the medicines for those who have developed resistant viruses! . . . This means, you won't get medicines every day. The CD4 [level] won't rise, and every day there will be opportunistic infections. So, guys, let's strain ourselves to take the medicines well. A resistant virus is dangerous! Here we have cheap medicines. . . . Those wealthy people over there [pointing toward me, presumably as a representative of "the Global North"] take medicines that perhaps are better. But us, we cannot take these better medicines, they are sold at a very high price . . . and our country is poor. So, once you've developed resistance, you get yourself into big trouble! (Nurse Katherine, 15 May 2009)

In order to avoid treatment failure and a relapse into destitute health, patients were routinely reminded that there was no excuse for deviating from the timing schedule of their drug intake.

When you're told to take the medicines at eight o'clock, it's eight o'clock sharp that you have to take them, and at eight at night, you have to take them [again]. If it's seven, it's seven! There's no, "I'm on a journey," "I was busy with work," or "I've been at a wedding." These medicines don't know "wedding," they don't know "burial," and they don't know any "kitchen party" that could ever prevent you from taking what? Your medicines! Have we understood each other?! (Nurse Hidaya, 23 December 2008)

Taking the pills every day at the right time had to become "second nature," an unreflected-upon, implicit part of everyday life, like getting dressed in the morning. Some nurses equated the medicines with life itself (*dawa ni uhai*—the medicine is life) and even went as far as to identify the medicines with the patients themselves (*wewe ni dawa, dawa ni wewe*—you are the medicine, the medicine is you).

Moreover, the provision of ARVs was depicted as a bilateral agreement between medical professionals and patients. According to the often-employed concept of a "lifelong contract" (*mkataba wa kudumu*), it was the clinicians' and nurses' role to provide the pharmaceuticals and appropriate medical care, while the patients' responsibility consisted of adhering to the treatment regime and always collaborating with the health professionals in order to receive the biomedical technology that, though very costly, was "generously provided by the government."

If you enter in there [pointing to the room where patients' readiness for treatment was individually evaluated after their completion of the adherence classes] we make what? What is it called? A contract. "I will take the medicines throughout my whole life." We put our signature. I put my signature [confirming] "He/she has agreed with me." The day you get lost, I ask them to tell me where you live, so if you don't come [here], I come to your place to find you. I'm not getting tired. When I get out of work, I will follow you to your home. I'll find you. (Nurse Katherine, 15 May 2009)

Even though this remark sounded almost like a threat, the nurse's tone of voice suggested that she rather meant to assure the attending patients that someone would look after them in emergencies. Nonetheless, it implied a particular power relation between the nurses and the patients, in which rather than meeting eye-to-eye, patients were subordinated to health workers' surveillance and control.

On other occasions, nurses made it much more explicit that the only authority capable of making any treatment-relevant decisions was the prescribing doctor:

Whenever you have symptoms [of negative side effects], come to see the doctor. . . . You took the medicines in the afternoon and you got problems. The following morning you say, "I have to go to the doctor!" . . . Listen well, all right? You must not stop taking the medicines! . . . Even if you get a problem, you have to take them. And the following morning, when you wake up, where do you go? To the doctor! . . . The doctor is the one who decides. It's not you who decides to stop taking the medicines! All right? Not even one day, not even one pill you decide to skip it! (Nurse Elizabeth, 14 August 2009)

Indeed, the surrender of decisive power to medical authorities was reflected in many patients' accounts and seemed largely uncontested. Even though she was the leader of various (self-)support groups, forty-six-year-old Alika (fourth year of ART), for instance, did not dare to openly disagree with her doctor's decision to stop ART while treating her acute tuberculosis. "It's difficult," she explained, "because she is a doctor and I am a patient. Especially to tell the doctor, 'Listen, this is not allowed, don't do that . . .' is very difficult. You can't talk to a doctor like that. . . . We are just supposed to be quiet" (Interview, 29 January 2009). However, even though Alika felt silenced, she nevertheless decided to travel hundreds of miles across Tanzania in order to consult the doctors at her home region's hospital, whose decisions fortunately coincided with her own ideas about the appropriate management of her situation. She thus accepted the prevailing hierarchy between her and the doctor in Tanga, but also demonstrated a subtle form of unruliness that went unnoticed by her clinician. In more overt cases of deviance from the prescribed treatment regime, such as the deliberate interruption of therapy, however, patients were usually considered in need of more education and obliged to attend another cycle of adherence classes before resuming treatment.

In the context of Tanzania's highly diverse therapeutic economy and the resulting competition between multiple healing traditions for therapeutic authority over HIV/AIDS (see Chapter 8), most nurses accentuated the superiority of biomedicine over other healing domains and cautioned against healing prayers in one of the local churches, rituals against malevolent forces like witchcraft or sorcery, and herbalists who claimed to cure HIV with plant-based medications.

> Once we start [ARVs], we should not see any *mganga* [healer] who will deceive us and tell us "AIDS is what? AIDS is curable," and we stop taking our medicines. . . . Neither should we see any pastor telling us, "In the name of Jesus, the virus is gone," or any sheikh who will read the Quran and disperse the virus. (Nurse Hidaya, 23 December 2008)

On another occasion, when a patient asked about the use of herbal medicines as a supplement to ARVs, the nurse replied in an equally determined way:

> Woman in audience: There are some people who say that there are local medicines [*dawa za kienyeji*] . . . that work [*zinafaa*]. So, if I take those medicines and these [ARVs], will that be a mistake?
> Nurse Christina: Those local medicines, what are they for?
> Woman in audience: They say they treat malaria. Others treat what? The diseases of AIDS.
> Nurse Christina: It's a mistake. Because those local medicines are not provided in a well measured way [*hupewi kwa kipimo maalumu*]. . . . That's why you will destroy your liver. These medicines [ARVs] contain toxins [*sumu*]. That poison is filtered in your liver. And those local medicines contain toxins too. But they are not delivered in controlled

portions. So, you are not supposed to take which medicines? Local medicines. If they really could cure, a lot of people by now would have been what?

Audience: They would have been cured.

Nurse Christina: If the traditional medicines really had worked . . . the problem [of HIV/AIDS] would have been finished, but there is no traditional medicine at all that what? That cures. And there is no such thing as sorcery (*uchawi*). You bewitch yourself if you don't take [ARVs] well and the virus wakes up again and it attacks; opportunistic infections come with speed. . . . So, the main thing for you is to concentrate on your medicine! (Nurse Christina, 12 December 2008)

Nurse Christina did not make an effort to address the issue of the complementary use of biomedical and nonbiomedical medicine in any detailed manner. Like several other nurses, she rather took the question as an opportunity to generally warn her audience against relying on any type of alternative treatment. Other nurses, however, supported at least the use of the herbal medicine that the TAWG offered to patients who were not yet eligible for ART. In contrast to the herbal concoctions provided by privately practicing traditional healers, these nurses argued, the dosage of the TAWG's medicine was at least well calculated and supervised by biomedical experts. A few nurses, finally, did not pass definite judgment on the possibility of there being a cure for HIV through traditional medicine or religious rituals and prayer. Nonetheless, they demanded that patients who engaged in any such practices always continue to take their ARVs, and that they should maintain an open dialogue about their alternative treatment attempts with the CTC staff.

The Imperative of Disclosure
Aside from the frequently repeated instructions regarding the correct lifelong drug intake and accepting the doctors' and nurses' authority, the adherence classes also constituted the central forum for the instillment of a patient's "positive identity." This was predominantly understood as a patient having a positive attitude toward him/herself as a person living with HIV and a particular way of relating to others resulting from this positive self-understanding.

First of all, the nurses encouraged patients to develop an attitude of "living positively" (Dilger 2001, 2005, 180ff), which, aside from the unconditional acceptance of their HIV infection, comprised the desistance of any feelings of guilt and extraordinariness. In order to guide patients' trajectories away from doubt and skepticism toward a "full mental embrace" of both their health condition and their ARVs, the nurses repeatedly reminded patients of the epidemic's widespread scope. By pointing out that HIV/AIDS has affected almost every family in Tanzania, they implied that the disease was anything but exceptional. The nurses further attempted to "normalize" HIV by pointing out that through the availability of ARVs, it had become a disease like any other medically manageable chronic condition. Therefore, patients should not worry about exposing their health status to others by publicly taking their ARVs. And while, in contrast to Nurse Katherine's quote below, nurses usually acknowledged that HIV was still stigmatized among large parts of the population, they nonetheless encouraged patients not to frantically hide their health status from others. Ultimately, they argued, one of the most important steps in fighting societal stigmatization around HIV was to cease "self-stigmatizing."

> Let's not be afraid of taking our medicines! . . . Take it as any other medication! . . . All people are taking medicines. One is taking *amoxini* [Amoxicillin], the other is taking *septrini* [Septrin, i.e., Cotrimoxazole]. So, if anyone asks you, just tell him/her, "I'm sick". . . . Nowadays, the only problem with stigmatization is us HIV infected persons ourselves! It's not the others; it's us! People feel like if they tell a relative, they don't know what it will be like . . . but you know what? If my relative knew, he/she would support me! (Nurse Katherine, 15 May 2009)

Similarly, many nurses stressed the importance of patients' openness about their HIV infection as an indispensable strategy to garner social support. Only if the persons in their social surroundings knew about their problem and the necessity of taking drugs would they be able to help them by reporting to the hospital if they got sick and could not pick up their drug refills. Relatives or friends would also be able to remind the patient to always take their medications, which would be particularly useful in the long run, when the patient might start to feel a certain treatment fatigue.

Finally, aside from this personal advantage of disclosing to others, not hiding their condition from those who could care for them was depicted as each patient's contribution to the decrease of HIV prevalence at the population level. By openly communicating about their illness, Nurse Ruth once argued,

> you will teach the society members around you the truth about AIDS, which are the ways to transmit it, and what it is like to live with HIV and AIDS. Now, once you've taught them . . . stigmatization will decrease. But if we keep the infection secret, infections will increase very quickly. Because . . . if people aren't open about it, someone may fall ill in her/his home . . . and when she/he has already experienced stigmatization there, she/he will hide her/his problem. Those who will nurse her/him can get infected by this patient. . . . So, my fellows, what I insist on is to ask you to decrease self-stigmatization, let's get rid of it altogether. . . . If you are open, you are free, guys, have you understood me? Christians say when you know the truth, it sets you free. So, once you have got to know the truth about AIDS and the virus, you are absolutely free. (Nurse Ruth, 24 December 2008)

Disclosure thus was depicted as serving varying purposes, including the attainment of freedom and the moral high ground in a Christian sense (cf. Nguyen 2009b), and patients were strongly encouraged to develop a positive self-image that would facilitate their openness.

At the very least, however, they were asked to disclose to one relative or friend. In fact, in contradiction to the national guidelines, which did not consider the lack of a treatment assistant a criterion for precluding any person from ART (NACP 2008, 225), the nurses had made this a *sine qua non*. Without a treatment assistant, patients were usually not initiated on treatment. If they vehemently refused to disclose to any person within their social environment, they were urged to enroll on an HBC program so that one of the HBC providers could become their treatment assistant. In a few cases, CTC nurses living in their neighborhood were asked to take on the task.

Responsible Sexuality and Reproduction
A further important element of instilling patients with a "positive identity," besides encouraging them to be open about their health status, consisted of teaching them how to practice "responsible" sexuality. In this case, responsibility was first and foremost defined in the sense of reduction and abstinence. The discourse around sexuality in the adherence classes thus predominantly focused on several modes of restricting *ngono zembe* (*ngono* = sex, *zembe* = slack, idle, negligent), the Swahili term used to refer to multiple concurrent

sexual relationships. First of all, patients were told to reduce their number of sexual partners to one trusted person, which mostly implied having sex exclusively within (monogamous) marriage. And even when sleeping with their wives and husbands, patients were instructed to always use a condom.

Secondly, within their long-term, stable partnerships, patients were instructed to reduce the frequency of sexual intercourse to a maximum of once per week. The nurses often claimed that sexual intercourse consumed the same amount of energy as walking several kilometers. Reduced sexual activity was therefore a way of preventing the loss of valuable physical energy and, in a second step, preventing the decrease of one's CD4 level. On the other hand, of course, there was a public health benefit to patients' sexual abstinence. It not only reduced the risk of spreading the virus across sexual networks,[5] but also prevented patients from becoming reinfected with new and possibly treatment resistant viral strains. The following passage of an adherence class given by Nurse Sanura (18 December 2008) provides a sense of the didactic style that nurses adopted in conveying to patients how and why they should regulate their sexuality.

> Nurse Sanura: If people make love, they get infected. What kind of lovemaking are we talking about here? It's not like if today I made love with my husband, I will already be infected, no, all right? It's about having *ngono zembe*, have we understood each other? *Ngono zembe* is making love but . . . it is making love with more than one person, okay? Without using condoms. You are a man, and you have perhaps three women at the same time, and you don't use a condom. . . . That's what we call what?
>
> Audience: *Ngono zembe*.
>
> Nurse Sanura: . . . To have only one partner is good, okay, eh?
>
> Audience: Yes.
>
> Nurse Sanura: *Jamani*, truth or lie?
>
> Audience: Truth.
>
> Nurse Sanura: Only having one partner will lead to more faithfulness than having many. Because if you have three partners, today you have slept with Kahdija, but Mariamu wanted you to sleep at her place today. So, possibly Mariamu will sleep with someone else until it is your turn again to sleep with Mariamu. Is that a lie?
>
> Audience: It's true.
>
> Nurse Sanura: So, to have one partner gives you the calmness not to get reinfected and not to infect another person, because [pointing to a

married couple sitting in the first row and taking them as an example]
you have Zeina, and she knows, "I have Juma."
Audience: Yes.
Nurse Sanura: . . . For your health, plan it yourself: "I will only [have sex]
once a week." Or in a month, I'll do it how many times [showing one
index finger to the audience]? Once!

Nurse Sanura's explications are exemplary of how gender stereotypes were actively reproduced in the HIV clinic. It was often men
who were blamed for contributing to the spread of HIV infection
due to their "inability" to restrain their sexual lust and reduce their
number of sexual partners (cf. Mfecane 2011). To some extent, this
was a reflection of public discourses about—mostly older—men who
engage in unprotected, cross-generational sex with younger women
in exchange for gifts—a phenomenon that was also readily taken up
in the discourse of transnationally organized AIDS campaigns, such
as those of PEPFAR.[6]

For many patients, the issue of sexuality was highly relevant, particularly because of their fertility desires. The topic of having children, however, was much less frequently addressed by the adherence
nurses than the importance of sexual abstinence and the prevention
of unplanned pregnancies.[7] In fact, throughout my research, I met
several patients who had attended three adherence classes but had
never heard that there were ways for HIV-positive mothers and parents to have an HIV-negative child. And even if nurses did address
the question, their explanations usually remained quite short and
limited. They explained that an HIV-positive person had the right to
have children just like anyone else. But similar to their instructions
about where the decision-making authority lay with regard to their
treatment regimen and interruption, they put it straight: the timing
was solely in the hands of the doctors, who would decide if the
prospective mother's physical state (predominantly based on her
CD4 count) would allow a pregnancy.

For some health professionals, the question of how to counsel
women with fertility desires, during the adherence classes but also
in their personal interactions with patients, posed a serious moral
dilemma. They acknowledged how important having children was
for women and men, not least due to cultural expectations, but they
also could not edit out the real risk of the child being HIV-positive too.

The following clinician's quote illustrates the inner turmoil this could cause.

> [The mothers'] main question has been, "Can I have another child?" . . . They seem to be stuck. And I won't lie to you, even for me it's a challenge to tell a mother, "You know, you are HIV-positive, yes? Your CD4 may be good, therefore your viral load may be low, but [still] you shouldn't be moving around getting pregnant with another child because you are spreading the infection." At the same time, she wants the child, so you are stuck. . . . How do I tell her that it isn't good for her to have a child again, because definitely that child may end up being positive? . . . How to tell an African woman, "No, don't have a child!"?! Ah, it's a problem! (Dr. Olivia, 2 October 2009)

Dr. Olivia sometimes referred what she termed "particularly difficult cases" to a colleague with more experience in counseling, who would, she assumed, "probably discourage them from getting pregnant, and tell them it's to their advantage, and [ask them:] 'Why [give birth] to the child who will end up suffering?'" As drastic as such directive counseling may seem, from the perspective of medical professionals, it was certainly justified in light of Tanzania's high rate of perinatal HIV transmission. Although PMTCT programs had been implemented in several health centers in Tanga at the time, the risk of infecting a child before, during, or after delivery was far from negligible. The Tanzania Commission on AIDS reported that the "mother to child transmission rate for Tanzania . . . is estimated to be 26 percent . . . due to the low efficacy of the regimens used, and the long duration of breastfeeding" (TACAIDS 2012a, 24).

Healthy Nutrition and Lifestyle
Facilitating patients to take appropriate care of their bodies in terms of eating a balanced diet and abstaining from alcohol and other drugs constituted another important pillar of the adherence classes. In quite significant detail, the nurses explained what a balanced diet (*lishe kamili*) meant according to biomedical criteria and instructed their audience to make sure to eat at least five times a day. It was particularly important to always eat a substantial meal before taking the ARVs, because that way, potential adverse drug reactions could be diminished. There were also a number of dietary restrictions that patients were told to stick to. They should not drink milk for

at least thirty minutes before and after taking their ARVs, because this was said to interfere with their body's ability to absorb the drugs' active ingredients. Secondly, the nurses suggested abstaining from any food that is hard to digest. Furthermore, because caffeine and theine impede the absorption of nutrients in the body, patients were told to abstain from products like coffee, black tea, cola, and the like. Finally, the consumption of alcohol and any other type of drugs was strictly prohibited to patients, because it was said to decrease the ARVs' effectiveness and constitute an unnecessary burden on the body. Additionally, the nurses argued that under the influence of drugs, people become more imprudent and engage more easily in unprotected sexual intercourse than they would otherwise.

The didactical design of the adherence classes very much resembled a school-like set-up, in which teachers drilled the correct answers to their questions into their students until they could reproduce them perfectly. The extent to which the content of the class was tailored to the living realities of the patients at times seemed of lower priority. Although the nurses occasionally made an effort to account for patients' limited economic means by suggesting that they optimize their food spending habits by buying healthier natural products like oranges that were cheaper than less healthy processed products like orange lemonade, enjoying a meal, no matter how small, five times a day remained an idea far removed from many patients' living realities. That no patient ever really questioned this discrepancy between the nurses' instructions and his or her living conditions is unsurprising, considering the latter's positioning as undisputed authorities and the particular atmosphere of the adherence classes that in my view hardly encouraged patients to raise any controversial issues and disagree with the health workers. Perhaps even more than in the adherence classes, medical professionals' strategies to establish clear power hierarchies became evident during the "readiness assessments" that constituted the next element of the treatment enrollment procedure.

Consolidating Authority—The "Readiness Assessment"

After their participation in three adherence classes, the patients had to prove their newly gained knowledge in an individual "readiness assessment" (also termed "adherence panel"), from where, in case they gave an unsatisfactory performance, they could be sent to attend further classes before being provided with ARVs. The adherence panel was also the first stop for treatment defaulters, who were obliged to pass through it when, after having interrupted ART for a certain period of time, they wished to continue treatment.

The panels were supposed to be conducted in a confidential setting that would enable patients to talk openly about their living situation in order to assess their individual barriers to consistent treatment adherence. Often, however, this was not the case. At the Bombo Regional Hospital, at least two to three patients with their treatment assistants were routinely present in these "individual" assessments. Additionally, the assessments were often interrupted by other patients or personnel who entered the room in order to ask something, or by ringing mobile phones—including those of the nurses. Furthermore, it often occurred that while one nurse was conducting an adherence assessment with a patient, another one would be flipping through piles of laboratory results in the same room and handing them out to other patients waiting by the open door.

The situation in and the quality of the panels varied significantly from one CTC and health worker in charge to the other. They ranged from actual individual exam-like assessments to monologic group "counseling" sessions, after which a so-called "adherence checklist" was ticked without any further questioning of the patients. Although the level of patients' assessed comprehension of the treatment varied just as much as the structural configuration and content of the panel itself, I rarely witnessed patients being sent back to class if they were unable to provide the expected answers. Whether or not the patients "passed" the assessment, however, did seem a rather random decision by the nurses in charge. The assessments of "deviant" patients who had interrupted their therapy or had not shown up at the right appointment date were a clear indication of this arbitrariness. A woman who repeatedly failed to get her ARV refills on the indicated day was told that she would have to attend further classes. "I say forgive me," the woman implored. But the nurse refused: "Ah, I don't forgive you. Don't you see? I have taken you here [to the panel]!" The patient insisted: "Mhm, now I ask for your forgiveness, may you forgive me!" "Ah, it's not about asking for forgiveness, you have to understand the importance of the medicines, about the correct intake of the medicines," the nurse instructed her. Only after the woman further apologized and assured her goodwill was she finally allowed to see a doctor and continue with the treatment. "If you forget another day, we will throw you out (*tutakufukuza*)!" the nurse warned her at the end of their tense conversation (Adherence panel, 27 May 2009).

Once patients had passed the adherence panel, they had to report any possible afflictions to a clinician who, after a quick physical examination, reassessed their treatment readiness by asking them a few questions about the correct intake of the ARVs before providing them with the prescription. With this, they had to move on to the CTC's pharmacy, where a pharmacist once more reminded them to take their pills at the right time and never to interrupt their intake without a clinician's advice, before finally handing over the first two-week ration of ARVs and whatever other drugs they had been prescribed for the treatment of opportunistic infections (Figure 4.1).[8]

Finally, at the so-called "exit desk" (Figure 4.2), nurses or peer educators once more controlled the patients' understanding of the rules of drug intake, provided them with the date of their first refill,

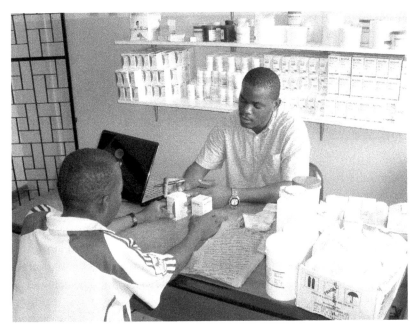

Figure 4.1. Handing over of ARVs, Pharmacy, CTC, Bombo Regional Hospital © Dominik Mattes 2009.

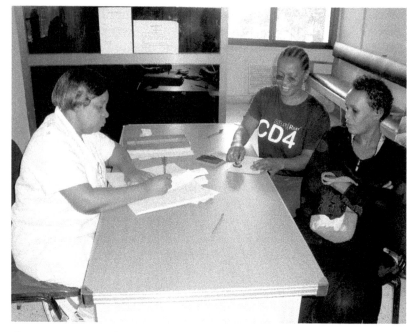

Figure 4.2. Exit Desk, CTC, Bombo Regional Hospital © Dominik Mattes 2009.

and insistently suggested that they participate in an HBC program, before releasing them with small plastic bags full of pills.

"Three Days Are Not Enough for Edna!"—A Morning Class Incident

Facilitating satisfactory treatment literacy among patients, and their readiness to follow nurses and clinicians' prescriptions in the long run, was not only an important part of treatment preparation. At every visit to one of the CTCs, patients were urged to participate in early morning health talks given by nurses or peer educators. These talks, which at the Bombo Regional Hospital were called "morning classes," did not have a fixed curriculum, but usually covered topics similar to the adherence classes and the readiness assessments. The health talks also largely consisted of teacher-centered teaching; that is, the nurse or peer educator stood in front of the patient crowds squeezed onto the benches and delivered monologues about how patients were expected to behave. Even though a few nurses delivered the classes with quite some humor and managed to create a rather pleasant atmosphere, the health talks thus constituted another platform for consolidating health workers' authority over patients.

One episode during a health talk that I attended in late 2008 demonstrated the strong hierarchy of authority that characterized the professional–patient relationship in the CTCs particularly well. As was often the case in the morning classes, on that particular day, volunteer peer educators joined the nurses in instructing the crowd of approximately sixty persons, and they were also referred to as role models of how to live positively with HIV and ARVs. Similar to the nurses in the adherence classes, these peer educators urged the patients not to create an atmosphere of silence and secrecy around their medicines, but to freely take them in public just like aspirin or paracetamol. Furthermore, they strongly recommended that patients join one of the (self-)support groups that were mushrooming in most of the city's neighborhoods, in order to gain further knowledge about how to live with the infection and to become part of a network of mutual support (see Chapter 7).

At some point during the discussions, a peer educator handed one of the blue patient cards to the nurse in charge and whispered something in her ear. The nurse paused for a moment and then spontaneously produced what could be called a "didactic play" in front of the audience. The card belonged to a patient who had supposedly imitated the pharmacist's signature on the card several times in order to make the nurses believe that she had followed the treatment regime as required. The truth was that she had not collected her drug refills for at least three months. Ignoring the fact that this could only have happened on the basis of severe failures in the control mechanism of ARV administration, the case greatly aroused both the nurse and the audience. An animated discussion about the woman's behavior unfolded, until the volunteer could no longer restrain himself: "So what do we do with this person whom we have here among us?!" he asked indignantly before he suggested that "her punishment is that today she begins the adherence class [again] and she has her CD4 count tested again. That's the first thing."

It was at this point that the nurse commanded: "We want to know her! . . . Edna Ramadhani, stand up!" Hesitantly, an approximately twenty-year-old woman, her *kanga* (long piece of cloth worn by many Tanzanian women as a skirt, dress, or a kind of cape covering the shoulders and head) drawn over her face, her gaze directed to the ground, rose from one of the benches in the center of the room. A reproachful murmur ran through the audience: "Why, Edna?!" some asked her. The nurse ordered her to come up to the front and explain her motivations for her malefaction. The intimidated woman was barely able to defend herself. She muttered something about an uncle of hers who used to collect her drugs at the CTC and send them via motorbus to her village some 50 km from Tanga. She claimed that it was he who had falsified the signatures. An HBC provider who was present recognized her and revealed to the audience that she had started ART a few months ago, but once she had regained an acceptable state of health, she had stopped the treatment and taken herbal medicines instead. Now she had come back because opportunistic infections had started to plague her again. Edna continued to try to defend herself, but her words were swallowed up by the loud utterances of the agitated audience. Someone proposed that she be handed a paper and pen so that they could find out if she herself had falsified the signatures, but the nurse did not bother. "We won't give her paper nor a pen, and I will personally hold the class she will attend. . . . Three days [of adherence classes] are not enough for Edna, three days are not enough for Edna!" she concluded, and ordered her to attend adherence classes for two weeks in a row before she would be allowed to continue with the treatment.

This incidence of the public exposure of deviance certainly constitutes a rather extreme attempt to cultivate patient compliance. In many other cases, ART defaulters were subjected to disciplinary measures in a less performative and instrumentalized fashion; after an individual discussion with a nurse or clinician, for instance, and without other patients becoming aware of it, they were simply obligated to attend more adherence classes. Treatment defaulters' reassessment and reeducation, however, was always a procedure that very clearly demonstrated the power hierarchy prevalent in the CTCs, which subordinated patients to the authority and discretion of the medical professionals.

As I hope to have shown up to this point, the social practices involved in treatment enrollment and surveillance in Tanga's public

CTCs diverged significantly from the practices of patient empowerment that HIV activists and policy documents envisioned as essential for the success of large-scale ART provision. In reference to Nguyen's definition of therapeutic citizenship "as a set of rights and responsibilities" (Nguyen et al. 2007, S34), one could say that in these treatment settings, the focus on conveying to patients a sense of their responsibilities—or rather obligations—was much stronger than any efforts to instill in them a self-image as a subject with any right to self-determination with regard to their treatment and therapy-related domains of life, such as nutrition, sexuality, and reproduction (cf. Hardon 2012; Rasmussen 2013).

Ownership and Partnership? A "Field Visit" from AIDSRelief

One morning in mid-August 2009, the Bombo Regional Hospital's CTC received an expected visit from the "technical assistance team" of AIDSRelief, which was scheduled to conduct one of its quarterly four-day field visits. As I should learn on that day, these visits constituted a central element of the "surveillance of patient surveillance" and clearly exemplified the frictions arising in the endeavor to implement transnationally propagated ideas of ownership and empowerment in local institutional practice.

The AIDSRelief team supervised the management of PEPFAR funding, the implementation of ART and PMTCT programs, and the capacity building of CTC staff in twenty-two facilities in the region of Tanga, as well as many others in three further regions. After a warm welcome by the CTC staff and brief conversations about how things had been developing over the previous three months, the five clinicians and public health experts divided themselves up. Each team member proceeded to one of the different "stations" of treatment enrollment and patient management in order to observe the extent to which in their everyday work, the CTC staff were able to implement the protocols laid down in the national guidelines. Of particular interest to the supervision team was gaining an insight into what information the staff provided to patients on HIV and ART, and how they interacted with them. Furthermore, they scrutinized the quality of the administration of patient data on a sample basis.

When I entered the room for the adherence class, it was already running. Sitting in the first row, Claude, one of the AIDSRelief experts, was listening attentively to the instructions of the nurse and the two assisting peer educators. Toward the end of the class, he intervened by complementing the nurse's explanations about HIV-positive persons' risks of contracting TB. When the class ended and small groups of patients were consecutively called to attend the readiness assessment in the room next door, Claude asked the peer educators to share their experience of teaching and following-up fellow patients. Repeatedly, he reminded them how important they were for the improvement of patients' treatment adherence, as they functioned as a connecting link and mediator between the CTC and patients' communities.

Claude then turned toward me and explained that in his view, the Bombo Regional Hospital's CTC was performing comparatively well. Nonetheless, he criticized the fact that patients with varying levels of knowledge were being mixed up in the classes, whose content he considered overwhelming. Furthermore, he was concerned about the maintenance of patient confidentiality during the adherence panels, one of which was taking place while he was voicing his critique. Through a windowpane, we could see that, as was often the case, several patients' understanding of ART was being assessed simulta-neously. Claude did not raise these concerns directly with the nurses and peer educators. Rather, he explained, all of his and his colleagues' critical observations would be discussed in a final feedback meeting with the CTC staff on the last day of their stay in Tanga.

Claude's conversations with the nurses and peer educators were very amicable, and, as far as I could observe in other parts of the CTC, the other team members had established equally good rapport with the CTC staff. Frequently, their conversations and interactions were enriched with jokes and laughter, and it seemed that the CTC personnel and their supervisors had found a way of meeting eye-to-eye in their common struggle to raise the quality of service provision. During the final feedback meeting, however, which was attended by a representative of the hospital management, three CTC clinicians, a representative of the hospital's laboratory, and a number of nurses involved in the HIV care, this impression of equity, harmony, and a spirit of fighting together for a common cause was somewhat obfuscated.

Dr. Oscar, the leader of the "technical assistance team," opened the meeting with a PowerPoint presentation of the current statistics on the patients being treated at the CTC and in the hospital's PMTCT program. He then turned to the main points that had been identified as in need of improvement. On the basis of the team's sample of patient files, only 60 percent of patients had had their baseline CD4 count determined before beginning ART, and only in 40 percent of cases had their CD4 level been checked as a control measure six months after treatment initiation. Furthermore, the rate at which children were being enrolled on treatment was too low in view of the national target that stated that at least 20 percent of all patients on ART should be children. Finally, the rates of patients lost to follow-up were still too high, despite all previous recommendations on how to reduce them.

After raising these issues, Dr. Oscar invited the participants' ideas on how to tackle these shortcomings, but his encouragement was met with silence. Only after repeated requests did one of the CTC representatives finally issue a brief comment. In a rather enervated and somewhat reproachful tone, she explained that the number of patients lost to follow-up was in fact not that high. Most of these patients were simply continuing their therapy somewhere else. Another clinician involved in the provision of pediatric ART then refused to take responsibility for the insufficient routine of determining patients' CD4 counts. Over and over again, she complained, they told caretakers to have their children's CD4 levels checked on the Monday following their appointment at the children's clinic, which usually took place on the last Saturday of the month (when the hospital's laboratory was closed). The pediatrician of the AIDSRelief team immediately added for consideration that this was very difficult for caretakers to realize given the fact that they then had to take their children out of school. Upon the CTC clinician's suggestion that, as a solution for this problem, the laboratory would have to open its doors during the Saturdays when the children's clinic was held at the CTC, the present lab technician uttered a deep sigh but did not pass any comment. With this, the discussion ebbed away.

The CTC staff remained equally reserved when the other points Dr. Oscar raised were to be discussed. Only at one point did one of the clinicians voice a critical concern with regard to the demands of meeting the reporting and quality requirements of AIDSRelief, as well as the two other donors supporting program implementation at the CTC. The clinician suggested that all of these supporting organizations should coordinate their activities and assess the CTC facilities together. In this way, the staff would not have to spend a disproportionately large number of working hours preparing reports for the three different organizations, and they would achieve a clearer sense of the exact requirements that they were expected to meet.

From the few comments that the CTC staff issued during the meeting, I got the impression that rather than being interested in evoking productive discussions about the shortcomings identified by the AIDSRelief team, they predominantly tried to rebuff the critiques with which they were faced. Some of the interviews I conducted with CTC staff during the weeks following the feedback meeting confirmed this. One staff member was particularly outspoken in this regard. Her remarks pointed particularly to the problems arising from the power hierarchies within the CTC, but also from an implicit power imbalance between the CTC staff and the AIDSRelief supervision team, which, after all, represented the CTC's major donor. "The feedback meeting is not an ideal place for me to talk about the problems of [the Bombo Regional Hospital]," the clinician explained.

> When AIDSRelief comes, it is a matter of showing up the good part of your own facility. So . . . I was not supposed to complain. There were a lot of things I wanted to say there, but I held back. I didn't say them because . . . as I was asking the question about the CD4 on Saturday, Dr. [name of one of her superiors who also participated in the feedback meeting] nodded to me, kind of like, "Say it later" or "Don't say it." See? So, it's not easy to talk about it. And I don't blame them [her direct supervisors] much because I do have some criticism about AIDSRelief and, what do you call it, NACP. . . . When you are in the field, things are a lot different from when you are setting up the rules and regulations. And unfortunately, when they do come from their big offices, they . . . come for a week or for three days. It's not enough to assess what we do. It's not enough, not at all! . . . it would be good if they organized themselves [in a way] that one person comes and stays for like a month working with you and seeing the problems. . . . They are good, they have to do their jobs, yes. But sometimes I think their criticism is not good. That is why the facilities to which they go, they take the meetings . . . like a defensive thing instead of being open to listen [to] what they have to say. (Dr. Mary-Ann, 2 October 2009)

In order to discuss difficulties in care provision more productively, without the additional burden of having to perform well for a donor organization, Dr. Mary-Ann argued that regular internal staff meetings at the CTC would be helpful. With frustration, however, she recounted her attempts to suggest such meetings to her colleagues. When I asked her if there was any possibility to raise critical issues with her supervisors, she replied:

> No, you can't, and . . . this is Africa, it's a corrupt society—the more you criticize it and the more you talk about it [referring to critique of the working routines at the CTC], the less likely is it to have your contract renewed. So, it's not something you talk about unless you have a job somewhere else waiting for you. . . . I remember AIDSRelief came and insisted that we need to have meetings to discuss problems that are there and which you can solve right here at the hospital, which could have been the opportunity for me to complain. . . . Immediately after AIDSRelief was there, they wanted to have a meeting on Tuesday at one o'clock. I went there. There was nobody. When I went to ask, "Is there a meeting?" [They answered,] "We will let you know." I waited until three o'clock, and I went like, "Okay, is the meeting going to be tomorrow?"—"Ah, probably tomorrow." Until today, it has been "tomorrow," and the meeting hasn't taken place. (Dr. Mary-Ann, 2 October 2009)

Only a few days after my conversation with Dr. Mary-Ann, I had the opportunity to conduct an interview with Dr. Oscar. We were sitting on a beautiful restaurant terrace with the afternoon breeze coming from the nearby ocean. While constantly checking his mobile phone for incoming messages, Dr. Oscar freely acknowledged the observations I had made during the AIDSRelief field visit. In fact, he enumerated many more critical issues than those he had brought up for discussion at the feedback meeting. The lack of documentation of patient data, poor communication within the CTC and between the CTC and other hospital departments, routinely insufficient physical examinations during the doctor consultations, a lack of transparency of CTC routines for patients, the inefficient scheduling of patients' routine control visits, and hardly any existing platforms for individual patient counseling were only some of his concerns.

But then he adopted a conciliatory tone, pointing out that the improvement of all these issues needed time and that the CTC staff was making good advances. And after all, one could not simply force people to work in a particular manner. In fact, he explained that AIDSRelief's approach to "on-site mentoring" was to include local health personnel in all processes of decision-making. Sustainable change should come from within the health facilities themselves, he explained, implicitly drawing an analogy to AIDSRelief's (and many other donors') approach of helping HIV-positive people to help themselves through the establishment of (self-)support groups.

The awkward atmosphere that prevailed during the feedback meeting at the Bombo Regional Hospital and Dr. Mary-Ann's above remarks suggest that the approach outlined by Dr. Oscar did not always work out as intended. Despite all efforts to avoid top-down decision-making and foster a sense of ownership and self-responsibility among health staff, the relationship between CTC personnel and their supervisors ultimately remained that between a donor and its recipients, in which the former sets the rules and requirements by which the latter have to abide in order to keep the funding flowing. As a consequence, the staff rather strove to deliver the best possible performance of their daily work routine during the four-day field visit, instead of proactively pointing out the challenges they experienced in their daily routines.

In "showcasing" the quality of their work and their adherence to their supervisors' instructions during the AIDSRelief team's field visit, but not implementing suggestions such as the establishment of regular staff meetings, the CTC's superiors displayed a subtle unruliness similar to the above example of Alika, who performed adherence to her clinician's directions while secretly following the advice of other doctors. As the following section illustrates, in one of the private HIV treatment facilities, which were also partly funded but much less intensely supervised by AIDSRelief than their public counterparts, the resistance to AIDSRelief's representatives turned out to be much more overt. Consequently, particular strategies used to increase patients' treatment adherence and retention were not considered. This did not carry too much weight, however, as patient surveillance at the private CTCs was anyhow organized to a significantly lesser degree than at governmental HIV clinics.

ART Management in the Private Sector

Only two private medical institutions were providing ART in Tanga in 2009. One was the Tanga Healthcare Center, a larger health center with several departments situated in the vicinity of the Bombo Regional Hospital. The other was a much smaller private doctor's practice called Tanga Afya, located in a densely populated neighborhood housing many small shops and several street markets. Both institutions began delivering ART services in late 2007. By September 2009, they reported having 77 and 106 patients enrolled on HIV care respectively. While the incurring costs were partly shared by public and private funding bodies, ART provision in the private sector was still explicitly implemented as part of the public treatment program and thus equally supervised by the NACP. The ARVs themselves were obtained from the National Medical Stores Department through the same "Supply Chain of ART Commodities" that was used to deliver pharmaceuticals to the public institutions. ARVs, HIV test kits, and specific types of laboratory reagents were paid for with governmental funding and provided free of charge to the private institutions. Additionally, the private CTCs were entitled to send their patients' blood specimens to the Bombo Regional Hospital's laboratory to perform CD4 count analysis. The costs for the provision of any additional medical services, however, were carried by the private facilities themselves, unless they passed the costs on to their patients, which was often the case.

The procedures of patient enrollment, management, and surveillance at the Tanga Healthcare Center and Tanga Afya differed in many respects from those in the public treatment units. Neither facility had buildings that were specifically assigned for the treatment of HIV-positive people, and no visible signs within the institutions referred to the treatment of HIV/AIDS. In fact, a doctor at Tanga Afya told me that the patients had asked the nurses to remove any such indications from the doors of the consultation rooms, "So no one would know 'this one is entering for this thing'" (Dr. Daniel, 6 September 2009). A high level of confidentiality was furthermore achieved within both institutions by not managing HIV patients collectively—for instance, in the form of designating one specific day of the week as "medicine day" (when patients were appointed to receive their first dose of ARVs or refills) or "CD4 day" (for drawing the blood of a predetermined number of patients)—as was the case at the public HIV clinics. Instead, HIV-positive patients could make use of such medical services whenever they wished, with the result that none of the other patients sitting in the waiting area would know that they had HIV. Moreover, the comparably low numbers of patients under HIV care at the two facilities spoke for the possibility of a more confidential handling of patients' concerns than at the overcrowded governmental institutions.

Another advantage of having only comparably few ART patients was that treatment preparation and education could actually be delivered in individual conversations between patients and adherence nurses. As the focus of my research lay on governmental CTCs, I never conducted participant observation of the treatment preparation process at the Tanga Healthcare Center or Tanga Afya. At both institutions, however, the adherence nurses told me that they handled the process of treatment preparation in a rather flexible manner. They explained that only a few patients needed several educational talks over the course of several weeks before they were ready to start the therapy. Most understood everything quite quickly and could promptly be provided with their first ARV supply, often after a single educational session of one to two hours. While the nurses recommended that patients share their health status and the fact that they would have to live with ARVs for the rest of their lives with a family member or other close person, they did not insist on it.

The monitoring and surveillance of patients was also conducted in a less systematic and restrictive way than at the public CTCs. Dr. Mkonge from the Tanga Health Care Center told me that they were thinking about establishing their own HBC team or, alternatively, engaging in a cooperation with the TAWG or TRC in order to organize the follow-up of treatment defaulters. At the same time, however, he doubted whether this would be effective, since most of the health center's patients came from far away, and no HBC service could cover the costs of tracing patients beyond Tanga. Dr. Mkonge was also skeptical about the option of systematically involving peer educators in treatment preparation, which would establish closer ties at least to patients residing in Tanga. The patients themselves did not want this, he assumed, because this would possibly mean that a person from their own neighborhood could get to know about their health status, and they had chosen to seek treatment at the private practice precisely to avoid this.

While the measures of patient follow-up at the Tanga Healthcare Center thus remained restricted to making phone calls, Dr. Deodatus, the owner of Tanga Afya, explained that at his practice, one person was assigned with the task of actually searching for patients who had missed their appointments and could not be contacted by phone at their home. Due to economic and time constraints, however, only defaulting patients who resided in nearby neighborhoods were actually traced. Like at the Tanga Healthcare Center, many nonlocal patients could only be called in order to enquire why they had not shown up for their appointment.

When I asked Dr. Deodatus what he thought about improving patient follow-up at his practice through the inclusion of community care providers who were mentored by AIDSRelief, I had apparently struck a nerve. Rather than merely voicing careful skepticism like Dr. Mkonge, he decidedly rejected any cooperation with AIDSRelief. His subsequent remarks about governmental health officials and the AIDSRelief supervisors as their cooperation partners revealed a considerable degree of frustration and disappointment with regard to his cooperation with the (quasi) public sector. He generally complained that much of the designated funding hardly ever reached those who really did the daily medical and caretaking work on the ground. Additionally, Dr. Deodatus felt excluded from the supply of medical commodities that private healthcare providers involved in ART provision were legitimately entitled to receive from the government, and, secondly, from local health officials' decisions concerning ART provision in the area, which had a significant impact on his and his staff's working conditions.

Dr. Deodatus's relationship with AIDSRelief seemed to be particularly tense. Obviously, AIDSRelief had never provided concrete advice and practical support on implementing ART provision at his practice to the extent he had expected. Instead, according to him, his cooperation with the organization had always been limited and one-sided. In fact, he explained, AIDSRelief had hardly done anything other than enter his practice once per quarter in order to request patient data. Dr. Deodatus was so annoyed by this that at some point, he decided to kick the AIDSRelief team out of his practice. "When they come here, they just look for that [statistics for their reports]," he explained grumpily.

> They sit in this room with their computer, they collect data. That is why I chased them out. . . . I said "I don't want to see you here! Go to your boss and tell them Dr. Deodatus has chased you out and he has reasons for that. Because your duty is not to come and collect data. You have to come and see how we are giving service, which problems we are facing!" (Dr. Deodatus, 8 September 2009)

While I do not know how AIDSRelief reacted to Dr. Deodatus's refusal to grant peer educators access to his practice, shortly after my interview with him, I coincidentally learned that his decision had raised considerable indignation, not only among the peer educators themselves but also among nurses at the Bombo Regional Hospital's CTC. Unaware of Dr. Deodatus's problematic relationship with AIDSRelief, they suspected that he was afraid of granting outsiders insight into his practice because he was illegally selling ARVs and not conducting adequate treatment preparation. Notwithstanding such dramatic allegations, Dr. Deodatus's refusal to even consider the inclusion of peer educators in treatment preparation and patient management at his practice did imply the maintenance of a lower level of control and patient surveillance than was the case at the public CTCs. As was shown in Chapter 3, most of the peer educators were also simultaneously the leaders of (self-)support groups in their respective neighborhoods, and thus played a crucial role in establishing contact with patients who were lost to follow-up.

In summary, in the case of the Tanga Healthcare Center, peer educators were not included in the system of tracing treatment defaulters out of respect for patients' desire for anonymity. At Tanga Afya, in turn, peer educators were denied access due to the conflict-laden relationship between private and public healthcare providers. Notwithstanding these specific reasons for noncooperation, it is reasonable to assume that it was the resulting lower degree of patient surveillance, together with less insistence on patients' disclosure to others and the generally more confidential and less burdensome routine work procedures, that made ART enrollment at both of these facilities rather attractive, particularly for more affluent people living with HIV. Indeed, large proportions of both institutions' clientele were reported to belong to higher social strata than those undergoing ART in the public sector. Even some businessmen of Arabic and Indian descent were enrolled at the private institutions, nurses explained. In contrast to most of my respondents receiving ART at public institutions, who did not earn even the Tanzanian monthly minimum wage of 65,000 TSH, these private clients could afford to regularly pay 4,000–6,000 TSH for laboratory analyses and privately purchase the pharmaceuticals they needed in addition to ARVs. Having money thus equaled higher confidentiality and lower levels of adherence surveillance, and all of the private institutions' ART patients seemingly preferred to pay this price over risking disclosure by seeking help in the public CTCs in their own communities.

Chapter Conclusion

The social interactions that evolved during treatment enrollment and long-term patient monitoring at Tanga's public HIV clinics hardly resembled the dynamics between medical professionals, patients, and activists that were interpreted by Robins and Nguyen as the formation of a new kind of health/therapeutic citizenship. In particular, the connotations of active claim-making and patient empowerment seem to be at odds with the observed medical authorities' endeavor to establish and maintain clear-cut power hierarchies within the clinics and to control and discipline the conduct of the rapidly growing patient masses. Patients were enclosed within a frame of conditions that rigidly determined access to medicines and aimed to extensively modify the way in which they understood themselves, cared for their bodies, and interacted with others in a manner that was considered "appropriate" and "healthy." The instillment of patients' self-transformations within the hospital setting can be viewed as a particular exertion of biopower and a far reaching process of medicalization (Conrad 1992; Lock and Nguyen 2010, 67–71; Zola 1972); inasmuch as through the propagated technologies of self, patients were supposed to realign many central domains of their life in relation to biomedical rationality.

Oftentimes, "responsibilizing" patients was thus not understood or implemented in the sense of enabling them to make well-informed decisions on the basis of a more profound biomedical understanding of their bodies and therapeutic processes. In fact, some issues, such as the possibilities of avoiding perinatal mother-to-child HIV trans-mission, were usually not explained to patients in a manner detailed enough for them to make a decision that could even approximately be called "informed" (cf. Moyer 2012, S73f).

Moreover, the degree to which health workers *wanted* patients to make their own decisions can be called into question. The strongly hierarchical relationship between professionals and patients, as well as the systems and strategies that were established to foster and con-trol the latter's "obedience" to the former, rather suggested patients' disempowerment through particular mechanisms of stimulus and punishment that aimed for the full subjugation of their "docile bodies" to medical authorities (Foucault 1977, 135). Patients were not *enabled* to choose how they wanted to deal with their treatment, disclosure, and sexuality in terms of what they deemed in their best interest with regard to their living conditions and particular social environment. Rather, they were compelled "to make 'the right' choices to ensure the success of ART and to prevent further trans-mission of HIV" (Rasmussen 2013, S537; cf. also Moyer, Burchardt, and van Dijk 2013, S435). This closely resonates with the shift "away from rights and individual liberties, moving toward a greater emphasis on control and public good" that Lisa Ann Richey (2006, 5) observed in the "global development perspective" in relation to global ART provision.

It is difficult to determine the degree to which the health care providers' generally authoritative attitude was ascribable to the enormous pressure on them (and their felt ethical obligation) to perform well and contribute to a satisfactory intervention output in the form of high treatment adherence rates, or to their professional identity in a context where—in contrast to "Western" discourses of equitable professional–patient relationships—health workers are conventionally ascribed a position of authority and power over those seeking their help (cf. Rasmussen 2013, S547). In any case, I often had the impression that the power dynamics prevailing in Tanga's public treatment centers hindered patients from openly discussing critical ideas, doubts, and fears about the treatment with medical professionals. In fact, patients hardly ever voiced any critique with the clinicians, nurses, or other CTC staff, which made it difficult to discern anything like a "claim-making attitude" among them—an important dimension of health and therapeutic citizenship, as described by Robins and Nguyen. Instead, the majority of ARV users did not seem to be driven by a politically motivated urge to claim what they conceived of as a human right. They considered the biomedical treatment simply as an additional—and sometimes the last—option to remedy their desperate health situation (cf. Beckmann and Bujra 2010). Once enrolled in the treatment program, they then found themselves clamped into a rigid system where necessary basic knowledge and medicines were only provided if they adhered to a range of rules and exhibited a precisely predetermined behavior, which—at least in theory—was tightly controlled. My short account of ART provision in Tanga's few private HIV clinics, in turn, showed that the option for people in need of ART to actively decide to undergo treatment in a setting that not only promised a higher degree of confidentiality but also implied fewer restrictive measures of patient surveillance and disciplining was closely contingent upon their economic capacities.

Susan Whyte and colleagues (Whyte, Meinert, and Twebaze 2014, 58) have proposed the term "therapeutic clientship" as a complement to "therapeutic citizenship" in order to better describe the kinds of social relationships that are forged between health care providers and patients (or clients) in the context of HIV treatment programs in Uganda. To some degree, I hold this term to be apt for describing the power relations governing ARV provision in Tanga's governmental CTCs. Firstly, it places particular focus on the dyadic interpersonal relationships between patients and providers, rather than those between patients and abstract international polities; and in my view, it was precisely the particular quality of these dyadic relationships that was most relevant for people in successfully negotiating access to ARVs. Secondly, clientship (or patronage) describes a category of social relationships in which "vital resources are accessed through enduring social relationships to a powerful authority, with expectations by both parties about the morality of exchange" (Whyte, Meinert, and Twebaze 2014, 58); that is, it accounts for the significant power imbalance that characterized the relationships between health workers and patients in Tanga's HIV clinics.

However, I also see a certain discrepancy between the notion of clientship and the power dynamics, social relationships, and interactions in Tanga's public CTCs, for it implies a general sense of endurance, continuity, and reliability that I often found difficult to discern in the interactions and relationships between patients and providers. In innumerable situations, I rather felt that the "emotional texture" and the concrete outcome of particular encounters between individual patients and clinicians or nurses were entirely contingent on unforeseeable factors, ranging from the provider's mood at that moment to the degree to which the structural and social apparatus of the CTC (including, for instance, the technological equipment and colleagues' willingness to collaborate) was functioning on that particular day. The resulting contingency and personal arbitrariness that significantly shaped individual treatment trajectories and that patients simply had to cope with considering their lack of alternatives, is a dimension of ART provision in these settings that, in my view, is glossed over in the notion of clientship, which usually refers to more stable and long-term relationships of loyalty and exchange (cf. Whyte et al. 2013, 150).

Quite apart from the consideration of the degree to which the theoretical notions of therapeutic citizenship or clientship apply to the social dynamics that I observed in Tanga's CTCs, however, the most pertinent question that arises is regarding the impact on patients of the techniques deployed to propagate the "biomedical truth" of HIV and ART and instill corresponding patient subjectivities. The following chapters will explore in detail how people living with ARVs conceived of, communicated about, and lived and struggled with this medical technology that intruded into the most intimate spheres of their lives. This will open up the view to the socioeconomic, cultural, religious, and moral circumstances that shaped their subjectivities and determined what they considered to be the central concerns in their lives, just as much as—and at times far more profoundly than—the biomedical treatment regime and the technologies of self that were so vigorously promoted by the medical professionals.

Notes

1. This meant that every day over the course of six months, the patient had to self-administer anti-TB pills in the presence of a health worker.
2. Parts of this chapter have been published in Mattes (2011) and Mattes (2014a).
3. According to CTC statistics, in December 2008, 66 percent of the patients enrolled in the treatment program were female. However, at the adherence

classes in Tanga's public CTCs, I observed an even more unequal female–male ratio of about 4–1.

4. This particular description refers to the spatial situation at the Bombo Regional Hospital. As outlined above, however, a general feature of all Tanga's public CTCs was a significant lack of space for the management of the large numbers of patients.

5. At the time of my research, discussions about the reduced risk of contracting HIV from a person whose viral load is undetectable due to successful antiretroviral treatment (through mother-to-child transmission or via sexual intercourse) have only begun to evolve in the scientific community. In the communication of medical professionals and patients I witnessed, this question was never brought up. Aside from this, the national guidelines did not entail any recommendations in regard to the sexuality of ART patients.

6. http://www.pepfar.gov/press/119789.htm. Last accessed 15 December 2015.

7. This reflects the prioritization of the National Guidelines for the Management of HIV and AIDS, which contain elaborate sections on family planning services and HIV-positive women's use of contraceptives (NACP 2008, 52f, 196f), but no indications about how to deal with patients' fertility desires other than these few lines: "Although family planning is part of a comprehensive public health strategy to prevent MTCT [mother-to-child transmission], it has been neglected in most programs. Having children or not is every woman's or couple's right. The use of [family planning] should respect and respond to reproductive rights of a woman and her partner. HIV infected women should receive information about preventing unintended pregnancies, the risks of MTCT of HIV infection and consequences thereof, thus enabling them to make informed decisions" (NACP 2008, 196f). This suggests that from a public health policy perspective, efforts to discourage HIV-positive women from having children were prioritized, even though, and again perfectly in accordance with the neoliberal logic of the new public health, in the end, it should be the woman herself who makes the final "informed" decision. In practice, however, it was rather the "informed" clinician's decision as to which women were to subordinate their reproductive desires.

8. Throughout my research, though I witnessed hardly any stock-outs of ARVs, medicines for the treatment of opportunistic infections were often unavailable and patients were obliged to buy them in private pharmacies.

Chapter 5
Diverging Trajectories of Reconstitution
Living with ARVs and the Pursuit of "Normalcy"

This chapter shifts focus from the context of medical institutions to ART patients' everyday lives. Through close observation of their quandaries related to living with ARVs in local moral worlds, I intend to shed light on these individuals' transitions to living with HIV as a supposedly "chronic illness."[1] Transition is understood here as "a person's adjustment towards incorporating the illness" and their treatment regimen "into their lives, within themselves (self), in their identity and interactions with others, in their daily routines and their future outlook" (Russell and Seeley 2010, 375). Put differently, I question the extent to which one can indeed speak of a "normalization" of HIV when it comes to the subjective experience of those concerned. Considering that biomedical institutions, professionals, and discourses become an important part of patients' local moral worlds—but in most cases only constitute one among many other factors that shape their behavior and desires—I also inquire about the alternative discourses, social frames of reference, and moral concerns that determine people's practices and ideas related to their therapy beyond—and in contrast to—the biomedical understanding of ART.

As argued above, health workers used the concept of "normalcy" in the attempt to engender patients' "ideal" behavior, in the sense of being adherent to the treatment regime and adapting their lifestyles in order to facilitate their medicines' full efficacy. If patients adhered to "the rules" of the treatment, so the principal message went, they would eventually recover a "normal" state of health, meaning regained physical strength and an unobtrusive bodily appearance. As will be demonstrated in the following sections, however, for patients, "normalcy" entailed a lot more than bodily transformations. It implied leading a fully functional life in terms of rehabilitated social and economic relations, resumed sexual activity, and a reconstituted sense of self (cf. Beckmann 2013; McGrath et al. 2014; Moyer 2012).

Strategies of normalization (i.e., the moves made in the endeavor to reestablish a sense of ordinariness in one's life) have long been described as central to the illness management of people living with chronic disease (Charmaz 1995). Anselm Strauss delivered one of the first detailed theorizations in this regard:

> The chief business of chronically ill persons is not just to stay alive or keep their symptoms under control, but to live as normally as possible despite the symptoms and the disease. How normal they can make their lives (and their families' lives) depends not only on the social arrangements they can make but on just how intrusive are the symptoms, the regimens, and the knowledge that others have of the disease and of its fatal potential. ... When regimen, symptom, or knowledge of the disease turns out to be intrusive, then sick persons have to work very hard at creating some semblance of normal life for themselves. ... Furthermore, even when normalization tactics are working well, various ups and downs of symptoms ... and the hazards of the trajectory itself, combined with any changes of relevant social contingencies, all potentially threaten whatever arrangements have been established for maintaining a near-normal life and social relationships. (Strauss 1984, 79)

It is important to note that in the context of adapting to living with chronic disease—as in all other social contexts—"The idea of the 'normal' is in itself a value judgment based on the moral-ity of the society in which any of us live, thus, any anomaly only becomes pathological in relation to the 'milieu' in which it lives" (Marsland and Prince 2012, 463). Many people who had suffered from "full-blown" AIDS before initiating ART may have had to learn the hard way about the close connection between being perceived as "deviating from the normal" and others' corresponding derogatory judgments and discriminatory behaviors. In an ideal scenario, the uptake of ART, the subsequent disappearance of the discrediting bodily indices of AIDS, and the eventual restoration of health should prevent people from further negative experiences and facilitate their attempt to "regain control, create order, reduce dependence on others, and to 'feel normal' again" (Russell and Seeley 2010, 375). As the case studies in this and the following chapters show, however, the pursuit of continuity and normalcy in this comprehensive sense was not a linear process and was susceptible to diverse forms of adverse interference. Despite experiencing positive transformative effects from taking ARVs, many patients had to cope not only with the "ebbs and flows" (Manderson and Smith-Morris 2010, 16) of their (now) chronic illness, but also with *new* uncertainties evoked by the very drugs that were meant to restore certainty and continuity to their lives. How divergent the process of reconstitution and normalization after the commencement of ART could be for individual patients over the course of time is illustrated by the first case study of two sisters by the names of Furaha and Imani. Among all my interlocutors living with ARVs in Tanga, Furaha impressed me most with her irrepressible optimism, humor, and confidence in her medicines, which was not even dampened during phases in which she suffered from severe side effects. The story thus begins on a rather positive note, before it moves on to Imani's and other patients' more problematic experiences with HIV treatment.

Case Study A: Furaha and Imani

> Nurse: Now, the results are showing that you are infected with HIV.
> Furaha: [whispering] All right.
> Nurse: Have you understood me?
> Furaha: I have understood you very well.
> Nurse: All right, just take time to let it settle.
> Furaha: I'm not worrying. . . . Now I know about my status and I know how I will [be able to] live. . . . If I will get medicines, I will take them. So, I'm not worried at all. I will just feel as if I had malaria.

Two days before Christmas Eve 2008, fifty-year-old Furaha received her positive HIV test result at the Bombo Regional Hospital. She had come with her neighbor Ruth, who also wished to know if she had "this disease" (*ugonjwa huu*). Together, they received pretest counseling by a nurse, who in a very warm and careful way explained the details of the HIV test, before she squeezed a blood drop out of their index fingers and asked them to wait a few minutes outside.

While my research assistant Edna and I discussed the dangers of occupational exposure to HIV with the nurse, two black lines slowly appeared on the quick test strips, indicating that both Furaha and Ruth were HIV-positive. The nurse called Furaha in, asked her what she would do in case the test was negative/positive, and finally disclosed the result. After reacting in an impressively composed manner, Furaha immediately started to conceptually normalize HIV, comparing it to diabetes, tuberculosis, and malaria. When the nurse enquired about how she felt after receiving the test result and how she planned to go on with her life, she explained that in the case of these other illnesses, you also had to take medicines on a daily basis, at least for a certain period of time. When it was Ruth's turn to receive her test results, she reacted with equal equanimity. After both women had been informed about the further procedure of receiving ARVs and were encouraged that they would be able to live many years with the medicines, they left the hospital with the instruction to come back a few days later in order to check their eligibility to start ART.

Two and a half weeks later, after Furaha had been enrolled on treatment and had already been taking ARVs for one week, Edna and I visited her at her sister Imani's house. She awaited us on the street and warmly asked us to come in. Following her through a narrow passage between Imani's and the neighboring house, we reached the large concrete building's spacious patio, from which seven rooms could be accessed. Several women were doing all kinds of household chores, and a bunch of children were running around, laughing loudly. Cheerfully, they greeted me (the *mzungu* researcher) and Edna, as Furaha led us across the patio into one of the adjoining bedrooms. In the presence of her sister Imani and two of Imani's daughters, all of them sitting on the floor next to us, Edna and I launched into a long conversation with Furaha.

Furaha had completed primary school and soon after had married. But long ago, she told me, her husband had left her, and she now lived together with her youngest child in Muheza, a town some 40 km from Tanga. Her other five adult children had already moved out. Some of them worked in Dar es Salaam, and while she occasionally sold chapatis (flat bread) and tea in Muheza, she predominantly lived from the financial support she received from her own and some of Imani's children.

In 2002, Furaha's mother died of AIDS. She had been sick for a long time, and Furaha and Imani had already been caring for her for eight years when she was finally tested and discovered that she was HIV-positive. Shortly afterward, she succumbed to the disease. Furaha believed that she had been infected with HIV through nursing her mother, as did Imani, who at some point during the conversation told me that she was also HIV-positive and undergoing ART at the Bombo Regional Hospital. Both sisters lamented that during the time their mother was sick, they did not know very much about HIV. They had never taken any protective measures while taking care of her. In the year of her mother's death, Furaha's own itinerary of suffering began. She fell sick more and more often, and every time, it took longer to recover her health. In 2008, she stepped on a sharp stick while working in the fields. When the wound got infected and would not heal for three months, she reminded herself of her mother's fate and finally picked up the courage to test for HIV.

She decided to test and enroll in ART at the Bombo Regional Hospital, because she had had previous negative experiences at Muheza's district hospital. Several times, she said, she had been stigmatized and treated in an unfriendly manner by its health workers. "In hospitals like the one in Muheza, you can wait until you vomit bile, and you're still not attended to," she explained. Her subsequent eulogy to the services at the Bombo Regional Hospital, by contrast, indicated that her ART enrollment had gone smoothly. Two things about medical services were particularly important to her: routine and affectionate treatment by health care providers. At the Bombo Regional Hospital, she found both. Apart from that, she added with a laugh, she took my presence and that of other researchers as an indicator of the hospital's high quality services.

Furaha's attitude toward her ARVs was very positive. "They reduce the fierceness of the AIDS virus," she declared, reproducing one of the central messages of the adherence classes, "and you can do your work for many years . . . so you live with hope." She alluded to other women she had seen at the CTC whose spotless skin and corpulent bodies she took as proof of the medicines' efficacy. Despite the medicines' bothersome side effects, such as intense bouts of vomiting, the sensation of a burning heat in her body, and a profuse production of saliva, she eagerly expressed her readiness to take her daily dosage without fail.

Fortunately, Furaha had no problems maintaining balanced nutrition, unlike many other patients I got to know. Apart from her children's regular financial support, she explained that she also had a few cattle in her *shamba* (a piece of land for cultivation), which allowed her to even eat meat every now and then. As long as there were no unforeseen negative incidents, she therefore did not see any obstacles to her successful therapy.

When I asked Furaha and her sister what would happen if they interrupted their treatment, a discussion evolved between them. While Furaha stressed the absolutely essential obligation of taking ARVs every day for the rest of one's life, Imani was convinced that one could cease the therapy after a while. "It all depends, you hear?" she tried to convince her sister.

> Imani: There are some people . . . who were in a very bad situation. They have taken the medicine until they felt that they got strong again. Maybe after one, three, four, or five years, they have seen that they got their strength back. Without seeing a doctor, they can decide that at this point, I can [stop the medication] and only eat [well] or take another medicine like aloe vera.
>
> Furaha: Now, I tell you something: you take these medicines until you die. What you're saying here is gossip from the streets!

Imani insisted and referred to people she knew who had interrupted their therapy even upon the recommendation of their doctors. But even when Furaha countered that these must have been unqualified doctors and advised her sister to "go back to [adherence] class," Imani could not be dissuaded from the idea that soon, the doctors would also allow *her* to stop taking ARVs and to continue only with daily doses of aloe vera extract.

One week after this conversation, I met Furaha again at her first ARV refill at the hospital. As during the enrollment procedure, she was accompanied by her niece, Imani's sixteen-year-old daughter Jahaira. Her health state had deteriorated throughout the week. She looked very exhausted, walked with difficulty, and her face was covered with dark and painful bumps. She also had a high fever and stomachaches, and strained to speak even at a whisper.

I sat down with Furaha and Jahaira in the crowded hallway and waited with them for the consultation with the doctor. As was often the case, on that morning, the CTC was packed with some sixty people in need of assistance, but the procedure of processing patients seemed to be stuck. After a while, one of the clinicians rushed out of his consultation room. With irritation, she reprimanded the nurses, urging them to get things going. Finally, Furaha was called into the clinician's consultation room. With a weary look on her face, the clinician inspected Furaha's skin, quickly asked her if she had any other problems, and wrote a prescription for a different ARV regimen than the one that Furaha had been taking. The clinician cautioned her that these medicines could cause other side effects, such as heavy nightmares, and advised her to always eat enough. Wordlessly, she then wrote another prescription, handed the little pieces of paper to Furaha and sent her to the pharmacy. Entering the pharmacy, we were welcomed by the sounds of a US action movie, which blared out from an electronic notebook on the pharmacist's desk. After glancing at Furaha's prescriptions, he gave her two bottles of ARVs, a small plastic bag with pills for her rashes, and another one with pain relievers. He told Furaha that he did not have the last drug that she had been prescribed in stock and quickly explained how to take the drugs he had given her—all the while continuing a conversation with another visitor. Outside, I asked Furaha if she had been able to follow the pharmacist's instructions. Neither Furaha nor Jahaira had understood which medicines were for which affliction, nor how many of each she was supposed to take and at what time of day. While Jahaira returned to the pharmacy for clarification, I agreed to accompany Furaha again for her second refill one month later.

Two days before that appointment, I paid a spontaneous visit to Furaha at Imani's house. She welcomed me with a wide smile on her face. Her whole appearance had changed. The spots on her skin had disappeared, and she looked younger than when I had last seen her. Enthusiastically, she told me how good her medicines were, that they did not trouble her at all anymore, and that she had regained her strength and enormous appetite.

At her refill appointment, she appeared in an equally cheerful mood. She told the clinician that her hands were often numb at night, but obviously she did not consider this to be a serious disturbance. Instead, she happily registered that she had gained 4 kilos since starting the therapy. The clinician instructed her to discontinue taking co-trimoxazole (Septrin), a prophylactic antibiotic that most patients were instructed to take in addition to their ARVs for the first month. In its stead, she was prescribed another drug for neurological disorders. The clinician's tone was a bit more friendly than at Furaha's first refill, but the communication between the two still had the form of a one-sided interrogation about the medicine's physical effects followed by further medical instructions.

Three and a half months later, I met Furaha at Imani's house again for a follow-up interview. She was full of energy and joked a lot during our conversation. She explained that, after staying at Imani's house for a month, she had returned to her house and her everyday activities in Muheza. During the past two months, she had fallen sick with malaria and had taken a course of medication. Apart from that, she had had no further health problems. "I eat, Domi. I eat so much!" she told me enthusiastically, as if she could not believe it herself.

> In the morning, I have two cows that I milk. . . . Now . . . when I wake up, I peel three or four oranges and eat them. Then I boil half a liter of milk and drink it. Then I cook chapatis and eat them. Apart from that, we have a lot of green vegetables (*mboga za majani*), herbs, okra, and whatnot at our house, so I add my *ugali* [a dough-like dish made of cornmeal] to the vegetable I have already prepared. . . . I can eat a whole plate of vegetables, and when it comes to *ugali*, don't measure it! I eat it all!

Eating large quantities of a balanced diet certainly played an important part in Furaha's revived physical strength that enabled her to resume her day-to-day work. Every morning, she got up at 6 a.m., swept and mopped the floor, and washed her clothes. She also took care of two of her grandchildren. She washed them, prepared breakfast, and walked them to school. Moreover, she proudly told me that three times a day, she walked to the nearby river in order to fill a twenty-liter bucket, which she would then carry back home on her head. She also took care of her cows and sheep again, and planned to revive her small street shop, which had gone down during her sickness.

Furaha also enthusiastically referred to her transformed physical appearance. She now had more beautiful hair than her friends, she claimed, laughing out loud, and the skin of her face no longer had the slightest defect. Several people who had seen her when she was seriously sick could not conceal their amazement and told her that they could hardly recognize her anymore.

While Furaha said she now needed no assistance to accomplish her daily tasks, she appreciated the help she had received from her family during her illness episodes and before starting ART. Apart from Imani's support, Furaha particularly stressed the support of her other younger sister Majida. When Majida was notified about Furaha's situation, she traveled more than 300 km from her town to Tanga in order to take care of her at Imani's house. She only returned home when Furaha was starting to feel better. When I asked Furaha if she considered compensating her sisters for their support by any means, she referred to the unconditional reciprocity and solidarity that she took for granted among kin.

> We usually help each other with many things, you understand? [Majida] is my relative, the mother who gave birth to us is one person. Although each of us has another father, we help each other very much. Even if I heard that she got a problem, I would need to get on a bus and look after her. . . . If I hear that Majida's child fell sick or that Majida has been admitted to the hospital, I must get on a bus to Morogoro and see her. And if she cannot look after herself, I stay there and help her, and once she will get strong again . . . everybody returns to his/her place—that's how we do it. So, it's not like I pay her a salary, and if I [for example] get hold of a good piece of clothing, or if I have the capacity to buy something for her, I will give it to her. If one day I see that I have a good chicken, I will tie it up and tell her, "My friend, I brought you chicken!" Kin, that's what you're told, are not there to look similar; they are there to help each other.

The persons to whom Furaha had disclosed her HIV infection were confined to a small circle of consanguine family members who "stemmed from the same womb" as her (*tumbo moja na mimi*): her mother and aunts, her children, her siblings and their children. She had not told any of her friends or neighbors in Muheza. Nonetheless, she said that in the future, she would counsel acquaintances who were sick and whom she suspected of being infected too. In order to dispel their hesitancy and anxiety about getting tested for HIV, she would then refer to herself as a positive example and tell them that even if the test should turn out positive, with the medicines, they could live well for many years.

Furaha's exemplary adherence to the "sociomoral regime" of ART also manifested itself in her determined rejection of healers who claimed that they could cure HIV. "I've never had the idea of going to a traditional healer (*mganga wa kienyeji*)," she explained, "and nobody can deceive me [about their curative powers]." She had seen people who had taken traditional medicines for HIV and then died. After all, she reasoned, the healers would be rich if they really had a cure for HIV at their disposal. Absolutely convinced that ARVs were the only available effective drugs against her affliction, she wholeheartedly declared that she would take them, as she had been told at the hospital, until the end of her life, that she viewed her HIV infection as any other disease, and faithfully put her fate in God's hands.

"To a Certain Extent, I Also Hate Them": Adverse Drug Reactions, Persistent Pain, and ART Interruption

Furaha's mostly positive experiences with ARVs and her resulting exemplary adherence to the treatment regime contrasted considerably with her sister Imani's experiences. Imani was forty-eight years old and, like Furaha, had completed seven years of primary school. She was married, had six children between the ages of eleven and thirty, and made her living by selling plant seedlings that she grew on a piece of land that the local police authorities had placed at her disposal. For the last twenty years, Imani told me both proudly and complainingly, she had been at her garden every working day from 7 a.m. to 6 p.m. While during the rainy season, she made up to 300,000 TSH per month, her income during the dry season from September to April was significantly lower. The monthly profit her husband made as a freelancer in the small-scale timber trade was even smaller and, above all, more irregular. Imani was therefore the main provider for her household, which comprised of her husband, three of her children, two of her children's friends who lived with them, one nephew, and two grandchildren.

After Imani and I initially met during my first interview with Furaha, I ran into her again in mid-June at the Bombo Regional Hospital's CTC. She had not taken her ARVs for the previous ten days, she told me. Obviously, she had also confided her "offense" to some of the nurses, who had consequently obliged her to attend three adherence classes before they would allow her to resume treatment. When I asked Imani about the reasons for her treatment interruption, she just laughed and suggested that we talk about it on another occasion.

Three weeks later, I visited her in her garden. She was busy preparing *ugali* and beans on a fireplace. Crouched between light green plant seedlings, eating her lunch, and serving a handful of clients now and then, she revealed her concerns about her health situation. Similar to Furaha, she had decided to test for HIV in January 2008, after having gone through frequent illness episodes over the previous months. Her husband had accompanied her to the health center in their neighborhood. While he had tested negative,[2] she was found to have "those problems" (*matatizo hayo*), which was a shock to her as she had thought that meant the end of her life. "I cried a lot! I worried about my children who are still so young. I was totally taken aback. I cried, and at night I didn't sleep." She was referred to the Bombo Regional Hospital, where she initiated ART in February. Over the following months, however, she got caught up in a maelstrom of side effects and further bouts of disease. She got malaria, which was followed by a severe urinary tract infection. Then things got even worse when she caught a tuberculosis infection and finally developed herpes zoster. Horrified, Imani remembered how she had vegetated in a state close to unconsciousness from March to July. Intermittently, she was admitted to the hospital in Muheza at her own request. Envisaging her imminent death, she chose that hospital due to its proximity to her home village. "If I die," she recalled her considerations, "they can take me [to the burial site] by bicycle."

During those difficult months, Imani had had to take large quantities of different drugs in addition to her ARVs. "I had a whole bag [of pills], enough for one person to be stuffed with. . . . It was a whole truck load," she lamented. In October, her situation finally began to improve. Similar to Furaha, she happily reported how her skin lesions had disappeared, she had regained vigor and corpulence, and her friends had commented on her wondrous transformation in amazement. At times, she even wore knee-length trousers, which she had never done before, so that others could see the flawless skin on her calves. And sometimes, she would even borrow golden earrings and necklaces from a friend in order to underscore and display her reappearing beauty even more. In her view, physical recovery went hand in hand with material well-being and social recognition. She underlined this idea by telling me that after having maintained a productive business during the rainy season, she could even offer small financial loans to those within her surroundings. "When it had lots of rain—they respect me a lot!" she laughed out loud.

But while her general condition had started to improve, the terrible pains in her legs that she had been suffering from ever since she had started ART would not go away. Sometimes, her legs were completely numb; at other times, they felt like someone was crushing her bones, she said with a tortured look on her face. These pains constituted a central concern in her life. On numerous occasions during our conversations in both of my field stays, she desperately repeated how much they were bothering her at all times of the day. The clinicians at the CTC told her that they were a side effect of her ARVs that she would have to endure. But in October 2008, even though her general health situation had started to improve, she could not bear the pains any longer and stopped taking her drugs. Instead, she began taking herbal medicines she got from a healer recommended by a neighbor. Over the following months, she felt rather good, so she assumed that the medicines had helped her and that she could now do without the ARVs.

The persistence of Imani's leg pains, however, affirmed her suspicion that rather than a pharmaceutical side effect, they were the consequence of evil forces. In order to have this verified by a specialist, she invested 75,000 TSH to bring a widely renowned healer from Dar es Salaam to Tanga. The healer told her that she had "these problems that can be treated at the hospital" (*matatizo ya hospitali*), but that she also had been bewitched by a person he could not specify. Imani had no doubt who her perpetrator was and launched into a long and complicated story about a conflict she had once been involved in. While many details of her story remained somewhat opaque to me, the main plot can be summarized in the following way: A friend of her husband had once been in a dire financial situation and had applied for a bank loan. As the bank would not give him the loan without any safeguarding, Imani's husband had "lent" him the deed of ownership for Imani's house. The friend, however, never repaid his loan to the bank, which is why—in an illegal transaction—the bank had sold Imani's house to a woman from another city. Once Imani had discovered what had happened, she sued both her husband's friend and the bank. After a long and consumptive court case, she finally won the house back. Even though the court settled the case, the woman who had bought the house would not surrender. Neighbors informed Imani that she had been talking to people in the streets that she would do something bad to Imani, and Imani was certain that her permanent pains were an effect of her bewitchment.

While the healer's rituals and medicines did not bring about the desired relief, Imani never doubted his diagnosis. Yet over the following months, she was torn between whether she should put her hope and confidence in ARVs or in the healer's remedies. In February 2009, she finally decided to return to the CTC—because "so many people believed in these hospital medicines"—where, after receiving a severe scolding from the staff, she was reenrolled on ART. Nevertheless, during our conversation in her garden almost half a year later, she once again seemed to be undecided about which therapeutic pathway was the best for her. In addition to ART, she was continuing her self-therapy with aloe vera, which she believed protected her from getting fevers. She had also heard of people who had been cured from HIV by traditional healers, some of whom even resided in Tanga, and she planned to seek them out too.

Two years later, I met Imani again in her garden to see how she was doing. Her situation had hardly changed. She still complained about her incessant pains, and she had again started a therapy with another healer, who once more had diagnosed her as having been bewitched. What else could explain the persistence of her pains, she wondered, despite taking all the medicines she received at the hospital, while other ART patients' similar discomforts usually disappeared some time after treatment uptake. Moreover, she believed witchcraft could be a possible cause for HIV, cancer, and TB, confirmed by the many stories she had heard about people with such diseases who had been cured in Loliondo (see Chapter 8).

While Imani asserted that she was now an obedient ART patient and at the most forgot to take her pills for a day only now and then, she still expected to be allowed to stop the treatment after she had taken them for a long time. Meanwhile, she had heard that a company in Dar es Salaam had just started producing ARVs, which at least decreased her worries about there being a sufficient and sustainable stock of the drugs in Tanzania. Ultimately, however, she also set her hopes on a more powerful type of future HIV drug that would be able to cure the virus. In sum, both traditional healers' therapeutic capabilities as well as scientific progress constituted sources of hope for her, despite her troubles with biomedical treatment thus far. Referring to how well her sister Furaha was doing, she once more mentioned her respective difficulties. "I thank God for these medicines; they help me," she said toward the end of our final conversation. "But to a certain extent, I also hate them, because sometimes they bother me. But *she* [Furaha] tells me that she'd love nothing better than taking them ten times a day!"

Bodily (Re)Constitution

Biological Markers of Physical Improvement

Furaha and Imani raised several issues that played an important role in ART patients' reconstitution. To begin with, they experienced this process in a deeply bodily manner. As exemplified by Furaha's enthusiastic and detailed explanations of her daily food intake, one of the most important ways of referring to bodily reconstitution was to mention one's regained appetite and ability to eat large portions of food. Accordingly, gaining weight was taken as one of the principal signs of improvement. Similar to Furaha, Imani also read her clothes becoming tight as a sign of being on the right track. This emphasis on body weight relates to a societal aesthetic norm that equates corpulence with wealth and well being. It was also affirmed by medical professionals, who cheerfully commented on patients' weight gain and encouraged them to keep eating well; or, in the opposite case, they asked patients, at times reproachfully, what kept them from gaining weight.

The decreasing frequency of illness events that Furaha observed after starting ART also reflects the experiences of other patients. "Since I started taking these medicines, I've only caught a fever once," explained Nasra, who had been taking ARVs for nearly three years and whose husband and eleven-year-old son were on ART too.

> Maybe I got a cold and that's it, but I didn't go to the hospital with malaria or so, no! . . . So, I think that the medicines have helped me a lot, because the way I was doing before and the way I'm doing now—that's quite a difference! . . . My body feels like, well, I feel like it's free again, as if I had no problem at all. I find myself doing just all right, like I've been

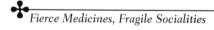
doing before, when I did not have this problem [HIV]. (Nasra, thirty-three years, 11 June 2009)

Like gaining weight, the increasing relief from repeatedly occurring bouts of disease constituted an important indicator of a person's reconstitution. This was particularly due to a common pattern with regard to the timing of patients' HIV tests. Most of my interlocutors undergoing ART had decided to get tested as a sort of last resort after they had unsuccessfully tried other biomedical therapies and/or self-medication for their frequently occurring illnesses, as well as consulting nonbiomedical health experts. Repeated unspecified fevers, diarrhea, nausea, rashes, herpes zoster, typhoid, and tuberculosis were some of the conditions that people were afflicted with until a close relative or a medical professional finally impelled them to test for HIV.

Unlike Furaha and Imani, many people were literally on the brink of death when they finally found their way to the treatment center and were initiated on ART. For them, the experience of bodily "resurrection" was particularly strong and impressive. Ismail, for example, had most dramatic memories of how he had been suffering before he started taking ARVs four years earlier. He had been so sick that he could not turn over in bed without assistance. Still horrified, he remembered the painful bedsores he developed. A rather muscular man and more than two meters tall, he had become emaciated to the point of weighing only 38 kilos. Even a short woman could easily carry him, he told me, making the gesture of carrying a child in his arms. His CD4 count was undeterminable when he was finally initiated on ART, and when he told me about what happened afterward, his face lit up.

> God took care of me! . . . When I started taking these medicines, my body gained weight until I reached a weight of 100 kilos. I gained so much weight that they started getting afraid. . . . Everyone [in the neighborhood] was amazed when they saw me come out of my house and drive away on my motorbike; they wouldn't believe it was me! (Ismail, thirty-five years, 12 June 2009)

Aside from weight gain and the decreasing frequency of illness episodes, there were also other changes in bodily perception on which patients based their positive appraisal of the medicines. At times, such indicators of regained bodily endurance and toughness could be rather particular, as in the case of Issa (Case Study B), who had only been on ARVs for a few weeks at the time of our first interview.

> I notice that my body . . . is perspiring sweat that is clean. I feel that the sweat is coming out well; when I walk around, my body feels comfortable! [Before taking ARVs] I was like—when I sat down, I was all hunched. I felt heat in my body, [but at the same time] I felt cold. But right now, even if you told me to get some water out of the freezer and to shower with it, I'd do it right away! . . . So, I am grateful, the medicines have really helped me. (Issa, forty years, 23 May 2009)

Socializing Biology: The Invisible Markers of Recovery

Another important indicator of physical reconstitution referred to transformations below the threshold of human perception: the increase or decrease of the CD4 level. As pointed out above, patients were familiarized with this measure of treatment progress during treatment preparation, where they were told that CD4 cells were the soldiers of their body's defense system. That the number of these microscopic fighters in the bloodstream did not necessarily correlate with individual perceptions of well being was a lesson that particularly those patients who had tested for HIV before developing AIDS-related symptoms had to learn.

Most patients responded well to the metaphor of CD4 cells being their body's soldiers. For many, the regular monitoring of their CD4 levels over the course of time became as important as it was to the health workers. Raised CD4 counts gave cause for joy, while stagnating or decreasing levels could cause great distress to patients, even if they did not *feel* bad or register any visible signs of their deteriorating health in their bodies. Many of the longer-term patients knew not only the exact outcomes of their CD4 measurements of the last years by heart, but even the dates when they had received the results. Often, they showed me the respective entries in their CTC card while talking about the progress they had made on ART.

On many occasions, people living with ARVs, but also those who had not yet started treatment but were enrolled in the program, established a causal relationship between their CD4 counts, their psychological state, and social occurrences in their lives. Quarrels with friends or family and "worrying/thinking too much," for instance, were viewed as having an immediate influence on their CD4 level. The following passage from Ahmed, a thirty-eight-year-old man, father of two children on ART, and husband of an HIV-positive wife whose too-high CD4 count, like his own, did not yet indicate ART initiation, illustrated this idea particularly well.

> This is the seventh year that I live with AIDS, you see, and I still haven't taken any medicine other than paracetamol! . . . And I haven't been hospitalized or anything like that, and I'm doing hard work. . . . I believe this protection comes from God himself. During all that time, the number of my CD4s has been growing. (Ahmed, thirty-eight years, 6 January 2011)

But then an incident happened that seriously endangered his family's already fragile living situation. In an attempt to demonstrate his political clout to the public before a pending local government election, Tanga's Regional Commissioner had managed to enforce a cleanup campaign entitled "Clean Tanga" (*Tanga Usafi*), which, amongst others, pursued the aim of eliminating from the townscape the innumerable hawkers trying to make a living on the streets. As a consequence, the police confiscated all the portable radios that Ahmed had been selling on the sidewalk of a busy commercial street and imposed a draconian fine on him that he could not pay. Referring to this rather threatening incident, Ahmed said:

> It made me very sad. Especially because I still owed the rent of one month and my children were sick. . . . I had managed to put aside some money, but all my savings were gone. It was a very difficult time and situation, and I was worried a lot. So, it simply had to happen: my CD4 count fell to 391. (Ahmed, thirty-eight years, 6 January 2011)

Establishing a correlation between the fluctuations in one's social circumstances and the number of CD4 cells in one's bloodstream, an act of "socializing" a scientific laboratory indicator (cf. Marsland 2012; Meinert, Mogensen, and Twebaze 2009), was a phenomenon that was co-induced by health workers at the CTCs. They stressed such interrelations both in the adherence classes and in individual conversations with patients as yet another way of encouraging them to develop a positive attitude toward their health status and life on ARVs. Jemima, a forty-eight-year-old woman living with ARVs and mother of two HIV-positive boys who were also on treatment (see Case Study E), recalled such a conversation with a nurse at the

Bombo Regional Hospital. She explained to me how her former neighbors had prevented their children from socializing and playing with her sons because, as they warned them publicly, they were "at the center," meaning the CTC, and "had AIDS."

> This has made me feel very low, and it was the reason why I decided to rent another house for ourselves. Doctor Elizabeth [referring to the nurse] also recommended that. When I arrived [at the hospital], she asked me, "What problem do you have?" And I told her I don't have a problem, but I'm surprised that every time I come here my CD4 level has decreased. "Yes," she told me, "so something has to be bothering you." When I explained about this issue to her, she told me, "Eeh [yes], that's it; find another house." So, I looked for a house for us alone to stay in, and I feel like I have a bit more peace now. (Jemima, forty-eight years, second year of ART, 2 June 2011)

Biological Contingencies

The majority of the patients I got to know had to deal with severe adverse reactions; headaches, dizziness, fatigue, lack of concentration, nightmares, neurological disorders, vomiting, diarrhea, erectile dysfunction, menstrual anomalies, impaired vision, and lipodystrophy were only some of the conditions that strained many people's physical and psychological reserves. Furaha's manner of enduring and forgiving her side effects with such fervent confidence and conviction was rather exceptional. Other patients expressed more skepticism about their new drugs. Yet, not least due to the counseling of medical professionals, they thought of these first difficult weeks and months of ART as a period of adaptation and patiently continued treatment.

Some vested the ARVs with agency and viewed it as a mutual process: it was not only their own body that had to get used to what were often referred to as "those fierce medicines" (*zile dawa kali*), but the medicines themselves had to "accept" (*kukubali*) their body too. Salma, for instance, had reacted so strongly to her initial ARV regimen that after a few days, she presented at the hospital in a state where she could barely walk or speak. During the subsequent four-week long hospitalization, she was switched to another regimen. "The first time when I took these medicines, they affected me to the extent that I was admitted to the hospital," she explained shortly after her return home.

191

> Those [new medicines] that I was put on right now, let's say, this is the second month, so I start to control them, I have to observe them, how they will muddle inside my body. . . . I've already seen that they have done what? That they have accepted me. . . . Once I've taken them for some five months, they will have settled well inside my body, they will have got used to it—and I will have got used to them. (Salma, forty-two years, first year of ART, 2 September 2009)

Amir, a particularly self-reflexive adolescent orphan who had already been living with ARVs for several years (see Mattes 2014b), expressed a similar idea of how the ARVs chose the people that were compatible with *them*, and not vice versa:

> These drugs select. There are two sorts of people: You find that one takes the medicine and develops wounds or he/she takes a certain medicine and starts coughing a lot. . . . So, these medicines—the patient's body and the medicines, they don't match. (Amir, sixteen years, eighth year of ART, 30 May 2011)

Other patients told me about their initial doubts about whether the ARVs would really effect the desired changes in their lives. Gradually, in correlation with the improvements they noticed in their own bodies, they developed more confidence in the drugs. Nasra's husband Juma remembered well how he felt during this initial phase:

> When I started taking these drugs—you know, when you start something new, you have these suspicions—I was like "*Dah* [expression of astonishment/doubt], will I really be able to return to the state I was in at the beginning [before falling sick]?!" . . . But then, with the passage of time, you notice, "*Kumbe* [expression of surprise]! I do certain things [again]!" At this point where I am right now, I also have some plans for later, because now I don't assume anymore that because I have that problem [HIV], I'll die tomorrow. (Juma, thirty-eight years, second year of ART, 11 June 2009)

In many cases, the intensity of the initial side effects decreased to a bearable level a few weeks after ART initiation. Imani's incessant pain in her legs that began with ART uptake, however, points to the need to acknowledge that some people do have to deal with bothersome and intrusive side effects for months, if not years. While Imani had decided to breach her "adherence contract," interrupted her ART, and had turned to several healers and nonbiomedical remedies in her desperate search for relief, others showed remarkable endurance. Michael, a thirty-four-year-old man who had started taking ARVs in 2006 (see Case Study D), recounted that for several years, he had been suffering from almost permanently occurring diarrhea and stomach pains. Only after a switch to a second-line regimen in 2011 was he relieved from these profoundly troublesome side effects.

The manifestation and severity of the ARVs' side effects were closely related to another bodily phenomenon: the intake of food. In contrast to the rather exceptional abundance of foodstuffs available to Furaha, for the majority of patients, providing themselves with sufficient and balanced food to go along with their medicines on a daily basis constituted a principal concern. Based on health workers' warnings and/or their own experiences, they knew that undernourished bodies were more vulnerable both to the medication's side effects and to recurring opportunistic infections. But they knew just as well that the implications of interrupting their therapy could be even worse. Issa was one of those who had to brace himself to adhere to the regimen despite the disconcerting consequences of taking his pills on an empty stomach.

> When you take these medicines, your body lacks strength. . . . Sometimes I'm short of food and I get problems. Sometimes there is no money, you go to bed hungry, then the medicine you take is very strong, you see? . . . There is food that builds up your body, so if you take these strong medicines and you don't have this food, that's a problem. (Issa, forty-two years, third year of ART, 20 July 2011)

But then he emphasized that even if his ARVs made him extremely weary every time he took them without eating enough food beforehand, he would not miss a single dose.

Others were affected so profoundly by taking ARVs in conjunction with insufficient food intake that they felt that the only option was to skip their doses during these periods. Joseph (Case Study D), for instance, regretted having to interrupt his therapy when he had serious problems feeding himself even one proper meal a day, but did not know how else to cope with the side effects. In the middle of an interview in the early afternoon, he once pulled a little piece of paper out of his pocket that contained two ARV capsules. Because he had not had anything to eat that day, he explained, he had not taken them. This was not an uncommon experience for him. Two unopened ARV boxes in his cupboard, each containing the doses for one month, provided silent evidence of how frequently he actually faced this plight. Referring to his treatment interruptions, Joseph explained:

> It happens that you swallow [the pills] and not even an hour and a half later, you feel bile (*nyongo*) coming up. You feel the urge to chew something in order to get rid of the bitterness in your mouth. . . . You wake up in the morning and you can't even walk because you're so dizzy! (Joseph, forty years, fourth year of ART, 21 January 2009)

That an enhanced sensation of hunger was itself a common side effect of ARVs—many patients stressed their ravenous appetite after starting treatment in a similar way to Furaha above—complicated the affair. Not only for Joseph, this vicious circle posed one of the most substantial challenges both to treatment adherence and survival (cf. Hardon et al. 2007; Kalofonos 2010).

From Experience to Representation, from Physicality to Sociality

As we have seen so far, it is at the level of "the individual body, understood in the phenomenological sense of the lived experience of the body-self" (Scheper-Hughes and Lock 1987, 7), that people become aware of the effects of ART in a most immediate and often very powerful way. This is unsurprising since the body is also the realm where the debilitating and disrupting impact of chronic illness is often felt first and most intensely.

> Chronic illness assaults the body and threatens the integrity of self. Having a serious chronic illness shakes earlier taken-for-granted assumptions about possessing a smoothly functioning body. It also disturbs a person's previous assumptions about the relation between body and self and disrupts a sense of wholeness of body and self. . . . Thus, chronic illness with impairment intrudes upon a person's daily life and undermines self and identity. (Charmaz 1995, 657)

In both Furaha's and Imani's narratives, the disappearance of physical defects and the reappearance of bodily beauty featured as important tokens of reconstitution and normalization. In both cases, the declining frequency in perceived periods of bodily dysfunction were equally important. And yet, the two sisters' differing experiences with the medicines' side effects show how diverse these reconstitution trajectories after ART uptake could be, even "simply" with regard to corporality. Imani's leg pain is only one example of how severe physical malfunctions—which may either be the result of irreparable damage to the body *before* ART uptake or an actual side effect of the ARVs themselves (this often remained obscure even to the clinicians in charge of therapy)—turned into sources of permanent distress, concern, and frustration. Moreover, certain side effects, such as lipodystrophy, develop only after long-term drug intake, which stands in stark contrast to patients' expectations of and hopes for things to become better and normalize with time. Temporality thus plays an important role, not only in terms of the time required for gradual health improvements to become discernible; there is also a negative side to it, as the downside of the therapy may only become apparent in its entirety after a significant amount of time has passed.

The challenges of living a life with ARVs based on such biological contingencies have garnered little attention in social scientific studies on the experiences of HIV-positive people in their transition to "normalcy" in sub-Saharan Africa, particularly in contrast to the social and psychological aspects of chronic disease management (but see Kyakuwa 2011, 142–55). Yet they offer equally important evidence of the "uneasy balance between overarching narratives of hope and promise generated by global discourses of ART scale-up, and local lived experiences of ART" (Bernays, Rhodes, and Barnett 2007, S6). In reference to the unequal global availability of ARV regimens due to the TRIPS agreement, such bodily contingencies further underscore the urgency for policymakers and pharmaceutical manufacturers to put greater efforts into creating a political–economic framework that allows for a faster decrease in the price of new drug formulas with fewer harmful secondary effects, so as to make them affordable for treatment programs in the countries that are carrying the largest proportion of the global burden of HIV/AIDS.

That the experiences of bodily change after treatment uptake shaped patients' personal attitudes toward their medicines, their sense of self, and their expectations with regard to their life as long-term ARV users does not come as a surprise (cf. Strauss 1984, 38f). Furaha's and Ismail's evident satisfaction when they told me of how incredulous their neighbors had been upon seeing them after they had regained their strength and healthy appearance, however, suggests that such experiences were crucial for them in another sense too. For most patients, recognizing physical recovery *in* their own body was of the same significance as displaying their reconstitution to others *through* their body. In other words, the representation of "normalcy" in their social surroundings was just as important as their lived experience of physical improvement and the related emerging confidence about returning to the routines of ordinary life. This was particularly so if, prior to ART, they had fallen victim to stigmatization and discrimination on the basis of their poor health and serostatus. Based on similar observations made during Whyte and colleagues' ethnographic study of the experiences of what they call "the first generation" of AIDS survivors (and ART patients) in Uganda, the authors note: "The lived body is also eminently social in that we are always both experiencing subjects and objects for others with whom we interact as bodies. Their gazes, their responses to our embodied selves, are part of our experience as subjects" (Whyte, Meinert, and Mogensen 2014, 224). Physicality, in this sense, is closely related to sociality and morality.

Moral and Social (Self-)Normalization

Demoralizing the Self

Furaha's comparison of the daily management of HIV with that of diabetes and tuberculosis that she made immediately after receiving her positive test result suggests that many ART patients brought to bear particular strategies of conceptual normalization even before starting treatment, and thus long before any concrete effects of the medicines on their bodies could manifest themselves. These strategies can be seen as a form of "identity work" (cf. also Charmaz 1995; Estroff 1989; McGrath et al. 2014, 306; Smith-Morris 2010, 25) that patients engaged in in their attempts to disassociate themselves from the discrediting attributes of immorality and deviance that, in their experience, were (and are) still widely associated with HIV. Furaha's first spontaneous tactic in this regard consisted of reducing HIV to its regimen: living with HIV meant that one had to take a certain number of pills every day, just as one had to do when suffering from other diseases. By implication, it was just as morally "neutral" as these other conditions.

Another strategy of moral self-normalization consisted of adopting the framework of what could be termed "quantitative normalcy" once people became aware of the enormous crowds of HIV-positive patients at the treatment centers.

> If you go to [the hospital], you find a great many people [living with HIV]. If you are here at home, you cannot know. You really believe that it is only me; but if you go to the hospital, you will understand that the disease has really spread widely. (Nasra, thirty-three years, third year of ART, 11 June 2009)

Yet another strategy was to emphasize one's commonality with HIV-negative people by invoking the general unpredictability of death in a world of multiple uncertainties, such as nutritional scarcity, high rates of fatal motor accidents, and less serious diseases that can be fatal in the context of deficient health care delivery. "Even those who do not have that problem die, and you survive them" (Juma, thirty-eight years, 11 June 2009), was a phrase I heard in many variations. Joseph, for instance, who had lost one of his brothers in a car accident, said the following:

> I will live exactly the amount of years that God has foreseen for me. . . . You can anticipate that I will die tomorrow, but *kumbe*: I won't die! . . . I still consider myself as the same as any other human being. (Joseph, forty years, fourth year of ART, 2 June 2009)

Some people went even further than merely reconceptualizing themselves as "the same as any other." They took their own decision to test for HIV and live with all its consequences as an implicit sign of their moral superiority vis-à-vis those who could not raise the courage to do so. This could also be a strategy of coping with the discrimination people faced in their everyday lives. Johnson, who also volunteered as a peer educator in one of the health centers, said:

> This issue of being stigmatized is there. . . . I myself am a teacher, so if anyone gives me many [discriminatory] words, I tell him, "Man, I have been tested, I have this virus, and I'm fine. But the one who has not yet tested and does not know his health. . . . At least I *know* that I am sick!" So, that's where you leave him with a question mark right there. (Johnson, forty-three years, fourth year of ART, 10 August 2009)

Finally, several patients emphasized the manifold ways of trans-mitting HIV, apart from sexual intercourse, in their attempts to rebuild (or maintain) a positive sense of self. They stressed that they had been infected by blood transfusions or dental extractions, pro-viding first aid in motor accidents, or, as we have seen in the case of Furaha and Imani, tending to another person suffering from AIDS, rather than from sleeping with an HIV-positive partner. Implicitly, they therefore did not question or critique the moral condemnation of those who become infected with HIV through sexual intercourse. On the one hand, this attitude can be seen as a reflection of a similar form of reasoning made by the health workers, who in this way tried to "normalize" HIV among the patient crowds, without considering that such an argument falls short of demoralizing HIV altogether. On the other hand, it conformed to the moralizing discourses about HIV/AIDS that were pervasive among various religious congrega-tions (see Chapter 8).

The Social Performance of "Normalcy"

"A sense of continuity is captured in ordinary routines of daily life, the mundane and comforting sameness of repetitive activities, such as drinking a cup of coffee with the morning newspaper. These activities give structure and logic to people's lives." So discerns Gaylene Becker (1997, 4) in a compelling study on how people in the US reworked their sense of self and tried to restore order to their lives after deeply disrupting life events, including the onset of severe chronic illness. The way in which Furaha outlined her daily activities to me, from sweeping the floor in the morning to taking care of her grandchildren, fetching water, and feeding her cattle, exemplifies how much Becker's observation also applies to people suffering from HIV in a social context as different as Tanzania. It was extremely gratifying for people to be able to resume the mundane activities of everyday life after they had gone through the experience of not being able to look after themselves, let alone their family or other household members. Patients' satisfaction thus arose not only from resuming their enjoyable daily routines, per se, but also from realizing that they could get back to work and fulfill their obligations to themselves and others (cf. Charmaz 1983, 179).

Similar to how the positive body transformations brought about by ARVs were not only important markers of physical recovery for individual patients but also visible "images of normalcy" (Russell and Seeley 2010, 379; cf. also Steuer 2012) for relevant others, the resumption of everyday economic activities and household routines functioned as an outward "portrayal of a recovery of stability and order, of predictability and control" (Russell and Seeley 2010, 379). When describing how the ARVs had affected her life, the close connections that Imani drew between her flawless physical appearance, occupational success, and social recognition are a case in point.

The importance of "passing," "that is, engaging in normal interaction because nobody will define him or her as nonnormal" (see also Goffman 1963, 73ff; Strauss 1984, 83)—often in spite of subjectively perceived continuous impairment, as Imani's case demonstrates— did not only accrue from its role in providing inner satisfaction and improved self-esteem. As will be shown in Chapter 6, not being able to "pass" could have rather concrete negative consequences both on patients' biological survival as well as their social existence.

The following section turns to the topic of sexuality and reproduction as a central domain of life that exemplifies the convergence of biological and social concerns perhaps even more clearly than the matter of disappearing (or stubbornly persistent) bodily markers of illness and the social repercussions in patients' local moral worlds. In order to provide an ostensive impression of how problematic the undertaking of achieving "normalcy" after commencing ART could be with regard to sexual practices and reproductive desires, let me continue with the story of Issa, a man whose problematic experience of enrolling on ART corresponded to those of many other patients and, according to my observations, represented the everyday reality at treatment centers more accurately than Furaha's case.

Case Study B: Issa

Treatment Availability vs. Treatment Access

In early May 2009, I spent another day at *Uhuru* Health Center to see how things had developed since ART services had been introduced three months earlier. The management of the roughly eighty patients who had been steadily turning up since 8 a.m. that day seemed to be equally challenging as on the first "outreach day." Numerous patient files were missing, and the insufficient stock of

ARVs did not allow for providing the more experienced patients with two-month supplies, as designated in the protocol. One of the two "adherence nurses" and the "data clerk" had still not undergone any training, and when a nurse informed the waiting crowd that no blood samples to control patients' CD4 levels could be taken that day due to the limited capacity of the Bombo Regional Hospital's CD4 machine, many patients sullenly expressed their discontent, for this had been their sole reason for coming. Processing the many patients took a long time and was just as straining for the engaged health workers as for the waiting patients. One elderly woman who had been waiting for hours suddenly collapsed with a dull thud to the ground. Nurses heaved her into a wheelchair and rolled her away.

In the small and stuffy room labeled "Pharmacy," two nurses filled little plastic bags with ARVs and prophylactic antibiotics. Each patient received exactly the number of pills that would suffice for the days or weeks until their follow-up visit. Due to lack of staff, there was no "exit desk" that day, so the nurses also had to provide the patients with the dates for their next visit.

When I entered the "consulting room" at 12:30 p.m., the two nurses (who had come from the Bombo Regional Hospital to support the *Uhuru* team that day) and the clinician who prescribed ARVs were exhausted and hungry. They did not want to take a break, however, for too many patients were still waiting their turn. They called them in three by three. The nurses hardly made any eye contact with the patients while filling in and handing over the prescription forms. The clinician did make an effort to talk to the patients, cheer them up, and inquire about their afflictions. None of the patients with thrush or other visible complaints were physically examined.

Shortly before 3 p.m., an emaciated man, approximately forty years old, with scabs on his arms and face, entered the room. He was visibly weakened, stood shakily on his feet, and his hunched posture resembled that of his aged father who accompanied him. Desperate and with tears in his eyes, he told the clinician that he had been at the Bombo Regional Hospital in the morning, but, for reasons he did not understand, the nurses would not open a file for him there. Various times, he complained, he had been referred back and forth between the Bombo Regional Hospital and *Uhuru* Health Center. The two nurses and the clinician expressed their compassion and encouraged him to try once more on the following day. They even gave him their phone numbers in case anything would go wrong again.

Three days later, on a Friday morning, I ran into Issa, which was the man's name, and his father again at the Bombo Regional Hospital, where they were about to join the morning class. Issa told me that he had gone back the other day as he was told, and that his blood had been taken in order to check his CD4 level. Today, he expected to receive the results. After the morning and adherence classes, the patients, including Issa, were nevertheless told that they could not be provided with their CD4 counts because the machine had broken again. In order to save Issa and his father from the inconvenience of having to travel once more to the hospital on another day in order to repeat the test, I suggested to the responsible nurse that I take him to the headquarters of the TAWG to see if they could check his CD4 level there. At the TAWG, however, we learned that the only technician who could run the machine was sick, and we were told to come back after the weekend. Issa was extremely discouraged. Already so weak that he could barely walk, he feared that he would not be capable of once more undertaking the journey from his sister's house where he was temporarily staying, some 17 km from Tanga, to the hospital. But he assured me that he would try.

On the following Monday at 8 a.m., Issa and his father indeed appeared again at the CTC. Hoping that they had not come once again in vain, I hurried to the TAWG, where I was told that they would call me as soon as the technician had shown up. On the way back to the CTC, I also passed by the Bombo Regional Hospital's laboratory, in order to inquire if the CD4 machine was working that day. The receptionist told me that they did not yet know, but so far, no technician had appeared to do the necessary repairs. She suggested that I call later if I really needed to know.

Back at the CTC, I convinced Issa that, in case the TAWG technician did not show up, he should try once more to have his CD4 level tested at the CTC. I maneuvered him into the long queue of people waiting to have their blood drawn. About an hour later, Issa and his father, both confused and exhausted, entered the CTC's laboratory, where I had been observing the nurses' working routines. Issa's desperate plea for assistance was answered by a nurse's rough reprimand to get out and wait like everyone else. Finally, at 10:30

a.m., I received a phone call: the technician from the TAWG had arrived. Once Issa was finished having his blood taken there, the technician said he could receive the results back at the CTC on Wednesday. Once more, Issa and his father would thus have to make the effort to return to the hospital.

Two days later, they both participated silently in an overcrowded adherence class. Afterward, Issa finally received his CD4 results, and even the results of his liver and kidney function tests that had apparently been done using one of his earlier blood samples. Since his CD4 level was 23 cells/µl—which he had never been informed about throughout the enrollment process—he was called to the "readiness assessment," which he passed without difficulty. During the assessment, he explained that he was married and had two children, aged seven and twelve years. Neither his wife nor the children had been tested for HIV, but Issa claimed that his wife intended to do so and that they also planned to have the children tested. After the assessment, at 1 p.m., Issa and his father were told to wait for a consultation with the clinician.

Shortly before 2 p.m., Issa was finally called to the consultation with Dr. Ndovu. His father, Edna, two other clinicians, and I entered the room together with him. There was nothing in the room besides a desk, two chairs, and a hospital cot. Without paying any attention to Issa, the three clinicians began a detailed discussion about a woman who had interrupted her ART in favor of herbal treatment for one year. Finally, after the two clinicians left, Dr. Ndovu asked Issa in a rather unfriendly manner about his past diseases and where he had gotten tested. Issa seemed intimidated and answered in such a low voice that I could barely hear him, despite standing right behind him. Finally, Dr. Ndovu asked whether he preferred to start ART right away or to be referred to the *Uhuru* Health Center, which was much closer to his sister's house. If he decided for the first option, she added for his consideration, he would also have to return for control visits for the following six months before he could be referred back to *Uhuru*. Unable to make a decision, Issa asked Edna and me for advice. Worried that there could be further obstacles for him starting treatment at *Uhuru* that could ultimately prevent him from starting treatment altogether, I suggested that he start right away. He agreed, and Dr. Ndovu gave him the prescription for his first dosage of ARVs and the date for his first follow-up visit two weeks later. About an hour later, after having passed through the pharmacy and the exit desk, Issa and his father finally left the hospital. What hardships they had to endure, I thought to myself, in the struggle for this little plastic bag of medicines that would hopefully steer the course of Issa's life toward the better. How many others in Issa's place, without the steady support of a relative or other close person, would have ceased in their attempt to be enrolled on ART at some point in this straining itinerary? There could hardly be a better example of the difference between treatment availability and access.

"My Body Is Fresh"

Ten days later, Edna and I took one of the jammed minibuses running to the village where Issa was temporarily residing in order to see how he was faring with his new pharmaceutical lifelong companions. Walking down the dirt road toward his sister's house, we could already discern him from afar. Just a few hundred meters away from the *Uhuru* Health Center, he was waiting for us, standing underneath a small canopy that also provided shade to some fruits and vegetables that his sister sold to passersby. Issa greeted us with exuberant expressions of gratitude and invited us into a mud house that had seen better days. His sister Zawadi welcomed us equally cordially and took a seat with us in a dimly lit bedroom just large enough to accommodate a bed, a small table, and two chairs. Four large arms of a banana tree, each carrying several bunches of fruit, lay on the floor. Zawadi sold them for 1,500 TSH each, she explained, while I got my recorder ready.

At the beginning of our conversation, Issa mentioned that he actually lived in Tanga. He had only come to his sister's house that day because he had been informed by a friend whom we had contacted that we wished to interview him there—based on my misunderstanding that he lived in the village. Issa then told me more about himself. He was forty-two years old and had completed primary school. He lived with his wife in one of Tanga's extensive poor neighborhoods, where he also worked in a workshop repairing electronic devices. His wife contributed to their household income through an auxiliary job at an auto repair shop. Issa's two children stemmed from a former marriage. They stayed with one of his brothers in Mwanza, some 900 km away. Issa lamented that he could only contribute a minor portion of their school fees and living costs, while his brother covered the majority. Due to the large distance and high travel costs, he did not see his children very often. His brother who was taking care of his children had also financially supported him during the previous three months, when his health state had not allowed him to go to work.

When he had first started to feel sick and weakened, Issa recounted, he had wondered whether it had to do with the "electricity" that always surrounded him at his workplace. When his situation steadily deteriorated, he embarked on an exhausting journey to seek help. It led him to three different health centers and included the diagnoses of typhoid and malaria—and the intake of the respective courses of medication—until one of his *mjombas* (mother's brothers) took him to the *Uhuru* Health Center, since his wife was absent at the time and at least his sister lived nearby and could take care of him. He got tested for tuberculosis, but the test was negative. When the health workers tried to convince him to come back the next day and test for HIV, Issa refused. An HIV diagnosis was like a death sentence, he said, explaining his refusal to me. Over the following weeks, his situation worsened, and he eventually did return to the health center. When the doctor got ready to take his blood again, Issa became suspicious. He explicitly told the doctor that he did not want to have an HIV test. "If you test me for HIV, the answer will be yours alone! I don't want to hear anything about it," he warned. The doctor told him to calm down, and that he was only going to take another tuberculosis test. But when the doctor saw the results, Issa explained, he started to nervously wander around without letting him know the outcome. Finally, he sent for Issa's father, who shortly thereafter arrived at the health center and entered the doctor's room. After half an hour, he called Issa inside too. In the presence of his father, the doctor informed him that he was HIV-positive, emphasizing that it now lay in his own hands to neglect or accept it. "Don't be afraid," he tried to comfort him.

> You are infected, but if you want to keep going, you need to take medicines. You will live a happy, normal life. The opportunistic infections like malaria, and the pain in your chest that has been bothering you, will not bother you anymore as long as you give those bugs [HI-virus] their dose.

Then he explained to him that he needed to start ART at the Bombo Regional Hospital and that at a later point in time, he could continue his treatment at *Uhuru*, if he wished to do so. Apart from this, Issa did not receive any further posttest counseling.

Issa was "very surprised" and shocked upon hearing his diagnosis. But he decided to make the best out of it and to go to the hospital with his referral letter. Unfortunately, enrollment in the treatment program turned into another odyssey. On the first day, he was told to sit in the hallway and wait until he was called. After he had waited for six hours, it turned out that his referral letter had not been put in the right place and, consequently, no one had paid him any further attention. He then had to return another three times, as his laboratory results repeatedly turned out to be invalid. It was during his fifth visit that I met him and tried to get his CD4 test done at the TAWG, as described previously.

When asked about the effect of the ARVs on his physical condition, Issa broke into a spontaneous laudation:

> I'm looking good now! I'm totally well. I walk; I shower myself as normal; I don't have any problems. I take my medicines. At 7 a.m. in the morning, I take one of these [pointing to one of the pill bottles on the table in front of him]; at 7 p.m., I take two of these [pointing to a second one]. That's it. I don't have any problem with my body; I don't have any complaint that they did not help me [with]. These swellings and all that—gone! . . . Don't you see, my body is "fresh" (*iko freshi*). I'm doing great!

Issa was so impressed by how much the medicines had already helped him that the side effects he had experienced during the first days seemed to carry no weight. He had to vomit, felt dizzy after taking his daily doses, and at times his legs felt numb. But this did not prevent him from becoming the sort of patient that the adherence nurses wished for: every morning and night, after brushing his teeth, he explained, he took his pills, and nothing could prevent him from doing so. Why would he not want to take them, and thus fall sick again and die, he wondered.

Navigating Difficult Terrains: Disclosure, Sexuality, and Hope

Issa only knew of two other persons in his neighborhood who lived with ARVs. "The others hide themselves; they don't want to be known," Zawadi interjected. Only at the hospital could one see who was HIV-positive, Issa confirmed: "If someone finds out that you're like this [HIV-positive], they say, 'Ah, that one is infected . . . that one will die any time soon.'" Both Issa and Zawadi then confirmed to one another how people living with HIV/AIDS were despised (*kudharau*), not respected (*kuthamini*), and verbally abused (*kukehebi*) in their neighborhood. "So, this is the moment when you retract (*ndio pale utakapojikunja*)," concluded Issa, "[and the reason why] people want to take the medicines secretly, so that no one else gets to know about it."

> Dominik: So, you yourself, how many people have you told [about your infection] so far?
>
> Issa: This sister here knows and my father. . . . And my wife. But my wife, I told her that I have chronic TB, so they gave me these pills. . . .

At this point, Zawadi interjected and advised him to tell his wife about his situation in order to give her the same chance to take care of her health: to take an HIV test, and, in case of a positive result, live a good life with ARVs just as he did. Issa, however, preferred to find an indirect way of disclosing to his wife that he was HIV-positive. He explained that he had already suggested to her to get tested for tuberculosis—obviously assuming that she would automatically be tested for HIV too. Once she received her positive result, he was then going to tell her that he was "just like her." He claimed that he would even tell her if her test should turn out negative. But, he added, then he would really not know where his own infection had come from. He feared that if he told her directly, she would get worried to the point of getting sick and not be able to go to work. In the meantime, he did not intend to have sex with her. He had already told her that he had tuberculosis, that she might become infected with the disease and that she should first get tested; meanwhile, he was going to take his medicines.

If his wife should turn out to be HIV-negative, Issa claimed that he would simply stop having sex with her or make sure to always use a condom, as he would be afraid of infecting her. He considered living with an HIV-negative wife to be a great problem (*taabu sana*). Not only would he always be worried about her health status, but he also expected to receive less support in regularly taking his medicines if his wife should not have to take the medicines herself. If she should be HIV-positive, on the other hand, he did not see any necessity to use condoms other than for the purpose of preventing pregnancy, and he expected the two of them to mutually support each other in being adherent to the therapy.

When I asked Issa if he wished to have a child with his wife, he affirmed that he would like to "add" one to the two he already had. He also said that he would hold on to that plan even if she did test HIV-positive. "It will be necessary that we go to see a doctor and get advice how we can manage to get a child and care for it in a way that will be safe," he added, referring to the health professionals' instructions. Returning to the issue of using condoms within a sero-concordant relationship, it turned out that he had never heard of the danger of an HIV reinfection. Our conversation therefore ended with explanations from my side, as I felt he needed this knowledge in order to take every measure possible to protect his wife and himself from further affliction.

In the following weeks, I met Issa twice at the Bombo Regional Hospital's CTC. The first time, roughly two weeks after our first interview, he had come because he had developed severe rashes on his extremities. A clinician switched him to another ARV regimen. On this occasion, Issa happily told me that he had already resumed his work and felt no limitations at all. Another three weeks later, he showed up at the CTC for his first ARV refill. He complained about a persistent cough, but the clinician did not pay attention to it, and he simply received his next drug supply. The almost 4 kilos that he had gained since starting ARVs were taken as a proof of the therapy's success.

Roughly four months after Issa's ART initiation, I visited him again at his sister's house for another long conversation in the presence of Zawadi. Although he once again reported drug side effects, such as painfully cracked lips, repeated disturbances of sensitivity in his arms and legs, and a bothersome urge to have a bowel movement every time he ate a larger portion of food, he was still enthusiastic about his ARVs. In the meantime, he explained, he had also disclosed his health status to several of his friends and even convinced some of them to test for HIV. He did not, however, exhibit the same openness toward his wife. While he claimed that he had made sure to always use a condom when he slept with her, he still had not found the courage to tell her about his health status.

When I asked Issa about his future prospects of his life with ARVs, he expressed his expectations of being able to lead a good life.

Whether this expectation was based on a profound inner conviction and trust in the medicines, or simply on the lack of an alternative to taking the drugs, remained open to interpretation. His account of how he had known or heard about several people who had ceased their ART and succumbed to their recurring opportunistic infections spoke for the latter. But Issa was also anxious about the drugs' long-term effects on his health condition. It turned out that Issa had not fully understood why the virus could at one point "not listen to the medicines" any more, so Edna and I made an effort to explain to him the causal connection between irregular drug intake and the development of resistance. In the end, he proclaimed that he was even more convinced that he would never stop taking his ARVs, not even miss a single dose. "When my hour has come, I take my medicines. It's one pill. If it was necessary, I'd swallow one hundred per day, but it's only one! . . . How could you not manage?!"

Being a Long-Term Patient and the Disturbances of Life

After this visit, it took almost two years until I met Issa again, during my second field stay in late July 2011. This time he welcomed me to "his house," which consisted of one bedroom in the side wing of a large but simple concrete building. The room was untidy, laundry was piled up on the bed, and a pungent stench of urine hung in the air. Issa left the door half open and, right after we had taken a seat, put his Triomune 30 bottles (ARV regimen) on the small table between us. A few minutes later, when other people kept passing by his door, he hid them under the table again, laughing somewhat bashfully. Instead, he gave me his CTC card, which indicated that his CD4 count had only slowly risen to 220 cells/µl since treatment initiation. Once it had even decreased between two tests.

While I was still studying his CD4 trajectory, Issa told me that in the meantime, his wife had died. I was shocked and stumbled my condolences. He passed me some papers from the hospital stating that his wife was twenty-eight years old when she died of "severe anemia" in March 2010. She was pregnant at the time, Issa explained stoically, and there had been a complication. She was admitted to the Bombo Regional Hospital and scheduled for a cesarean section. Two days later, she passed away before she could be operated on.

Three months before her death, Issa had managed to persuade her to take an HIV test. Even though she had persistently asked him why he wanted her to test without receiving a satisfactory answer, she gave in to his pleas and finally tested HIV-negative. Issa never found the courage to tell her of his own infection, as he had envisioned two years before. Instead, when his wife inquired about his medicines, he found an excuse:

> I told her that I used to smoke many cigarettes, that these medicines . . . removed the smoke from my chest. . . . If I had told her that I was [HIV-positive], she would have died because of her worries. . . . If you have already been tested and discovered you were with this problem—there are people who hang themselves or who drink poison, so I thought to myself that it's better not to tell her.

Issa also made sure to always hide his CTC card from his wife; and when it came to the question of having sex, Issa first resorted to abstinence and later to further excuses:

> I also stopped making love with her. Then I got to the point that I told her, "Listen, I don't make love like this, let's use condoms." She really got angry, and I told her, "We'll be given an undesired pregnancy—this is not the [right] time to have a child." She agreed, I put on a condom, and we made love.

That she fell pregnant was an accident, Issa explained. "It's not like I wanted to give her a pregnancy," he said. "The pregnancy happened by bad luck." They had reduced their sexual intercourse to once a week anyhow.

At various points during our conversation, Issa came back to the topic of his and his wife's serodiscordance. He found it so disturbing that after living together for years, only one of them had contracted HIV. Ultimately, he believed that she must also have had the disease and that her test outcome was flawed, for he held her to be the most plausible source of his own infection. He claimed that in his entire life, he had only had sexual intercourse with her and his former wife. In his desperate attempt to know where his infection stemmed from, he had even contacted his first wife to ask her if she was HIV-positive, which was not the case. Issa recalled how she had even showed him her latest test results. The only alternative source for his infection he could think of was a situation when he had a tooth extracted, which involved heavy bleeding.

While the irresolvable question of his infection's origin posed a psychological problem for Issa that often occupied his thoughts, he also had more concrete difficulties. Due to the frequent power cuts during the previous months, he could not work as usual and recorded a significant reduction in his weekly income. He could thus not afford to buy enough food, which in turn strengthened the side effects of his ARVs. He estimated that for more than six days per month, he did not have enough food to go along with the medicines. On these days, the drugs made him particularly weak and sleepy, and yet he assured me that he had never missed a dose. With the consent of a clinician, however, he explained that he had discontinued taking the Septrin because it had caused open wounds in his mouth.

Rather than receive support from his sister Zawadi in this precarious situation, he explained that it was now he who was responsible for her and her children's livelihood. Zawadi had never gone to school, he explained, implying that she had no prospects of ever making enough money to make ends meet. Apart from this, his children were now also staying at her house (both of them, Zawadi herself, and her own children had tested HIV-negative), and she had to take care of them in addition to her own children. He had been sending them 25,000 TSH every week, but due to his own financial straits, he now had difficulties maintaining this support. He no longer mentioned his brother in Mwanza, and said that he did not receive any support from any other relative. Only his friends occasionally helped him out with minor amounts of money here and there. He had joined a (self-)support group in Zawadi's village (where he viewed social cohesion to be stronger than in the city), but had had such a bad and disillusioning experience seeing the unjust distribution of donations that he had stopped going to the group meetings.

Issa's attitude toward disclosing his HIV infection within his social network seemed to have changed too. He was very careful about to whom he disclosed, he said. Since we had met last time, he had told a few more family members and some "friends" at work. The latter, however, would not believe him that he was HIV-positive. Issa's relatively stable physical condition apparently diverged too much from their imagination of someone living with HIV. Apart from these people, he would not tell anyone.

It can happen that you're discriminated against, that you're sitting with your friends and you're told "Ah, that one has AIDS!" That's what they do in the neighborhoods. I don't want this, so I keep everything absolutely secret (*nina siri kubwa sana*). . . . I keep quiet—I don't want anyone to know about my situation (*sitaki mtu mwingine aelewe niko vipi*).

Issa did not have a new partner and was hesitant to engage in another relationship. He did not want to have an HIV-negative partner because, as with his deceased wife, he would always be afraid of infecting her, and he did not particularly like the idea of always using condoms, especially not within marriage. He rather wished to find an HIV-positive partner with whom, in his view, unprotected sex posed no risks. Yet he wondered how he could find such a partner given that he could not know the HIV status of a woman he might approach in advance, and it was such a difficult topic to bring up in conversation.

At the end of my final interview with Issa, I asked him again what he thought about living with ARVs for the rest of his life. This time, his answer sounded a lot more skeptical than two years earlier:

I cannot know which impact these pills will have on me. Some people say, if you take pills like these, you will not get sick or anything, [but] you will be shocked, one day, when you will have fallen asleep, you will be dead. Really, you will find that you have died. . . . Others say that . . . it's better not to take these pills at all. . . . These pills kill!

ART and Intimate Relations: Sexuality and Reproduction

The Quandaries of "Safe Sex"

Issa's story addresses various relevant issues for understanding ART patients' struggles to lead as "normal" a life as possible. It is particularly revealing with regard to the intricacies that many people face in resuming their sexual lives and childbearing plans. It begins with the fact that disclosing his HIV status to his wife constituted a tremendous hurdle for Issa. In fact, he had not managed to tell his wife about his HIV infection for a period of roughly two years before her death. He was too worried about the impact his disclosure would have on her psychological well-being (cf. Bohle, Dilger, and Groß

2014). Perhaps Issa also held the truth back because he anticipated accusations and rejection from his wife. The fact that she turned out to be HIV-negative only exacerbated the situation. Not only did their serodiscordance constitute a source of constant psychological distress for Issa, since he could not come to any conclusion about how he might have contracted the virus if not through her; it was also the reason for his permanent apprehension that he could infect her. Consequently, he was obliged to permanently find excuses not only for his regular drug intake but also for his initial sexual abstinence and later for his insistence on using condoms, despite her reluctance and the resulting tensions in their relationship.

Revealing their health status to sexual partners and negotiating the use of condoms constituted a source of immense concern for many other patients too. With respect to both problems, gender-related differences were observable. Women more frequently voiced anxieties about being rejected and left by their partner upon disclosing their HIV status. Mwanahamisi, a woman who also lived in a serodiscordant relationship, told me she had only told her husband about her infection after she had already been taking ARVs for a while. Finally, she made one of her husband's aunts her accomplice in revealing her status to him: "I didn't want to tell him on my own," she explained to me. "You know how men are. . . . If I had told him myself, he perhaps would have beaten me or who knows what" (Mwanahamisi, thirty-seven years, third year of ART, 2 July 2009). In order to avoid the threat of being divorced, other women would wait until they became pregnant and would then tell their husbands that the health professionals at the reproductive and child health care unit had obliged them to test for HIV and to bring their husbands for a test too. They speculated that once their husbands had tested positive too, they would not put the blame for their infection exclusively on them.

Negotiations about safer sex practices and the use of condoms did not only constitute a matter of great concern to persons who concealed their health status from their partners. In fact, most patients living with ARVs pondered a lot about condoms, whose persistent use was so vigorously advocated during treatment preparation. Outside biomedical institutions, however, condoms constituted the object of a discourse in which anxiety, responsibility, power, desire for sexual gratification, trust, scientific reasoning, and piety converged in a complicated amalgam that allowed for a great variety of ways of thinking about and using them. Hodari's difficulties in persuading her HIV-positive husband to use condoms reflected sexual power differentials that prevented women from protecting themselves from risky sexual activity, and have been observed elsewhere (e.g., Sarna et al. 2009, 784).

> My husband has no education at all about protection, so that means arguments, arguments, arguments. . . . When it comes to condoms, he does not want them at all. He says it is a sin towards the Lord to use condoms. That is the reason why I sometimes even think about running away from him . . . because the doctors say there is the problem that there are all kinds of different types of these bugs [HIV], so that one can catch the bugs of someone else on top of your own. That's what exhausts and worries me. But still, he refuses, and he's also attended the [adherence] classes! . . . He says he cannot use "medicine" with the wife he's married to; he cannot use protection. (Hodari, thirty-three years, first year of ART, 28 July 2011)

It was not only women who reported difficulties in agreeing on the use of condoms with their sexual partner. Forty-three-year-old Johnson (fourth year of ART), for instance, related similar problems, albeit for a different reason. His girlfriend refused to engage in protected intercourse because condoms made her feel uncomfortable.

> Johnson: My lover does not like them. . . . When I wear them, it hurts her. . . . She's also at the CHICC [HIV testing and information center in Tanga], she gets education; but concerning condoms, she does not like them at all. So, I can tell you, I'm really puzzled about what to do. Sometimes I ask her, "You are afraid of getting pregnant, right? So why do you not want us to use condoms?" Then she says that she does not feel pleasure with condoms.
>
> Dominik: So you don't use condoms. But she understands about the issue of reinfection?
>
> Johnson: She understands everything, everything! But what am I supposed to do with her? She simply doesn't want to. I also asked her about that issue once. . . . She just laughed.

It turned out that Johnson did not consider his girlfriend's refusal to be a very serious problem, due to his own misconceptions about the risk of reinfection. Ultimately, he reasoned, that danger only existed in places "as far away as Asia," where other types of HIV were prevalent (Interview, 10 August 2009). Johnson's superficial knowledge of reinfection lay somewhere in the middle of widely discrepant levels of understanding among patients about HIV reinfection. On the one hand, there were people who had fully understood the implied dangers and a very clear-cut opinion about unprotected intercourse. Ismail was one of them.

> I have been taught that you can meet with a partner whose viruses are fiercer than yours, and you can get another infection; or you give her/him the ones that are fiercer than hers/his and they destroy her/his medicine. So when I meet someone with the problem [HIV], I must use a condom. I cannot go like that. I'm also afraid of sexually transmitted diseases. . . . If you catch an STD, you have [another] calamity. (Ismail, thirty-five years, fourth year of ART, 12 June 2009)

On the other hand, there were many patients like Ally or Haruna and Zahra (see Introduction), who had not comprehended the risk of HIV reinfection and considered unprotected intercourse between two HIV-positive persons unproblematic and safe. Often, the pivotal reason for not using condoms was that people did not want to counter their religious leaders' prohibition on condom use.

This takes us to religion and piety as another factor that profoundly influenced some people's stance toward condoms. Similar to Haruna and Zahra, other patients across both Muslim and Christian denominations reported their religious leaders' unmistakable instructions and did not question them. "To use a condom within marriage is a sin," said Olivia, referring to the sermons of her Roman Catholic pastor. In her subsequent remarks, the cleric's sweeping decry of condoms conflated in an interesting manner with the notion of male dominance within marriage, which seemed to be just as natural a fact to her (and the pastor) as the immorality of practicing safer sex.

> A man has married you. He has paid money to your parents at home for you [referring to the bride price]. Eeh, he has paid money for you. To tell him, "Let's use condoms," is that possible? It's not possible. He will ask you why. He is the one who married you; he is the one who feeds and cares for you. Someone who questions this—for the pastor it is a transgression. (Olivia, forty-nine years, first year of ART, 5 July 2011)

Others, however, challenged prohibitive religious directions in a much more self-conscious and pragmatic manner. Ahmed, for instance, represented himself as a very devout Muslim who never missed his prayers. Nonetheless, he decidedly defied the condemnation of condoms by some of his brothers and superiors in faith:

> At our mosque, certain teachings are given that remonstrate against condoms. Such teachings exist, but I disregard them. Why? . . . Because I have learned that there are words from God and other words that are pronounced by humans in the attempt to impress one another. I knew, these [teachings] were of the latter kind, and I put them aside. . . . Because I have also been studying religion a bit . . . and I haven't found one place [in the Quran] where it says that [a person] who uses a condom will perish, or where God's prophets and ambassadors declared that in the future they will perish due to the use of what? The condom. I've come to see that as a lie. . . . Islam, or religion, does not prohibit a system of protecting oneself. . . . So, we use [condoms] as a measure of preventing reinfections. (Ahmed, thirty-eight years, 6 January 2011)

That the discourse about condom use within religious communities was by no means unanimous also became evident in Juma's explanations. In contrast to Ahmed, he seemed to view such discrepancies as problematic, as they implied a lack of orientation for him and other congregants:

> The leaders are split over the issue of condom use. There are those saying that by encouraging people to use condoms, you increase the problem because they will have more sex. . . . You know, our religion doesn't allow people to fornicate (*kufanya tendo la zinaa*). There are others saying "use this [condoms] to protect yourself," but the first don't agree. . . . So, up to now, the leaders haven't come up with one opinion. (Juma, thirty-eight years, 11 June 2009)

Reducing Sexual Activity

Aside from enhanced efforts to use condoms consistently—despite the often complicated and difficult negotiations that were related to it within and outside marriage—several patients adapted to their health situation by reducing their sexual activity. This was the case not only among those where fears of infecting their partner were involved, such as with Issa, but also within seroconcordant relationships where the use of condoms was a matter of course. In some cases, reducing sexual activity seemed to be a direct response to the health professionals' restrictive discourse on sexuality, which depicted frequent sexual intercourse predominantly as a waste of energy, detrimental to health, and therefore undesirable. Twenty-seven-year-old Mustafa, a man in his third year of ART, claimed, for instance, that in addition to using condoms, he had cut down the frequency of having sex with his wife to a maximum of three times per month. "You do so because these are the rules of that doctor," he explained. "It is the way we have been taught. The doctor said it was necessary because otherwise, we would endanger our lives" (Interview, 10 July 2009). The restrictions he subjected himself to had a further consequence on his life. As a Muslim, he commented, he had the right to marry several women. Not being allowed to have more frequent sexual intercourse, however, prevented him from living in polygamy, which would oblige him to a system of "taking rounds" in order to sexually satisfy his wives. Every three days, he would need to switch to the house of another woman in order to accomplish his conjugal duties and follow in the footsteps of his grandfather, who had had twelve children by three wives. "Now, how can you do this as a sick person?" he wondered with a tinge of disappointment.

Fadhila also claimed that she had significantly less sex since being on treatment. The way she delineated her interactions with her sexual partners revealed that, like many others, she felt a great responsibility to protect them from infection. Furthermore, the goal of getting on in life by finishing the sewing school that she was attending at the time I met her seemed to be a much greater priority to her than sexual satisfaction.

> I am a human being, and I have bodily needs. [I have sex] when I maybe feel overwhelmed. But first of all, I study. I care very, very much about my studies. Then, maybe one day, when I am overwhelmed—all right. When I'm together with my partner, I explain my special situation to him, then we use a condom. . . . Until the next time, even four or five months may pass. (Fadhila, forty-three years, fifth year of ART, 28 January 2009)

All of the strategies that patients had for adapting their sexual life after ART uptake in order to protect the health of their partners as well as their own—be it the reduction of sexual activity, complete sexual abstinence, or the consistent use of condoms—stood diametrically opposed to the potential desire to have children, a problem that I will turn to next.

The Dilemma of Reproductive Choices

Having children is of utmost importance for both personal and social identity in Tanzania, as well as in other societies of sub-Saharan Africa (Cooper et al. 2007; Smith and Mbakwem 2010). While being a mother or father is regarded as a crucial element of person-hood (Whyte, Kyaddondo, and Meinert 2014, 152) and of meeting one's obligations to society, having children is also of great relevance with regard to the support they are expected to provide to their parents over the course of time. This is particularly so in the context of societies where, in the absence of governmental arrangements, security in old age is predominantly a matter of intergenerational reciprocity (cf. Whyte, Alber, and Van der Geest 2008).

For ART patients in the process of reconstituting their lives, childbearing may additionally acquire a high priority, for it serves as one of the most powerful markers of "normalcy." "Having children is a necessary part of living a normal life in Africa for nearly everyone," states Eileen Moyer (2012, S76), "but for people living with HIV, having healthy children restores honor and respectability to the parents, allows them to distance themselves from [the] sick role and challenges deeply entrenched societal notions that 'AIDS = death' . . . ." Indeed, for Nasra and several other patients who already had HIV-positive children, the birth of an HIV-negative child became the ultimate "index of parental health and also social normalcy" (Moyer 2012, S74). To Nasra, it also constituted the decisive criterion when considering whether to disclose her health status to others:

> My plan regarding the issue of children is that first, I'll be without a pregnancy for two years. . . . Once I know that my CD4 level allows for getting pregnant, the Almighty Lord will take care of me, and I'll have a pregnancy without any problems. I'll give birth to my child, and it will have good health and look good and I myself will be fine. This is when I'll decide to inform the community that this problem is not the end of my life. (Nasra, thirty-three years, third year of ART, 11 June 2009)

Giving birth to a healthy child was paramount to some patients, not only because it was an utterly persuasive image of normalcy, but also because it brought relief to those who were already parents and who were tormented by feeling responsible for their children's HIV infection. Ismail, for instance, had been left by his wife shortly before I interviewed him for the first time, and lived alone with his five-year-old, HIV-positive son. Desperately, he explained:

> If I get work, I want to get married and have [another] child, because the child I have [now] is positive. . . . There is no difference [between a negative and a positive child], they are all children with the rights of any other child—but I pity him so much. I feel so sorry for the one who has had the problem . . . since birth. I feel so sorry for him, so sorry for him! (Ismail, thirty-five years, fourth year of ART, 12 June 2009)

Likewise, Zuwena, who had lost her husband to AIDS and not yet been initiated on treatment, also expressed her desire for an HIV-negative child. As her two children, aged eleven and five years, were both HIV-positive, she reasoned that another child without the disease would be more able to assist her, and not only in her old age. Aside from these pragmatic considerations, it was evident that Zuwena equally longed for a healthy child because she felt great anguish about having passed the virus on to her children during birth or lactation, even if she was aware that she had not known better at the time. "It hurts me a lot; sometimes I cannot bear it," she said.

> If it was only me who had got it instead of these angels, these beings of God who do not know anything, that hurts me a lot. . . . I also tell myself, it's not my fault, I didn't know [referring to measures of preventing mother-to-child infection]. But still, it hurts me, [and I ask myself] why? If there only was the possibility to ask God to release the children and to only leave me with the disease. (Zuwena, thirty-two years, 30 July 2011)

While people living with ARVs—the childless among them as well as those who had already experienced parenthood—had a great interest in the topic of childbearing, it nevertheless constituted a terrain that was difficult to tread. All patients were painfully aware that despite their lowered viral loads, there remained the risk of infecting their sexual partner or their future child during pregnancy and breastfeeding. Whether or not to engage in an intimate relationship and get pregnant and give birth thus posed a profound moral dilemma and stirred up a mix of emotions ranging from hope to anxiety and desperation.

At the beginning stood the difficult question of how to find a partner, if they did not have one already, and what the serostatus of this person should be. As has been reported from other parts of sub-Saharan Africa (and elsewhere) (Seeley et al. 2009), several patients resorted to the strategy of "serosorting": only considering HIV-positive persons as potential spouses or sexual partners. Juma, who could not imagine being married to an HIV-negative woman, explained that they recommended this strategy to patients at his treatment center. He found it quite reasonable. That way, he explained, his partner would always know when

> it is time for me to take my medicine, that I need a certain type of food, and even when we want to sleep with each other [we know] which way to do it [referring to the use of condoms]. But if she was healthy, the first thing is that she would not accept me [as a partner] because she would always expect me to infect her. [She would be thinking,] "If he infected me, it would be my death." ... Even her relatives would ask her, "How will you live with this man; will he not kill you?! You don't want to live like that!" (Juma, thirty-eight years, second year of ART, 11 June 2009)

Ismail ruled out ever having a sexual relationship with an HIV-negative woman because, like Issa, he would be too worried about infecting her. Furthermore, his explanations pointed to normative expectations that many HIV-positive people faced within their social environments with regard to their dating behavior:

> I'm afraid of even approaching a woman who has not the same problem, I absolutely cannot do that. If I get a lover, it is a person in the same situation as I. I sometimes go to that club. . . . I dance there, there are some girls who don't mind but I—my very personal soul (*roho yangu binafsi yangu*)—does not allow me to sleep with such a woman, not even for a single night. And . . . my mother has even made me swear, she has told me "My child, you have this problem, but if I should ever learn that you have taken a woman who doesn't have this problem, you and me, we will not see each other again until we stand in front of God!" (Ismail, thirty-five years, fourth year of ART, 12 June 2009)

In addition to nuclear and extended families, religious communities constituted social settings in which newly established rules governed partner selection, and patients were subjected to novel forms of normativity. Some patients thus reported that their religious leaders obliged prospective bridal couples to produce recent HIV-test results before they would proceed to bring about the marriage. If one of the partners should turn out to be negative and the other positive, they would refuse to wed them. The pastor of a local Pentecostal church explained the reasons behind such a practice.

> Here, we do not wed [serodiscordant] couples. We tell them, "Go to another church where they will wed you." Here, we cannot wed them, we rather . . . counsel them until one of them resigns. . . . We feel that we should not hold our hands [over them] in this way . . . while simultaneously we all teach the dangers of this disease at the church. We will contradict our own teachings. So, if they insist completely, we just ask them to look for another church to get married [in]. (Pastor Mary, forty-two years, 21 July 2011)

Other pastors, it was claimed, only recommended testing for HIV prior to marriage, but, given the consent of both parties, they would still wed serodiscordant couples.

Despite the benefits that many patients saw in establishing relationships with persons of the same serostatus, not all patients considered serosorting to be a satisfactory solution. After she had experienced the sorrow of losing her husband to AIDS, Zuwena, for instance, pointed to the continuous uncertainty and risk that this implied. In her view, she would always have to anticipate once more being bereaved in the case of her spouse's premature death. Her perception that the intake of ARVs by no means guarantees a long life left her with profound uncertainty over how to deal with her desire for a new husband who would take care of her and her children, and her wish for an HIV-negative child that would at least partially mitigate her sorrow.

As discussed in the previous chapter, in treatment centers, childbearing was postulated as the right of every HIV-positive person. The right to determine whether a woman's health condition allowed for a healthy pregnancy at all, and when, was, however, exclusively ascribed to health professionals. Many of the patients who held on to their procreation plans readily surrendered such decisions to the biomedical authorities. Nasra's quote serves as an example:

> I don't want to use any contraceptive medicine, but I use condoms in order to take care of myself until my CD4 [cells] allow me to get pregnant. . . . When they allow it, I will fall pregnant; when they don't, I'll wait until they make me merit [a pregnancy]. . . . But I cannot go like, "All right, let's get a child," and then, as soon as it's out, I'll get another one. . . . If I didn't have this problem [HIV], I'd just get [plenty of] children; but if you

have this problem, it is obligatory to plan one's births. You need to follow exactly the doctor's advice. (Nasra, thirty-three years, third year of ART, 11 June 2009)

The strategy that Ismail intended to apply in order to procreate with a prospective new partner who was HIV-positive like himself also illustrates the degree to which some patients had internalized medical advice. In an equal measure, it once more showed the great sense of responsibility that many patients felt for their partner's health:

> Once I have made sure that that woman of mine is sick [HIV-positive], we've gone to check that she does not have any venereal disease and I have no venereal disease, that will be the day to go a step further and say, "Let's have a child." Then we will pray to God that with one single act [of having sex], it will work out. If he agrees, fine, that's it, and I won't have sex anymore without a condom. (Ismail, thirty-five years, fourth year of ART, 12 June 2009)

All patients who talked to me about their considerations with regard to having children in one way or another had adjusted these plans to their HIV-positive status. Most people had done so in terms of drastically reducing the number of children they aimed for. Some, however, feared the prospect of having a (further) HIV-positive child so much that they did not dare take a chance. Hodari (thirty-three years, first year of ART) was a case in point. In tears, she recounted that the year before, she had had to interrupt the contraceptive shots that she used to get due to adverse reactions. She promptly fell pregnant but went to have an abortion because she could not bear the thought that the child might be HIV-positive.

While Hodari feared having another HIV-positive child to the extent of terminating her pregnancy, despite being aware of the procedures to reduce the risk of perinatal HIV transmission that were offered at treatment centers, other women were not conscious of the possibility of a healthy child being born to HIV-positive parents in the first place. I often met men and women who were just as eager to learn more about PMTCT, once I had mentioned it, as they had initially been anxious about the idea of childbearing.

On various occasions, finally, I observed situations where somewhat annoyed health workers admonished women who, from their point of view, had stubbornly become pregnant without taking any precautions. Whether these women's supposed act of resistance to the medicalization of sexuality and reproduction within the HIV treatment program (cf. Rasmussen 2013, S545) was rather the consequence of fragmentary comprehension of mother-to-child transmission, the perceived social pressure to procreate, a profound longing for self-fulfillment and social recognition, adherence to religious principles, or the outcome of a blend of all of these factors, could only be speculated.

In summary, being an individual with HIV, as a chronic but still infectious disease, constituted a significant impediment for many patients with regard to their sexual lives and reproductive projects, which endangered their acknowledgement and identity as a partner, spouse, parent, and community member. Patients had to reconcile multiple concurrent institutional and normative discourses on sexuality with their own values, aspirations, and anxieties. Some managed to tackle the task rather well and aimed for the strategies that involved the least biological risk for those involved. In so doing, they not only displayed their orientation toward pragmatic solutions but also a high degree of responsibility for others that disproves the fear that "successful treatment will lead to sexual disinhibition—that is, with the availability of successful treatment, people may eschew protective behaviors" (Smith and Mbakwem 2010, 346). Others, however, did not obtain sufficient information, were not in the social position, or were too apprehensive to take the "rational" choice to use condoms or inscribe into a PMTCT program in order to give birth to a hopefully HIV-negative child. Yet even if all scientific measures to protect oneself, one's partner, and one's prospective child are taken up, the risk of passing on the virus remains. Weighing one's personal desires and social expectations with this risk persisted as an ultimately insurmountable obstacle to "being like everyone else" or "doing just all right like I've been doing before, when I did not have this problem [HIV]," as Nasra put it (Interview, 11 June 2009).

Resuming satisfactory sexual lives and bearing healthy children constituted one of the most crucial signifiers of "normalization" and thus gained a high priority in the lives of many people living with ARVs. Yet, as we have seen, patients were dealing with many questions regarding these issues, at times over long periods of time, without coming to a conclusion.

As pointed out in the previous chapter, the topic of sexuality and reproduction remained relatively under-addressed during treatment preparation. In order to assist patients in finding an answer to at least some of their most pressing questions in this regard, it seems advisable that within health institutions, the sexuality and childbearing of HIV-positive people be addressed in a far more systematic, congruous, and detailed—but also less restrictive and tendentious—manner than I observed during patient enrollment. Instead of being given categorical advice to abstain from sex and to always use condoms, it is reasonable to assume that patients would benefit more from encouraging explanations of the opportunities they gained through ART to pursue their reproductive life projects and accurate explanations of all available options for leading a fulfilling sexual life and giving birth while protecting partners and prospective children. Furthermore, counseling offered to patients on these issues might benefit from taking greater account of the multiple factors (including, for instance, religiosity) that shape a person's reproductive desires and practices.

Anxiety and Aspiration: The "Trajectory Projection" of People Living with ARVs

All issues so far discussed in this chapter—the processes of bodily transformation, the more or less successful attempts and strategies to recuperate self-esteem and social recognition, and the hopes and dilemmas related to sexuality and reproduction after ART uptake— exerted a significant influence on how patients conceptualized their future, or what Strauss and colleagues have termed their "trajectory projection" (Strauss 1984, 69). While the case studies of Furaha/ Imani and Issa, as well as many of the quotes of other patients, reveal both the positive developments noticed after ART uptake as well as the new dilemmas that emerged for persons living with "chronic" HIV, in this section I would like to expand on the hopes and anxieties that people formulated, specifically with regard to their long-term drug intake.

As Issa's case has demonstrated, one concern that was expressed in this regard was related to the development of drug resistance. As pointed out above, health professionals explained to patients during treatment enrollment that there was always a constant risk that the

HIV "bugs" would get used to the medicine, which would then no longer manage to prevent their "procreation." Hodari was another of those patients who expressed her worries that this could one day happen to her. In order to come to terms with this danger, she resorted to a fatalism that other patients also drew on in the process of self-normalization:

> They say that you use these medicines until, in the end, they don't work anymore. So, when they stop to work . . . I try to comfort myself, "Don't we all have to die? Is there anyone who lives forever?" . . . So, when they fail to work and you die, that's how it is, your time has come, right? (Hodari, thirty-three years, first year of ART, 28 July 2011)

The idea of having to switch to another regimen whose effects on their body they did not know was a source of great anxiety, particularly to those patients who, after several attempts, had finally been put on a drug with bearable side effects. Due to the limited availability, higher costs, and more complicated intake of second-line medications, clinicians were somewhat hesitant to prescribe them to patients with insufficient immune responses to their first-line regimen. Patients' anxiety would certainly have increased had they been aware of this. But there were other ways in which the issue of multiple treatment lines could cause concern. To Hodari, the limitation of pharmaceutical variability posed a concern in itself:

> These medicines are told to exist in different grades. If you use this one and it brings you problems, you are switched to another one; if that causes problems, you're switched again to another one, so . . . isn't there [necessarily] a last grade? So, once you're given those of the last grade and they trouble you, what do you do then?! (Hodari, thirty-three years, first year of ART, 28 July 2011)

Another woman apparently had understood that there were differences in the mode of operation of drugs belonging to different treatment lines. In her view, there were also differences in the drugs' quality and efficacy, and she suspected that the social status of the patient decided who was provided with the best medications:

> Some people tell you that there are medicines of [different] grades. Some tell you that if you're given the ones of the first [grade], it's bad; if you're given the ones of the second [grade], I don't know; and those of the third [grade] are for those big ones [referring to the wealthy and powerful].

So, concerning this issue, we don't know—because you have no knowledge about the medicines, you cannot judge the grade you were given.
(Happiness, fifty-two years, third year of ART, 2 June 2011)

Half-truths and gossip were equally at play in patients' speculations about the long-term effects of their medicines. Occasionally,
the lack of knowledge about the impact of taking ARVs over the
course of many years manifested itself in sinister imaginaries. One
concern obviously accrued from the absolute imperative of consistent and punctual drug intake that health workers drilled into
patients at the treatment centers. Adhering to this directive while
pushing it to the extreme, a few patients apprehended imminent
death if they forgot to take their medicines for even a single day.

Issa's final remark quoted above—"These pills kill!"—was only
one example of a remarkable semantic reversal in which the life-
prolonging drugs themselves were characterized as potential killers.
While Issa was concerned about the possibility of sudden death
provoked by the medicines, other patients feared more prolonged
periods of agony once the phase of benefitting from the drugs had
been exhausted and they began to slowly "eat up" their inner organs.
Similar to Happiness's ideas about the different treatment lines, it
is likely that such fears were also partly based on health workers'
occasional comments about the detrimental long-term effects that
ARVs could have on physiological processes. Yet it is reasonable to
assume that they were also informed by prevailing rumors about
ARVs in Tanga's neighborhoods. Information material in print about
the drugs' availability, efficacy, and function was seldom available at
treatment centers and basically nonexistent outside of these facilities. Neither were there posters or public signboards visible in the
city or its outskirts that addressed HIV treatment. The two most
prominent signboards situated on the road leading to the Bombo
Regional Hospital instead contained deterring and moralizing messages that associated HIV with vices such as drug abuse and reckless
driving (Figure 5.1).

Those people who did not pay attention (or did not have access)
to the occasional informational radio or TV broadcasts about ARVs
thus largely had to rely on hearsay when forming their opinions about the medicines. They also drew conclusions from their
own observations of relatives, neighbors, and friends whom they

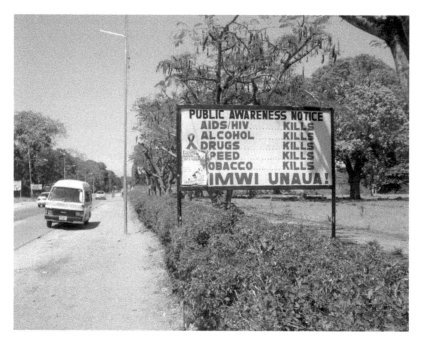

Figure 5.1. Signboard, Hospital Rd., Tanga © Dominik Mattes 2009.

assumed were being treated for HIV. This situation provided the grounds for a nonbiomedical discourse on ART based on biomedical half-truths and reinterpretations of ideas about drug resistance, adverse drug effects, and the rules of taking ARVs. A discourse that, in addition to the, at times, fragmentary and overly directive information provided at treatment centers, apparently also shaped some patients' attitudes toward their medicines and their related anxieties. Fadhila, one of the most "experienced" ART patients in terms of the length of time that she had been taking ARVs, was a case in point.

> Sometimes I wonder: "These medicines are for life." Why do they say that when you take these medicines for life, they become *chronic* [expression sometimes used instead of "resistant"]? How will things be later on? Is there the danger that [the medicine] will harm my liver, maybe because they need to be so powerful in order to work at all? I think a lot about these issues. . . . There are these rumors that any medicine, if you use it a lot, will turn into poison or destroy the liver. (Fadhila, forty-three years, fifth year of ART, 28 January 2009)

None of the patients who had expressed their doubts and apprehensions concerning their medicines' long-term effects had ever discussed these worries with medical staff. Ultimately, they explained, this was futile, for they had no choice but to take their medicines.

The idea of the necessity of taking ARVs for the rest of one's life, finally, constituted a source of unrest with regard to the treatment program's financial stability. Some patients were quite aware that the continuation of donor support was threatened by the global financial crisis. This evoked their profound concerns regarding the availability of treatment in the future and renewed fearful questions about long-term survival.

> I'm not growing tired of taking medicines for my whole life. But I'm thinking if one day there are no drugs anymore—and you are told that if you stop taking them for two years, the virus changes, right? So, when you use *ARV 30* [referring to his regimen Triomune 30] and then you use them again, they cannot put the virus to sleep anymore, because it has already multiplied itself and changed. And then, for example, suddenly there is no medicine, the donors say they won't provide them . . . and you were told, ". . . if you don't take the drugs—*dead!*" What will happen then?! (Johnson, forty-three years, fourth year of ART, 10 August 2009)

Imani had even heard about an ARV manufacturing plant in Dar es Salaam, but this did not dispel her concern about sustainable drug provision in the country. The thought that, sooner or later, the ARV supply could come to a halt and her premature death would not be preventable caused great anxiety for her, especially because she worried so much about who would take care of her children, the youngest one in particular.

Considering Imani's worries about the uncertain sustainability of ART provision, it is no wonder that time and again, she expressed her hope that one day medicines would be discovered that could cure HIV altogether. Her hope was nurtured by bits of information on innovations and scientific progress in the field of HIV research that she came across in newspapers or on the radio. "Why do I hear that over there, where was it again, medicines are available that cure [HIV] all the way?" she asked me once excitedly. Obviously, she had mistaken an article on experiments with a new type of ARVs that intervened in HIV replication in a different way than the current regimens as the announcement of the discovery of a cure for the virus. But even after I had explained to her what the article, which I had also read, was "really" about, she pleaded with me to inquire more about these experiments and inform her about the outcome.

Several other patients, and particularly the younger ones among them (Mattes 2014a), also expressed their hope of eventually being completely released from HIV and thus from the often bothersome necessity of daily drug intake. Like Imani, a number of patients did not restrict their hopes and related therapy seeking activities to the biomedical sector, but resorted to whatever other therapeutic experts and traditions they deemed promising (see Chapter 8). The hope of being cured of HIV that these patients immovably held on to, irrespective of the positive physical and social transformations that they may have realized after ART uptake, indicates that they did not quite perceive life on ARVs as a return to "normalcy" in the sense of a fully acceptable state of life.

Chapter Conclusion

Indubitably, ARVs had an immensely positive effect on the lives of people living with HIV in Tanga. As elsewhere, they granted people the opportunity to recover their health and reconstitute their lives after phases of often-profound physical, social, and moral disruption. Yet the way in which reconstitution took place after treatment uptake could differ widely from one person to another; and even if patients were grateful for the chance they had been granted in the form of ARVs to rebuild their lives and reimagine their future, even if they managed to retrieve their self-esteem, secure their economic existence, and meet social norms and expectations, there remained significant constraints on their lives.

The prospect of living a "normal" life was darkened by draining side effects, which were often exacerbated by insufficient nutrition. Even if some of these effects could be mitigated or decreased over time, community discourses about the toxicity of ARVs, the dangers of their long-term ingestion, and the ultimately uncertain sustainability of treatment exacted a great deal of psychological effort from some patients to sustain their confidence in the drugs and their hopes for long-term survival. The desire to resume sexual relationships and bear children further confronted patients with the basically irresolvable moral dilemma that reestablishing "reproductive normalcy" was only possible at the cost of accepting the risk of infecting one's partner or child.

While ARVs thus enabled people to survive, they also confronted them with some quite existential complications. Coming to terms with these complications required a person to have the capacity to pragmatically reconcile various, at times diametrically opposed, discourses and to balance personal priorities and desires with the responsibility toward others. It also required the strong volition to adhere to the treatment regime despite painful and troublesome side effects. Regaining and upholding a sense of "normalcy" in the light of such challenges implied patients' hard day-to-day work (cf. Scandlyn 2000). Ultimately, however, the question arises of what "normalcy" in this context means, and whether it is an appropriate term to refer to the experiences and concerns of people living with ARVs, such as those discussed above. Researchers who have studied ART-initiated processes of transition and reconstitution in Uganda have suggested that normalcy in this context can only signify a return to the "ordinary uncertainty and contingency" that marks everyday life in the context of widespread poverty (cf. Russell and Seeley 2010)—or, put differently, "a move 'from certain death to uncertain survival'" (Whyte, Mogensen, and Meinert 2014, 278). In light of the limitations, concerns, and anxieties of life that emerged in the narratives of Imani, Issa, and other patients, I see a need for even greater conceptual restriction, for even this interpretation does not account for the fact that some of the problems that people living with ARVs face are simply not resolvable through the use of medications, nor does it account for the fact that many of these problems are newly created by the regular ingestion of the medications themselves. Being HIV-positive remains, after all, a heavy burden for many people, even in times of ART.

Notes

1. Parts of this chapter have been published in Mattes, 2012 and 2014b.
2. Imani and her husband's serodiscordance did not seem to pose the same problems as we will see in the case of Issa, the protagonist of the next case study, and his wife. Imani assured me that she lived with her husband "like brother and sister," implying that they had no desire to have any more children and had ceased to have sexual intercourse.

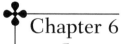

Chapter 6
Cohesion and Conflict
Living a Social Life on ARVs within Kin-Based Networks of Solidarity

This chapter shifts focus from individual patients' personal attitudes, ideas, hopes, and anxieties to the context of their kin-based networks in which they lived and "practiced" their everyday life with ARVs.[1] The nexus of sociality, communication, and day-to-day interaction within, and partly beyond, kinship networks are thus placed at the center of attention, rather than patients' individual subjectivities, although obviously neither can be considered independently of the other.

In concurrence with Moyer and Igonya (2014, 137), I propose that life on ART can only thrive in the long-term if patients are able to mobilize and receive care that "encompasses the[ir] physical, emotional, social, and economic needs . . . which generally exceed the efficacy of biomedical treatment." Patients' extended families constitute one of the most important social institutions where people living with HIV and ARVs seek these diverse forms of care and support throughout the years following their treatment initiation. This constitutes a continuation of a phenomenon widely observed during the first decades of the HIV epidemic, when no treatment for the virus was available, and relatives of people suffering from HIV/AIDS carried the greatest burden of caring for their loved ones. This was particularly the case in regions like sub-Saharan Africa, where specialized palliative medicine and care was largely unavailable to the average citizen—and remains so to this day. People diagnosed with AIDS were usually released from overburdened hospitals into the care of their kin, where they stayed until their mostly unpreventable death. Anthropological research has shown how straining and conflict-laden this situation could be for kin relations, but also what an indispensable source of assistance familial networks constituted for the sick and dying (Dilger 2005, 2008, 2010, 2013b; Whyte 1997, 2006).

The case studies in Chapter 5 have already pointed to the continued significance of kin-based networks as sources of social, financial, and material support for patients in the era of ART. In the cases addressed in this chapter, this will become even clearer. During the, at times, prolonged transition from acute suffering toward living with HIV as a long-term condition with the help of ARVs, most patients were heavily dependent on the support of their families. And even once they had recovered their health, many people living with ARVs could only survive with the help of their kin due to increasingly precarious living conditions. Moreover, patients' households, which were predominantly composed of consanguine and affine kin, were the primary locus of the practical management of ART on a day-to-day basis. Patients' specific treatment-related requirements, such as maintaining a balanced and substantial diet and getting sufficient rest, had to be met, and responsibilities of care had to be allocated and possibly renegotiated over the course of time. In many cases, this worked out well and patients managed to adhere to their treatment regimes and resume their life projects, counting on the steady and reliable support of their families. In other cases, however, kin-based household units and wider networks did not stand up to the pressures that the HIV infection of one or several of their members added to their already dire life circumstances.

While the case studies presented in this chapter illustrate the range of possible constellations of care and support within networks of extended kin, the story of Joseph (Case Study D) in particular points to the potential limitations of such arrangements. Moreover, it also points to patients' desire for a sense of belonging that goes beyond the security of being provided with "tangible" help such as monetary and material assistance in times of need. As will be shown, Joseph aspired to an "emotionally-charged social location" (Pfaff-Czarnecka 2011, 2), not only in the sense of finding his place in a web of reliable and resilient social relationships, but also in the sense of feeling morally respected and acknowledged.

My examination of how life with ARVs unfolded and how such multilayered needs and expectations were met within patients' extended families is oriented by three larger questions: How and to what effect was HIV and its treatment communicated about within kin-based networks and beyond? How and by whom was ART managed on a daily basis? And how did stigma and discrimination affect patients' treatment and social networks of care?

I will begin the exploration of how ART was inscribed in familial relations with the story of the Ramadhani family. This narrative lends itself as an opener because it illustrates particularly well how complex the communication about and management of HIV within a single family can be due to its members' multiple—and at times widely contrasting—attitudes and positionings toward both the disease and its treatment.

Case Study C: The Ramadhani Family

Fatuma

In the raging heat of an early afternoon in mid-December 2008, I met Fatuma at the TAWG headquarters. From there, we had agreed that she would take me to her house, where we could have a calm conversation. The week before, I had met Fatuma in one of the meetings of a (self-)support group facilitated by the TAWG. She was one of the first to walk up to me when I asked the group members if anyone felt ready to talk to me about their experiences of living with ARVs. One of the TAWG's drivers had to do some business in Fatuma's neighborhood and offered to drop us off at her house. The short drive of ten minutes was enough for the surroundings to change completely from the ample shady premises of the Raskazone peninsula to the one-storied, unrendered concrete buildings with corrugated iron roofs that, side by side, lined the dirt roads of Fatuma's and many other neighborhoods in Tanga's extended suburban residential areas.

When we entered Fatuma's house, she spread a straw mat on the floor in the hallway and asked me to take a seat. On both sides of the hallway, four doorways led to adjacent bedrooms; although most of the doors were missing and instead, large cloths, hung up for privacy, were swaying in the breeze blowing through the house. *Taraab* music could be heard from one of the rooms. Zeinabu and Halima, two of Fatuma's sisters, came in, presented themselves, and also took a seat as I started my conversation with Fatuma.

Fatuma was forty-nine years old at the time, lived separated from her husband, and shared the house with her mother, two sisters and three brothers, four of her in-laws, her own four children, eleven nephews and nieces, and four grandchildren. Each of her siblings' nuclear families shared one room in the house we were in, and another smaller building in the backyard accommodated more family members. Fatuma had graduated from primary school in 1972 and had spent her whole life in Tanga. Until 2006, she had worked as a kitchen helper in a local hotel. When her son was in an accident, she had to take some time off in order to care for him. When she came back to resume her work, however, she found that she had already been replaced. Since then, she had been unable to find another job. The money she made by occasionally buying second hand clothes and reselling them on the streets was not enough to get by, and she depended mostly on the income of two of her brothers, who were marketers and worked seven days a week.

Fatuma tested HIV-positive in 2005. She did not have any rashes, fevers, or other ailments, she emphasized. She just wanted to know her health status, because "the problem had already entered the family," she said, pointing to Zeinabu, who turned out to be HIV-positive too, and also because she suspected her husband of sleeping with other women. After Fatuma was tested at a nearby health center, she was referred to the Bombo Regional Hospital. Her CD4 count was too high to allow for ART initiation, so she was sent to the TAWG where she received herbal medicines to support her immune system.[2] Nevertheless, she was also enrolled in the treatment program at the CTC and was instructed to have her CD4 count checked every six months. Fatuma even voluntarily attended some adherence classes and joined the (self-)support group, where she gained further knowledge about ARVs. Moreover, Fatuma was mainly responsible for managing the ART of three of her brothers' children, who were three, six, and ten years old. She regularly went to the CTC with them in order to get their ARV refills or have their opportunistic infections treated. She also made an effort to always give them their daily medications, though she conceded that sometimes she forgot.

By taking care of her nephews' and niece's treatment, she became well acquainted with the routines of HIV treatment. Upon my question of why her brothers did not take care of their children's therapy themselves, Fatuma speculated that they were too afraid of being pushed into taking an HIV test themselves, the result of which they anticipated would turn out positive. Fatuma claimed that she often talked to her brothers about HIV. "I give them education. I teach them everything. I let them know every little thing, and I am completely open to them [about her situation]. But they don't want to [test]," she complained. Only once did she manage to persuade her younger brother Abdallah to come to the hospital with her and get tested. Unfortunately, the CTC was closed that day due to a donor visit, and they returned home without having accomplished their aim. Abdallah would not make another attempt, even though, as Fatuma assumed, "He knows very, very, very well" about the possibility of getting treatment.

> But he says the obligations [of ART] are difficult; he could never fulfill these obligations. . . . The difficult obligations he is talking about have to do with enjoyment (*mambo ya starehe*). . . . Aren't you told at the CTC that you're not supposed to have sex, so that you don't infect anyone and you're not [re]infected? [Don't they say that] it is not allowed to drink [alcohol] until you tumble over? Those are the rules that he finds difficult.

Other family members were more open to Fatuma's advice. "This little sister of mine has already tested," she said, pointing her finger to Halima. Halima's test had turned out negative, but she was told to test again after the "window period"[3] of three months. Even though Halima admitted that she did not know much about ARVs, she did indicate her confidence in the drugs and her readiness to start treatment should the next test turn out positive. Fatuma's mother had also tested upon her suggestion and was also HIV-negative.

Fatuma's openness and educatory activities apparently stopped at her doorstep. She categorically judged her neighbors, arguing, "They despise you here wherever you go if you try to educate them [about HIV]." Consequently, she never talked to any of them about her situation, and she did not know if any of them might have learned of her HIV infection in another way. In case of her involuntary disclosure, Fatuma was less worried about the consequences for herself than for her children. She suspected that they would be catcalled about having a mother suffering from AIDS when walking through their neighborhood. In her own family, Fatuma remarked gratefully, there had never been any discrimination.

Every single day for the previous three years, Fatuma had been boiling the herbs she obtained from the TAWG in order to prepare the concoction that was supposed to support her immune system. She was fed up with this and found taking pills a lot more convenient. She therefore wished to finally start taking ARVs; though at the same time, she regarded the medicines with a certain wariness:

> Some say these medicines have their problems. . . . Those patients themselves, some of them say "Exert yourself to continue with your 'roots' [traditional medicine]; don't long for ARVs." . . . Some say their legs are swollen; others tell you their heart is running fast; again others tell you they are hungry all the time. Some say your health is good, you look great, but then you die suddenly, they say that all of a sudden you die! . . . if you continue with them for a long time, they turn into poison, and if you interrupt your therapy, there will also be problems. You can suddenly drop dead. Now, I don't know what's better, I don't understand.

Her sisters added similarly frightening accounts about ARVs that they had picked up on the streets, and Fatuma admitted that to some extent, such comments made her fear the medicines. But then she claimed that she would still prefer to take them over boiling her herbs every day. In any case, she said, it was the doctor's decision when she had to begin ART. What would she do if the doctor told her to start ARVs, I asked her. "If you say [to the doctor] you won't take these medicines, they will throw you out quickly!" she replied. Furthermore, despite all the negative rumors about ARVs, she had seen many people in bad health states come back to life after starting ART, which is why she concluded that, ultimately, "they are a good thing."

When I asked Fatuma what she was aspiring to in the future, she did not have to think long before responding:

> I would like to have my own house to live in with my family. That's what I hope for in the future. As you see, we are all living in one place. I'd like to build my own place to live in with my children. I don't want to stay like this, with all the people here.

Fatuma's second priority, she repeated, was to have better nutrition and to start ARVs.

Zeinabu

Fatuma's desire to start treatment sharply contrasted with the experience of her sister Zeinabu, who had already been living with HIV and ARVs for many years. Zeinabu tested HIV-positive in 1991 in Mombasa, Kenya, where she was living at the time, and ever since then, she would spend several months of the year there. In 1995, she started taking herbal medicines; and in 1998, she said that she had been initiated on ART in a clinic in Mombasa. Conversing with Zeinabu was challenging. Often, she only indirectly and partially responded to my questions. On other occasions, she rambled using more or less incomprehensible sentences. I therefore did not manage to find out if she had been enrolled on treatment in the context of a medical trial or whether she had privately purchased the ARVs during the first years of her therapy, considering the fact that in Kenya, HIV treatment was only made available for free in 2003.

At any rate, Zeinabu told me that she had taken ARVs until August 2007. Then, she said, she "turned crazy" (*nilikuwa kichaa*), for which she offered only vague and incomplete explanations. At this point, Fatuma started to complement Zeinabu's answers for clarification. Zeinabu had returned to Tanga in order to inform the family about the death of a fellow Tanzanian who had lived with her in Mombasa. Together with relatives of the deceased, Fatuma and Zeinabu had travelled to Mombasa for the burial. On the way back, Zeinabu had started to act in a "weird" manner, for example, by shouting at the customs officers while crossing the border. During the following days, her unusual behavior increased to the extent that Fatuma and her family believed that "her mind was broken" (*akili zimeharibika*). They took her to a laboratory where she tested positive for malaria, and she was finally admitted to the hospital. The drips, injections, and medications she received there, however, had no effect. After one week, they removed her from the hospital against the physicians' recommendations and took her to a traditional healer. When his medicine did not help either, they readmitted her to the hospital, where she stayed for another two weeks. Zeinabu continued simultaneously to take biomedical medicines (including ARVs again) and "traditional" ones for almost a year. Only then did her situation improve. It was during this period when, in June 2008, Zeinabu decided to stop HIV treatment because, amongst other things, she ascribed her impaired mental health to the effects of the ARVs and felt like "taking a break" again.

Up to the day of the interview, Zeinabu had decidedly resisted Fatuma's appeals to resume therapy. Fatuma had even sought help at the TAWG, who had sent an HBC worker to speak to Zeinabu. "Just take the medicines," Fatuma recalled the woman telling Zeinabu. "Don't stop, because if you stop, you will get weak. Just continue taking them." She also addressed Fatuma and her sisters: "You need to force her to take them, even if her mind does not want to; just force her to take the medicines so that she does not stop." But every time the sisters tried to give Zeinabu a dose of ARVs, she would throw it away and accuse them of poisoning her. Zeinabu told me during our conversation that if she would continue treatment at all, it would be once she had found work that would enable her to buy more and better food to go along with the ARVs. She planned to return to Kenya in early January 2009. She intended to first look for a job before reporting her drug interruption to her doctors at the treatment center and resuming her therapy.

Aside from resuming treatment in the medical setting she was familiar with, Zeinabu had a perhaps even more important reason for returning to Mombasa: she had a "boyfriend" from Germany who used to come to Mombasa in order to spend a few weeks with her in a hotel every February and September. Their relationship had been going on like this for six years, Zeinabu explained. "He is Germany," she then said, switching from Swahili to broken English, "but so long time—he didn't see me for so long time because of my problem. He don't has any story about me. I just phoned but I didn't pick him." Zeinabu hoped that he would still come and see her again. Once, he had promised to take her to Germany and get "good treatment," even though he himself had tested negative and, Zeinabu assumed, did not really believe her that she was HIV-positive. Referring to this German boyfriend, Zeinabu had to think just as little as her sister when I asked her what she wished for in the future: "A good life" was what she aspired for. To her, this meant a life "with money [and] with somebody married."

Abdallah

In the midst of the conversation I had with Fatuma and her sisters in mid-December, their brother Abdallah came out of the room where the *taarab* music was playing, greeted me briefly, and slowly walked away again. Open sores marked his legs, and he seemed very exhausted. One month later, I returned to the Ramadhanis' house again in order to have an interview with Abdallah. I first received the good news that the week before, Zeinabu had been reinitiated on ART at the Bombo Regional Hospital. She had simply felt ready for it, explained Zeinabu, whose mental state seemed to be more stable than when I had last seen her. Abdallah, by contrast, seemed to be even weaker than the month before. We sat down in the hallway again to talk, and Fatuma and Zeinabu joined us. Abdallah declared that he would talk to me with pleasure, but he was apathetic and often absentminded. When he did not remember certain details or did not comprehend what I asked him, Fatuma helped out.

Like his sisters, forty-five-year-old Abdallah had no secondary school education. He had been married twice, but both wives had died of AIDS. At least this is what Fatuma assumed. Neither Abdallah nor his sisters could tell the exact age of his two children, but they estimated that one daughter was about twelve and the other about three years old. Like his two brothers, Abdallah was a marketer. Seven days a week, he sold fruits and vegetables at his neighborhood market. His income fluctuated significantly from one week to the other, but he estimated that the maximum he made per week was 40,000 TSH. The entire extended family living on the compound depended on his and his two brothers' income.

In 2005, Abdallah got herpes zoster and was admitted to the hospital, where he refused to test for HIV. Since then, however, he had repeatedly caught prolonged fevers. Because of this and because "this modern issue [HIV] has become [more present]," he reasoned that it was necessary for him to "check my health" soon. Moreover, his little daughter had tested HIV-positive and been put on ART, which is why Abdallah suspected that he might have the virus too. In a week or two, he would get the test, he assured me, but he did not seem very convinced himself.

Contrary to Fatuma's earlier contention that Abdallah "knew everything about HIV" but considered himself unable to come to terms with the rules of ART if he had to, he proved to know hardly anything about ARVs. The broadcasts on HIV/AIDS that he had heard on the radio emphasized the urgency of testing for HIV, he explained, but never addressed treatment. And even the fact that his own daughter and sisters were undergoing treatment did not lead to his greater understanding of the therapy. On the one hand, this was due to the fact that he had completely given over the responsibility of care for his child to Fatuma and his mother. They accompanied the girl to her hospital appointments, stored her medical documents and drugs in a safe place, and administered her daily medications. On the other hand, Fatuma explained that she did not consider it necessary to provide her brother with more detailed knowledge about ART as long as he was not enrolled in treatment.

> Even if I give him education about the medicines, and he is not taking them, it won't help anything, because the one you give education to about the medicines is the one who has already tested, who has already been educated [at the hospital]. [Then] I come and add to that.

Zeinabu, in turn, had also obviously never had a detailed conversation about her treatment with Abdallah, and, consequently, he did not know anything about ARVs apart from the fact that "they help her [his daughter] to have a good development (*zinamsaidia maendeleo yake yanakuwa mazuri*)."

Four months after my conversation with Abdallah, I met Fatuma at a meeting of her (self-)support group, where she told me that Abdallah's situation had improved. She assumed that he had secretly undergone an HIV test and that he was taking ARVs. She had never asked him directly, however, because she considered this to be "his own business." Halima had still not tested a second time. Zeinabu was back in Kenya and, Fatuma assumed, doing fine on ARVs. Fatuma herself was still desperately waiting to start treatment, but at her last control visit at the CTC, her CD4 count was still too high.

Negotiating and Navigating Hospital Procedures

A few weeks after I returned to Tanzania for my second field stay, in the early afternoon of 27 May 2011, I knocked on the Ramadhanis' door again. I had not seen them for almost two years. As I had expected at such an hour of the day, I found mostly female family members engaging in housework in the backyard. As their children bustled around their legs, they did laundry, ground coconuts, cleaned vegetables, fried chapatis, nurtured their babies, drank chai, and chatted. After a warmhearted welcome, we sat down on palm leaf mats. Fatuma recounted that the (self-)support groups facilitated by the TAWG only met sporadically, and that the herbal medicines that the NGO had been providing to patients free of charge for several years now had to be purchased privately.[4] After a while, I asked how Abdallah was doing, and Fatuma suddenly dropped her gaze. "He died two months ago," she said quietly. He had been on ARVs for quite some time, but, unfortunately, had not managed to regain his strength. During the last months of his life, he had been blind and dependent on the care of his sisters. One day, early in the morning, his situation had become so critical that they had rushed him to the hospital. Still in the car, Abdallah had succumbed to his disease. Struck by this sad news, I tried to steer the conversation into a more cheerful direction.

The other family members seemed to be all right, I was relieved to observe, except for Zeinabu. Emaciated and with a shrunken face, she was lying in the shade underneath a canopy. At regular intervals, she was shaken by bouts of hard, dry coughing. She had already been treated for tuberculosis, Fatuma explained, but she still had fevers, was very weak, and was molested by a persistent cough. They had not taken her to have a malaria test yet, Fatuma admitted, and I urged her to take Zeinabu to a laboratory as soon as possible.

One week later, I met Bassam, Zeinabu's son-in-law, in town. "Zeinabu has lost her mind again!" he exclaimed agitatedly and pleaded with me to see her. The next morning, the Ramadhanis received me as cordially as always. They offered me a chair in the backyard and indicated for me to wait. Suddenly, I heard Zeinabu roaring my name. A minute later, she stormed out of the house and walked straight up to me. Her reddish eyeballs exposed by torn open lids, she bent down and greeted me with pecks on the cheek. Nobody had ever greeted me like that in Tanzania. I was taken aback and intuitively retreated a bit. Rambling senseless phrases, Zeinabu sat down on my lap. She started playing with my hat and patting my face. While I was still puzzling about how to react, she had already stood up again. What followed was a long and terrifying demonstration of what seemed to be a severe psychosis. Her family members were apparently far less disturbed by this than I, and largely continued to do their housework.

At one point, Zeinabu spat at her sisters, and started attacking them. "She is bad. She has bewitched me. She wants our mother and me to die and seize our house for herself!" she screamed at

Fatuma, who stoically ignored the allegations. Zeinabu hit her mother's arm, which was stretching out toward her with a bowl of water. "Dirty bowl!" she shouted, prompting laughter from the others, and continued rambling incoherently. "Mombasa is a dirty place. They are all whores," I deciphered some of her words. She also rambled something about her German boyfriend, that he also had AIDS, that he cried so much, that all *wazungu* [white people] were so goodhearted and compassionate. With a shaking voice, she suddenly started intonating church songs, then switched from singing "Jesus will help me" to "In the jungle, the mighty jungle," before her singing turned into shouting insults again. When she tried to aggressively wrench her one-year-old granddaughter from Bassam's arms, he warned her not to touch his baby. Only when he raised his arm, ready to hit her, did Zeinabu finally release her grip on the child, who started screaming fearfully. "I have seven spirits, devils in me!" Zeinabu yelled, her hands raised to the sky. "Jesus will help me! Papa Hitler!"

The other children who had been playing in the backyard grew increasingly afraid of Zeinabu. They backed away and continued watching the scene from a secure distance. I felt compelled to do the same, but was glued to my chair. Tormented by horrible bouts of coughing, Zeinabu wrenched her mouth wide open, violently pushed her entire hand into her throat as if she wanted to tear out her lungs. Then she entered the house for a minute and returned with a small mirror in her hands. She looked at herself, made *me* look at my reflection. A second later, she threw the mirror with all her might at her sister. Fatuma managed to duck away and the mirror shattered against the wall. Everyone started shouting at Zeinabu, and she crouched on the floor.

Throughout this entire scene, Zeinabu fixed her attention on me more than anyone else. I tried to keep up with it by constantly telling her to calm down, that no one wanted to do her harm, that she would be all right, that she needed to rest, and whatever other soothing mantras I could think of. Finally, Zeinabu's aggression transformed itself into gasping exhaustion, and she collapsed into herself. "I'm tired," she said, and dragged herself to her bedroom on trembling legs.

Fatuma assumed that Zeinabu had never really resumed ART since 2008. In October of 2010, she had returned from Mombasa in a desolate condition. She had then passed through the first laboratory procedures of ART reinitiation (liver and kidney function tests), but the results had gone missing at the hospital. They drew blood once more, but when Zeinabu and Fatuma came to collect the results a second time, Zeinabu's entire file had been lost. Exhausted by the lengthy and unsuccessful stays at the CTC and annoyed by its mismanagement, Zeinabu and Fatuma would not return a third time. At least Zeinabu was under psychiatric care, Fatuma told me, presenting a bunch of small plastic bags containing multicolored psychotropic pills.

I was worried about Zeinabu's physical and psychological condition, but also about the security of the other family members in the face of her violent outbursts. I discussed possible options with Fatuma, and we decided to see to it that a psychiatrist reassess her current medication and that the family would make a final attempt to reinitiate Zeinabu back onto ART. In the meanwhile, I would try to utilize my connections to the CTC to Zeinabu's benefit. When I told a CTC clinician at the Bombo Regional Hospital about Zeinabu the next morning, she immediately shook her head in resignation. The whole family drove her to despair, she complained. Zeinabu had already interrupted her therapy three times. They had counseled her so many times, but back at home, they would "forget all they had learned" and "go straight back to see a healer," she lamented. Aside from this, they would arbitrarily decide that taking ARVs and antipsychotics at the same time was unbearable, and would thus instruct Zeinabu to discontinue her HIV therapy. "What in God's name are we supposed to do?" the clinician challenged me. Unconfident myself about whether it was really the right thing, I suggested that she be put on treatment again, and the clinician finally gave in to my stubbornness and grumpily led me to the psychiatrist's office. "*He* has to take a look at her *first* before you bring her to me," she instructed me and walked away.

Unable to communicate with Zeinabu on the phone, I rode my bicycle directly to her house. Drenched in sweat, I pleaded with her to immediately come with me in order to see the psychiatrist. Zeinabu was completely apathetic, but she signaled her consent to follow my advice. One of her brothers took her on his bicycle rack, and we hurried back to the hospital. The forewarned psychiatrist, who in his white uniform with large epaulettes looked more like a naval officer than a physician, called us right in and started his interrogations. "So, Zeinabu, how are we doing today?" he asked in a cheerful tone that seemed out of place. "Everything's good? How about your bad dreams? The snakes, the lions? Everything's gone?" Zeinabu said nothing for a while. "I have a cough," she eventually mumbled. "Splendid!" the psychiatrist concluded, filled in four prescription forms, and indicated that this was the end of the consultation.

Disillusioned, I walked with Zeinabu and her brother to the CTC. The clinician directed me to bring her Zeinabu's file. The volunteer in charge of the files started looking for it. After twenty seconds, she claimed that she could not find it. An obviously ill-tempered nurse came in. She commented on the volunteer's explanations concerning my desire with a deep sigh. She sifted through two of around forty file compartments without success. "A patient is waiting for me," she excused herself and left. The volunteer told me that she was incredibly hungry and urgently had to get something to eat. She left too, and I started looking for the file myself. Angrily, I flipped through hundreds of files. Of course, it was in the last compartment that I finally found Zeinabu's file, much to the astonishment of other nurses who in the meanwhile had entered the room and started discussing whether I would ever find what I was looking for. "You really exert yourself!" they commented on my efforts with a slight hint of irony. "Because of stuff like this, people interrupt their therapy and die!" I would have loved to yell at them.

Back in the clinician's office, Zeinabu and her brother received a severe telling-off by the clinician, whose lecture was tinged with allegations. Neither Zeinabu nor her brother dared to say a word. "The problem is their superstition!" the clinician said to *me* several times. She suspected Zeinabu of being resistant to the first line medications. "If she will interrupt the second line therapy, she will suffer an even worse impact!" she warned me, and explained that this was the reason why she and her colleagues had been so hesitant to put her on treatment again during the last couple of months. "We will kill her," she said, expressing her profound doubts right in front of Zeinabu. I was intimidated and could not answer the clinician's repeated question of what she was supposed to do. Finally, she wrote the prescription for the obligatory lab tests and some other medications. Simultaneously, she informed us that the machines at the hospital's laboratory were out of order and advised us to go directly to a private laboratory in town.

Approximately forty people were queuing in front of the barred counter window of the hospital's pharmacy. The stressed pharmacist glanced at the dozens of prescription forms that were held out in front of his face. "Have it, don't have it, have it, don't have it, don't have it, don't have it . . ." he exclaimed. I told Zeinabu and her brother that I would bring the medicines later and sent them home. One and a half hours later, I finally held half of the prescribed compounds in my hands, intake instructions carelessly scribbled on the plastic bags with a pen. Back at Zeinabu's house, I explained everything to them, repeatedly implored Fatuma to take Zeinabu to get the lab tests done at a private institution, and gave her 5,000 TSH that would pay for it. When I left the house, I felt exhausted and uncertain about whether insisting on Zeinabu's ART reinitiation had been the right thing to do.

Over the following weeks, I visited the Ramadhanis several times. Although her mother expressed her great gratitude for my engagement and said that Zeinabu had "calmed down a lot," I grew increasingly disillusioned, for at every visit, I ascertained that they had *still* not taken her to a laboratory, and *still* not returned with her to the hospital to check her CD4 count. For another period of several weeks, Fatuma kept telling me, "On Monday, Zeinabu will participate in the adherence classes."

On 1 August, Fatuma finally told me that Zeinabu had obtained all the necessary laboratory results for ART initiation. Her CD4 count was 200 cells/μl, but before she could start treatment, she would have to participate in the adherence classes again. Fatuma also explained that the week before, she herself had finally started taking ARVs too. The medicines made her dizzy and nauseous, she complained, before she excused herself and went to bed to take a rest. At my last visit to the family two weeks later, Fatuma told me that the side effects had grown even stronger. After they had started to make her vomit and her dizziness had increased to the point that she could no longer walk, she had been switched to another regimen. The new medications, however, provoked itchy rashes all over her body, she lamented, incessantly scratching herself. Zeinabu's state had thankfully seemed to stabilize. Yet she had still not attended the adherence classes, and shortly before I left the Ramadhanis after a long farewell, I heard her ask Fatuma in a low voice, "Should I not better wait and finish the medicine for my head before I take ARVs?"

Ambiguities and Limitations of Speaking Out about ART

The story of Fatuma and her brothers and sisters invites reflection on various aspects of how ART inscribes itself into and affects social relations within extended families. To begin with, I would like to take the Ramadhanis as an example of how HIV and its treatment are made the subject of verbal discussion. Fatuma's voluntary dedication to learn as much as possible about ARVs before she had even started the treatment herself was rather extraordinary, and she seemed to proactively and repeatedly appeal to her family members to get tested for HIV themselves. In this way, she could be viewed as an excellent example of how patients who are acquainted with the matter of HIV testing and treatment can function as "multipliers" of central public health messages within familial networks. Even though it cannot be claimed with certainty that Fatuma's "proselytizing" activities were the sole or principal stimulation for her sister, mother, and brother getting tested for HIV, it is reasonable to assume that her insistence significantly contributed to their decision to check their health status.

This assumption is supported by the fact that several other patients recounted that while they had been aware of the dangers of HIV and governmental health authorities' appeals to get tested, the decisive factor for actually taking the step to test had been the direct interaction and communication with a close person, who in most cases was a family member. These cases suggest that the expectations associated with the scale-up of ART across the globe were being met: that ever more people within the immediate social surroundings of people living with HIV/AIDS would witness the often dramatic transformation of their relatives (and/or friends) who had been on the brink of death, and would thus gain at least rudimentary knowledge about the pharmaceuticals that caused these wondrous reconstitutions. This, in turn, would prompt many people to increasingly conceptualize HIV as a manageable condition and to hesitate less before testing for HIV if they were sick, and to claim treatment if indicated.

Undoubtedly, such desired repercussions of treatment availability and accessibility were observable in Tanga during my research. However, the process of multiplying and transferring biomedical knowledge in a way that results in the behavior change of third persons is highly complex and nonlinear. It often remains incomplete, ambiguous, and fragmentary, and in other contexts, does not set in at all. The Ramadhani family exemplifies the fallacy of taking for granted the fact that living together with an ART patient will "automatically" foster treatment literacy and readiness to get an HIV test among those in the patient's proximity.

The case of Fatuma shows that the way in which people communicate about HIV and ART is not necessarily coherent. Even before Fatuma had started taking ARVs herself, she was the one in the family who was most optimistic about the drugs, best informed about their rules and benefits, and most closely tied to available community-based support structures. Yet her attempts to motivate her brothers to get tested for HIV were characterized by a peculiar omission of the topic of ART. She did not instrumentalize her knowledge about ARVs in a suggestive manner, based on the assumption that only those who have already tested HIV-positive need to know about and understand the therapy. Perhaps this was one reason why she did not succeed in prevailing upon her brother Abdallah to check his health status. Instead of discussing the benefits and disadvantages of ART with him, she simply assumed that he had already obtained sufficient knowledge about the therapy to decide that he was unable to adhere to the "appropriate" lifestyle of an ARV user. Later on, when his health condition apparently improved, she hypothesized that he had secretly begun treatment, but did not try to verify her presumption by asking him, for she felt that this was "his own business."

Whether such forms of deliberate noncommunication signaled indifference to one another's well-being, or should instead be interpreted as a specific form of care (cf. de Klerk 2012; Mogensen 2010) in the sense of sparing one another from having to talk about a topic as distressing as one's own HIV infection, was difficult to tell and certainly differed from one context to the other. In consideration of Fatuma's engagement in the care of her brothers' children and her great efforts to assist her sister in resuming ART, it is reasonable to assume that, in her case, the latter applied. In other cases, such as

Joseph's family (Case Study D), however, kin relations were already so strained by everyone's struggle to secure their livelihood that the matter of Joseph's HIV infection and related conflicts about familial responsibilities and economic resources seemed to be the last straw that led to the final breakdown of solidarity and mutual support. The near complete disruption of communicational ties between Joseph and his entire family suggest a mutual disinterest in how the others were getting by.

In the Ramadhanis' case, the peculiar communicative behavior and exclusive distribution of care responsibilities to specific persons led to a remarkable situation. While some family members were on treatment and regularly visited the hospital for control visits in different constellations, those who were not directly involved in the everyday routines of managing ART did not even develop a rudimentary understanding of how the therapy worked and what it implied. Abdallah's case is particularly striking in this regard. He had experienced the fatal consequences of AIDS through the loss of his two wives, who had supposedly succumbed to the disease. He was aware that one of his daughters was also living with HIV and was enrolled in treatment. His sisters lived openly with HIV, and one of them had been living with ARVs for several years. His own body bore the signs of an HIV infection, and he was obviously suffering. But all of these experiences could not induce him to get tested, at least not for a long period of time. Although the ingestion of ARVs and hospital visits were a daily routine in his household, he was excluded (or excluded himself) from the everyday care activities of his family members to the extent that he even did not gain any significant knowledge about the drugs that were keeping his own daughter alive.

"They Put Poison into Your Stomach": Selective and Alternative Discourses about ART

Fatuma's and her sisters' skepticism about the possibly detrimental effects of ARVs once more alluded to the impact of other patients' descriptions of persistent side effects, as well as recurring rumors and half-truths about the drugs, not only on prospective ART patients but also on those who had already been taking the medicines for quite some time. In the previous chapter, I showed the way in which such rumors shaped individual people's anxieties vis-à-vis their long-term daily medication intake. Fatuma and her sisters' concerns about

ARVs causing sudden death and turning into poison illustrated how negative appraisals of the drugs were interactively reproduced and effectively spread even among people with a considerable history of receiving education in the scientific "truths" about HIV and ART. It is reasonable to assume that such alternative discourses affirm the assumptions of patients like Zeinabu that the medicines cause significant damage to their physical and/or mental constitution and thus contribute to their decisions to terminate therapy.

Etiological understandings of ART and HIV that differ radically from biomedical concepts, such as those that associate HIV to witchcraft and spirit possession, certainly also have an impact on such decisions. While such conceptualizations will be dealt with in greater depth in Chapter 8, I would like to mention one further aspect that is related to Fatuma's assumptions about Abdallah's reasons for not getting tested. Fatuma believed that Abdallah was informed about the modes of behavior that were expected from ART patients, aside from mere regular drug ingestion. With regard to his personal lifestyle, she further speculated that these obligations seemed so unaccomplishable to him that he could not imagine himself becoming an ART patient, and therefore, in the absence of other treatment options, he had no reason to find out whether he was HIV-positive or not. Abdallah's own explanations, however, showed that he was rather uninformed about the obligations of being an ART patient. The fact that he later did get tested and started ART without telling Fatuma fortunately proved her assumptions to be mistaken.

Yet I encountered other cases, which did indeed point to the fact that health professionals' strong emphasis on patients' obligatory behavioral restrictions during ART preparation found entrance into lay discourses about ARVs, where they were amplified and at times had the unintended effect of putting people off from seeking treatment. Ismail's thirty-five-year-old sister-in-law Saada serves as an example. She explained that she had recently attended a burial, whose guests whispered with their hands over their mouths that the deceased had died of AIDS despite being on ART. Missing just one single day's dose had supposedly been enough to weaken him so much that he could not recover. As a consequence of such unsettling information, which was powerful enough to counter the positive impression that Saada had of ARVs after she had seen how they had brought her brother-in-law back to life, she admitted that she was still too afraid to take an HIV test and possibly live with the medicines herself. "If I was in that situation [of having HIV], I'd take the medicines," she claimed. "But honestly, it would also be a problem to me, and I would worry a lot. Every day, every single day for the rest of your life, you're supposed to take the medicines" (Interview, 7 July 2009).

As the above examples show, communication about ART within extended families and at the community level did not necessarily happen in such a way that those with little or no understanding about the treatment felt compelled to test for HIV and claim treatment for themselves. The causal chain between receiving suggestive firsthand information from closely related persons and the receiver's change of behavior was hampered in various ways. On the one hand, the information on ART that people passed on within their proximate social environments was always partial and fragmented—even within close kin groups, particular persons could be excluded from the flow of information. Moreover, positive depictions of ART were countered by alternative discourses emphasizing the negative sides of the treatment. These were often based on half-truths referring to the medicines' possible adverse effects or amplifications of negatively judged obligations concerning ART patients' lifestyles.

Such discourses certainly affected how both patients and others thought and felt about ARVs. The effects ranged from subtle but worrisome uncertainty and skeptical appraisals with regard to what it meant to take these medicines for a lifetime to outright rejection. In some cases, deviance from biomedical regimens, disregard of the biomedical claim to "exclusive therapeutic rights" over the body, and treatment interruption were the consequences. Regarding the people who had not started treatment because they had never even dared to take an HIV test, these discourses and communicational inconsistencies seemed in turn to contribute to the persistence of anxiety and a hesitation to do so.

"Kin Are Not There to Look Similar; They Are There to Help Each Other": The Provision of Care and Support in Practice

Despite the ambiguous and limited verbal communication about ART among the Ramadhani siblings, their example shows how indispensable and often irreplaceable familial support, solidarity, and cohesion are for people living with ARVs. It continues to be a common pattern that one or two breadwinners with more or less regular earnings provide for a large number of kin without sufficient income (cf. Dilger 2013b). As large parts of Tanzania's population have no regular job and depend on casual labor or subsistence farming, the position of breadwinner within the family is rather unstable. Inadvertent transformation from being the provider to being the receiver of familial assistance occurs, at times, surprisingly quickly.

Apart from receiving direct financial assistance, children are often sent to other households in order to live with relatives who are more affluent, and whose place of residence offers better educatory facilities (cf. Alber, Martin, and Notermans 2013). The moving of Haruna and Zahra's children to their uncle's place after Zahra's death (see Introduction), and Issa's children staying at his brother's and sister's places (Case Study B), are only two of many similar cases that are illustrative of the high level of mobility of children and adolescents within kinship networks (see also Alber and Martin 2007). While children's degree of mobility was already high before the HIV/AIDS epidemic, it has certainly increased in the times of AIDS, particularly during the time prior to HIV treatment when in many African societies, the disease pried away almost the entire generation of middle-aged adults, whose children were consigned to the care of their grandparents and other relatives (Evans 2005; Wolf 2010).

As the Ramadhani family evidences, children did not necessarily have to leave the household in order to be relegated to the care of persons other than their biological parents. Fatuma was thus mainly responsible for taking care of the health and treatment of Abdallah's daughter and her two other nephews. Accompanying them to the hospital to seek help for acute health conditions as well as for their routine control visits at the CTC was an arduous task and most often amounted to spending many hours at the clinic. The home-based part of managing her niece's and nephews' ART was a further challenge, particularly when the children called the necessity of their therapy into question and refused to take their daily medications (Mattes 2014b). This was the case with sixteen-year-old Abdul, another nephew of Fatuma who was also consigned to her care after he lost his mother to AIDS, and his father had gotten remarried to a woman who would not tolerate Abdul living in the house. In looking after her niece's and nephews' health, investing time in frequent and lengthy hospital visits with them, and making an effort to ensure that they took their pills, Fatuma unquestionably rendered her brothers a great service, which balanced the financial support she received from them.[5]

Provision of support and care in practice does not, of course, remain restricted to children, as Zeinabu's case shows. Despite her bouts of aggression during what I viewed as episodes of severe psychosis, which even posed a physical danger to her family, she was economically sustained by her brothers, while her mother and sisters fed and nursed her, accompanied her to medical laboratories and the hospital, supervised her daily drug intake, and were in charge of her ART-related and other documents. During my interviews and visits in patients' households, I witnessed and was told about many other ways in which people were taken care of and assisted over the years. The help given by grandparents, parents, husbands and wives, brothers and sisters, aunts and uncles, nieces and nephews, and, in several cases, also particular in-laws was essential for patients to successfully navigate the ups and downs implied in all stages of ART, not to mention the often strenuous and difficult times preceding treatment uptake.

Basically, all patients' narratives about their trajectories of suffering before initiating treatment thus included manifold explications of how they were cared for, encouraged, and supported by relatives. Issa's case (Case Study B) provides a good example: when his health had become affected to a critical point, it was his uncle who transported him to the health center near his sister Zawadi's house, where he found shelter during the following weeks. Ismail and his family offer another, particularly compelling example of how certain persons within the familial network formed situational therapy management groups (Janzen 1987; Nichter 2002), who steered "their" patient's itinerary of treatment seeking, always with the best of intentions, even when these eventually contradicted Ismail's ideas of what measures should be taken to his benefit.

Relatives' therapy (co)management, of course, did not stop at the doorstep of the hospital. As discussed above, it was often relatives who motivated patients to check their health status. In many cases, they also accompanied them to a clinic or VCT center in order to morally support them in actually taking this difficult step. During the subsequent lengthy ART enrollment procedures, it was again mostly patients' family members who functioned as treatment assistants, assisted them in negotiating with medical professionals, and spent hours with them waiting, wondering about, and discussing the at times incomprehensible medical routines. They encouraged them not to lose faith along the often burdensome process, and made plans with them for how to overcome possible obstacles. Issa's tireless elderly father, for instance, covered all of these supportive actions.

Furthermore, during the phase of treatment preparation, which implied regular visits to the hospital, patients were frequently accommodated by relatives who were living nearby, as we saw in the cases of Furaha and Issa. Many patients stayed for several weeks or months after treatment initiation. This initial phase of ART was particularly difficult to handle when severely weakened patients developed a so-called immune reconstitution inflammatory syndrome (i.e., "a transient worsening of the symptoms of infection at two to three weeks, and sometimes up to eight weeks after commencement of ART" [NACP 2012, 150]). The familial care during this phase did not only consist of physical nursing, but also included financial support, which compensated for patients' possible illness-related income loss.

Finally, and once more returning to the Ramadhanis, patients' family members played an utterly important role in the long-term management of the therapy. In the same ways as Fatuma reminded Zeinabu to take her pills, several other patients recounted how their drug ingestion was closely monitored and supported by their family members. In some cases, patients even reported that their young children below ten years of age reminded them to take their pills at the designated time of day.

The Limitations of Kin-Based Cohesion

The wide variety of all these actions in support of sick relatives undergoing ART, some of which implied considerable sacrifice and devotion on the part of caregivers, confirmed the prevalence of a great degree of reciprocity among kin, whose taken-for-grantedness Furaha so aptly described with the sapience that "kin are not there for looking similar; they are there to help each other." However, these positive examples ought not to reify idealized notions of the "African family" as a permanent, reliable harbor of security and unconditional kin-based solidarity (cf. Moyer and Igonya 2014, 139). There were also other familial setups that pointed to the limitations of kin-based cohesion. Processes of individualization were observable in households and wider families, in which each adult member more or less minded his or her own business and struggled for his or her own nuclear family's survival. Some of my interlocutors who found themselves in such a situation associated these dynamics to the fact that none of their family members had sufficient financial resources to share them. Olivia, whose husband had died of AIDS and whose son Anthony was on ART too, for instance, had a hard time providing food for her family and paying her children's school fees with the small income she made by trading fish in her neighborhood. But apparently, her brothers and sisters were even worse off.

> My sister and my small brother are farmers. They don't have any financial means (*hawana uwezo*). Their capacity is maybe that when they harvest maize . . . you may get one or two buckets. . . . But there isn't any help in the form of cents (*msaada wa senti*). This brother does not have work. Maybe once in a while, he can do some occasional jobbing . . . but it's not easy for him to care for himself and to satisfy my family too; it's not easy. (Olivia, forty-nine years, first year of ART, 5 July 2011)

Such precarious living conditions weighed heavily on kinship relations. Resulting tensions at times smoldered underneath the surface in the form of particular family members' largely unverbalized feelings that others were not meeting their familial obligations for care (cf. Dilger 2010, 2013b). In other cases, tensions steadily intensified to the point of sparking acute conflicts. Mutual solicitude was denounced, and the rupture of solidaristic relations left cracks in the social fabric of kinship networks of support (cf. Whyte 2005). HIV/AIDS and the growing inequality it evokes by enhancing the dependency of the afflicted on caregivers and supporters within their immediate social surroundings certainly adds to the pressure that social relations were already exposed to before (cf. Dilger 2005). Throughout the past three decades, the living conditions of large parts of the Tanzanian population have become ever more precarious as a consequence of structural adjustment, privatization, and cutbacks in public sector expenditure, including that on health care provision (Benson 2001; Lugalla 1995; Rösch 1995). The global financial crisis of 2008 significantly exacerbated this already critical situation by inversing the growth rate of the Tanzanian economy, enhancing unemployment rates, and evoking a steep increase in the price of everyday commodities (Lunogelo, Mbilinyi, and Hangi 2009; Tibandebage and Kida 2013). The following case study is illustrative of the way in which families struggled to maintain their cohesion in countering adverse living conditions. While constituting a contrast to the kind of support that was mobilized in the Ramadhani family, it simultaneously demonstrates the difficulty implied in disentangling long grown and often highly complex conflictive family relations in order to determine with certainty the degree to which the HIV infection of one or more involved persons played a decisive role in the conflict.

Case Study D: Joseph

In mid-January 2009, Edna and I took one of the *daladalas* (mini-buses) that depart from close to Tanga's main market in the center and travelled along the meandering dust roads through the city's extended residential belt. We got off at the final destination, where Joseph picked us up and led us to his place further down the road. We did not get to see much of the house he lived in, as he asked us to take a seat on a worn sofa in the sitting room we entered through the front door. Joseph's sister Grace was busy sweeping the red painted concrete floor in the hallway and only greeted us quickly before continuing her work.

Joseph was forty years old and unemployed at the time. He was not married, but had a fourteen-year-old daughter, who stayed with one of his sisters in another city, and with whose mother he had no contact. Joseph was one of eleven children, but three of his siblings as well as both of his parents had died. Joseph lived with his sister Grace and his younger brother Isaac in their recently deceased mother's house. In contrast to most of the other ART patients I got to know, Joseph had completed secondary school to the ordinary level. Nevertheless, he had not managed to profit from his level of education in the form of stable employment. Since he had finished school, he had first assisted one of his brothers doing farm work for some years, and then he occasionally worked as a bus and truck driver.

Joseph's trajectory before he tested for HIV in 2003 resembled those of many other ART patients. After suffering from repeated periods of persistent fevers and infections, he was motivated by his HIV-positive brother-in-law, Grace's husband, to check his health status. The result turned out positive, but since ARVs were not available at the time, he began taking the TAWG's herbal medicines, which helped him keep his health more or less stable for two years. Then his CD4 count decreased to 90. Fortunately, the national treatment program had been established in the meantime, and Joseph was initiated on ART in 2005. With the help of his new medicines, Joseph fared well for some time. His brother-in-law, in contrast, refused to start treatment at that time, because he did not want to take medicines every day. Shortly afterward, he succumbed to his disease.

In 2007, the next crisis occurred. Joseph's CD4 count had significantly decreased, and he tested positive first for malaria and a little later for tuberculosis. His eldest brother Benjamin, who lived some 300 km away from Tanga, arranged for him to be admitted to a tuberculosis clinic near where he lived and covered all related expenses. Joseph's left lung had been seriously damaged. He passed two months at a quarantine facility and another four months at Benjamin's house until he had finished his course of anti-TB drugs and fairly recovered. After his return to Tanga, however, Joseph's health steadily deteriorated again. He lost weight and grew increasingly weaker until reaching the point of hardly being able to do any physical work. From that point on, he entirely depended on Benjamin's financial assistance, just like the other members of his household did. Owing to the assistance and care that Benjamin gave to his siblings, and particularly to Joseph during his illness episodes, he played an important role in the family. "He has always been like a father to me," said Joseph, describing his relationship with Benjamin.

"Your Heart Grows Numb—It's Better to Die": The Shattering of Familial Solidarity

Despite all his good intentions, Benjamin's contributions to Joseph, Isaac, and Grace's household were barely enough to secure their survival, and any unforeseen event that would require additional financial resources posed an existential threat to the siblings. During this critical phase, Joseph's situation worsened even further due to a hereditary conflict about Joseph's deceased mother's house. Irene, another of Joseph's older sisters, intended to remove her siblings from the house and take over the property. A court case solved the dispute in Benjamin's favor, but the tensions between Benjamin and Irene increased, and the family was divided into two groups allying with one or the other of the two.

One day, when his daughter came to Tanga for a visit, Joseph was caught at the frontlines. When his daughter did not find her father at home upon her arrival, she went to see her aunt Irene, and Joseph later came to pick up his daughter at Irene's house. Somehow, Benjamin got to know about this and took Joseph's visit to Irene's place as a serious betrayal. As a consequence, he excluded him from his payments and strictly ordered Grace and Isaac to neither share any of the money he gave them with Joseph nor to support him in any other way. "Even cats have children," he replied disdainfully to Joseph's desperate explanation of why he had stopped by Irene's house.

After his abrupt exclusion from the household's cash flow, Joseph's situation became alarming. At the time of our first interview, he weighed only 45 kilos. He was barely able to provide himself with one meal per day, and while he was aware of the possible conse-quences for his health, he had only irregularly taken his ARVs during the previous month. As mentioned in the previous chapter, in the middle of our conversation, he explained that he had not taken his ARVs for two and a half days because he lacked food to go along with the medicines that would dampen their side effects. At that point, I interrupted the interview, gave him some money to buy enough food for the day, asked him to take his drugs, and agreed with him to continue our conversation on the following day.

Joseph's diction when talking about the conflict that divided his family and his own miserable situation revealed feelings of profound isolation and bitter disappointment. "They have finally ruined me. [My brother's] cruel and bitter words have entered my heart. . . . Your heart grows numb—it's better to die than to wait for anyone to return your heart [courage—*arudishe moyo wako*]," he stated. In an interview I had with Grace six months after my first conversation with Joseph, she claimed that she had advised him to reconcile with Benjamin. Apparently, however, his emotional wound seemed too deep to allow this. "I don't want to bow before anyone, even if he has money!" Grace remembered Joseph's reply.

In contrast to Grace's claims that she had attempted to mediate between Joseph and Benjamin and did not treat Joseph differently than any other person, Joseph recounted episodes that gave a different impression. At the very beginning, when Grace got to know about his test result, she took several of his clothes and burnt and buried them in the backyard because she was afraid that they could be contaminating. Later on, Joseph was always given his own plate to eat from, and while Grace took care of Isaac's laundry, she would not wash any clothes for him. Joseph also alleged that it was Grace who had told Benjamin about his visit at Irene's house, and once, he explained, she had even blamed him in front of Benjamin of intending to harm her and her children by witchcraft (*uchawi*), which evoked an intense argument between him and his brother.

Joseph suspected that Grace had always been jealous of his previously close ties with Benjamin. He also related her hostile behavior to her lack of education. "If she could, she would throw me out, but she can't, because it's not her house. It's all a matter of education. It's difficult with people who have no education. You better stick to your own business (*jua ya kwako tu*)," he reasoned. In Joseph's view, it was mainly Grace's envy that motivated her to influence his situation for the worse. His brother Isaac, in contrast, seemed to be rather indifferent about Joseph's situation and did not engage in his affairs at all. "He leaves the house in the morning at six and comes back at ten or eleven at night; he goes to his room and sleeps. He lives very much his own life (*maisha yake ye' mwenyewe*)," Joseph explained.

"Born from the Same Womb": The Danger of Social Proximity

Joseph's experiences in his wider social environment were equally pervaded by a strong undertone of frustration and alienation. There was such an intense dynamic of stigmatization in his neighborhood that another HIV-positive man had already strangled himself, he told me. Because Grace had spread the word, everybody knew about *his* HIV infection too, he complained, and described the serious impact this had had on his social standing. Not only had he become the scapegoat and target of public slander when, for instance, the mobile phone of a visitor to his house had been stolen, and the neighbors blamed him for the deed "because [they] saw that I'm in a difficult situation." He also saw other far-reaching consequences of his sister's betrayal in terms of revealing his health status in the neighborhood. No one would "invest" in him anymore because everyone knew "that this one is sick already" and doomed to die soon. This, he asserted, spoiled any possibility of finding partners with whom to start a new income-generating project in the surrounding area. In order to at least prevent further involuntary disclosure of his health status within his social environment, Joseph vehemently refused health professionals' prompts to be open about his condition and to be transferred to his neighborhood health center when the provision of ART became part of its portfolio.

The lack of solidarity and hostility that Joseph sensed in his neighborhood caused him to advance a theory about the disadvantage of social proximity that went beyond the specific causal link between HIV disclosure and social exclusion. "Since the 1980s ... I went to school here from the first class to the eighth grade. ... I know all young people of this neighborhood very well. ... I know every house, and the character (*roho*) of every person," he recounted. Even though he had no particular explanation for why people would not extend him a helping hand, he reasoned that this close social proximity between him and other community members was obstructive. Strangeness (*ugeni*), by implication, was empowering. "Everyone is afraid of you and ... thinks 'you can't know where this person came from. ... I better not start a quarrel with him ... .' It's different with a person who knows you right from the cradle," he reasoned.

Joseph was particularly consternated by the discord and disruption of solidaristic relations with his own closest kin who "were born from one and the same womb (*umezaliwa naye tumbo moja*)." Several times, he expressed his extreme disappointment about his siblings' unexpectedly cruel behavior, which led him to further distance himself from them. He spent as little time as possible at home, and when he met Grace or Isaac during the few hours he spent at his house, he avoided conversing with them. He no longer wished to enquire or know about their well-being, just as they did not care about his.

"You Never Know Where the Risk Is": Fragile Biosocial Collectives and Enclaves of Concealment

Based on his logic that social intimacy corresponds to vulnerability and disempowerment, Joseph developed the strong wish to move away from his neighborhood, find his own room, live peacefully and independently by himself, and build up new relationships with people who would respect him. "I don't even want to see the face of some people here anymore," he complained. "If I had the chance, I would have my own place far away." Eventually, he succeeded in establishing new social ties in the protective realm of strangeness that enabled him to at least spend his days far away from his own neighborhood. His friend Michael adopted him into the business of renting out bicycles on the opposite side of Tanga.

Michael was also living with ARVs and was in a similarly precarious situation as Joseph. He was thirty-four years old, unmarried, and had no children. He was born and had grown up in Tanga, but his life trajectory had been shaped by a high degree of occupational and geographic mobility. He had worked as an unskilled laborer in the mining, fishing, and timber industries, and had lived in many different parts of Tanzania. In 2002, he contracted a severe malaria infection that left him paralyzed on one side. This constituted a grave turning point in his life, and in addition, he tested HIV-positive only one year later. The relatives in the city he was living in at the time would not support him during the ensuing period when he suffered from multiple opportunistic infections, so he decided to return to Tanga and stay with his father, to whom he disclosed his problem. He shared a room with his father in a large rundown barrack on the margins of Tanga, which was occupied by a group of unemployed young men. Since then, the two of them had struggled together for survival. His father contributed to their household income through occasional short-term contracts as a plumber, and Michael added what he earned helping out at an informal bicycle rental stand in the neighborhood.

The relationship between Michael and his father, however, was tense. They frequently argued, and Michael complained about his father's ignorance of his critical situation and his reluctance to get tested for HIV himself. His father did not directly discriminate against him, Michael explained, but he was not interested in getting to know more details about his health situation and the requirements he had to meet in order to stay healthy. Perhaps this was the reason why, when he learned about Joseph's troubles with his family, Michael was also seeking to build a new survival alliance with someone else. Over the course of time, Michael and Joseph's friendship grew closer. Day by day, they sat together on the small dusty road passing by the barrack in which Michael lived, rented out his boss's bicycles by the hour, and kept the books for him. Even though Joseph was still sleeping in his mother's house, he spent each day until late at night with Michael at the bicycle stand. They shared their meager daily income of about 2,500 TSH, bought basic foodstuffs, and cooked and ate together. Furthermore, they took every opportunity to make some additional money. During my first interview with Michael in mid-January 2009, for instance, Joseph knocked on the door. Excitedly, he told us that a truck carrying vegetable oil had turned over and was spilling its valuable fright on a nearby road. People were running to the place to serve themselves, and Joseph was going to try and get a share too. Some two weeks later, he proudly told me that he and Michael could live off the money earned from selling the oil he had managed to steal for an entire week. After that, however, they had returned to their usual day-to-day paucity.

After Joseph had told me this, he took our meeting as a chance to ask me whether I was able to provide him with seed capital for a new income-generating project he was planning together with Michael. They had thought about purchasing a piece of land and growing veg-etables that they could sell. During our previous meetings, Joseph had made vague allusions to this idea on several occasions, but he had never asked me directly for assistance. I explained to him that for the sake of fairness vis-à-vis other research participants who had posed similar requests to me, I could not financially support him, but that I had already thought about giving him one of the two bicycles that I owned as a onetime present, which might help him in establishing a new economic project by being more mobile. A few weeks later, before I travelled to Germany for a few weeks, I met Joseph again, and he happily received the bicycle.

Joseph and Michael's collaboration was not limited to sharing their income and food. They also cared for each other during sick-ness episodes, and, most importantly, paid strict attention that no one from their friends and the other young men hanging around at the bicycle rental would overhear about their HIV infection. While it was important to Joseph to mention that these people had become his new peer group, where he could enjoy some unburdened and enjoyable hours each day, it was evident that he felt more closely connected to Michael due to their common, concealed biomedical predicament.

While the two allies' "biosocial microcollective" at least provided some form of income, it was still insufficient, and Joseph kept looking for further opportunities. He recounted an odyssey through Tanga's economy of nongovernmental social support. He asked the staff of an NGO about a job, but they shrugged their shoulders. He tried to join one of the TAWG facilitated (self-)support groups, which, as he had learned, provided access to a microcredit initiative conducted by another NGO called Action for Relief and Development Assistance (AFREDA, see Chapter 7). But he could neither pay the admission fee of 10,000 TSH nor the monthly members fee of 1,000 TSH. Promises of health staff at the CTC to help him find a job remained unfulfilled. They kept urging him to take his medicines instead. Joseph felt misunderstood and once more socially distanced.

> They always ask, "Why did you stop taking the drugs?" And I tell them, "I have stopped because I don't have enough food." Then they say, "You must not stop! . . . Eat and take your medicine!" . . . Their thoughts and my thoughts as a user (*mtumiaji*) are different. . . . They don't believe me . . . they don't understand me.

Joseph would not ask a private person for support because he feared further stigmatization; but about two months after our first interview, he did manage to find work as a night guard. He was assigned night shifts at the property of a high scale local authority. When he confided to his ward that he was HIV-positive and what a physical strain the job implied for him, he unexpectedly encountered a high degree of comprehension. He was offered to enter the house now and then during his shift to sleep for a while. He was treated "like his [the house owner's] child," Joseph expressed. Finally, with the help of an NGO staff member, Joseph also managed to join the TAWG's (self-)support group, whose admission fee and monthly contribution was waived. However, when AFREDA started recruiting the beneficiaries who would be granted microcredits, he faced the next hurdle. Like several others, he had no assets that could serve as a deposit in order to get the first credit of 100,000 TSH. It was private engagement again that enabled the destitute applicants to form a group and obtain the credit: a well-known HIV-positive woman who functioned as a peer educator in various health facilities agreed to take on full responsibility for them and to closely monitor their amortizations. With the credit, Joseph managed to buy two bicycles that he started renting out for his and Michael's benefit. Thanks to the profit and to Joseph's monthly salary, the situation of the two friends looked less somber for a while.

When I met Joseph for a follow-up interview at the beginning of June 2009, however, it was visible that working day and night was starting to exact a toll on him. He had fevers and skin sores, was utterly prostrated, and desperately longed for a week of rest. Furthermore, his microcollective with Michael had apparently reversed itself from an effective arrangement of cohesion and mutual assistance to yet another source of uncertainty. Michael was involved in substance abuse, he told me, and spent large parts of their money on drugs and women with whom he had affairs. Aside from this, Michael had supposedly not taken his ARVs for a considerable length of time. Dozens of unopened pillboxes were hidden in his cupboard.

Despite these problems, Joseph would not "resign the contract" with Michael:

> I won't let him down because he is my companion and I know that all the problems are ours together. He is a human and I am a human, and we were all built without knowing where the [next] risk is lurking. You can't let this one down and say, "This is your own risk," and then you find yourself falling just the same way.

This is how Joseph expressed his moral commitment, which underlined his perception of a constantly menacing uncertainty in life. However, he also articulated a more economic motivation for maintaining the relationship with Michael, in terms of a futile investment:

> I know, once we'll be in a fight, I will have destroyed the whole process. . . . I won't know where to start again; that's why I just endure it. . . . His behavior is incomprehensible. I don't know, is it a matter of his [lacking] education or what? But I have to accept him because he is my companion (*jamaa*) and he has offered me shelter (*amenikaribisha*). . . . We have made it up to where we are now, and I remember well where I came from.

. . . You never know where the risk for a person is; you can reject a person and all of a sudden he/she is your fortune.

While Joseph held on to his ties with Michael despite his disappointment about his irresponsible behavior in order not to spoil another carefully built source of support earlier than necessary, he would also not ask Benjamin for "forgiveness" for his "transgression." He prioritized his moral standard over resuming his proper position within the familial power relations, which could have possibly reopened the pathway to economic survival. His morally informed self-concept also emerged when he referred to a person occupying his room upon his sister's invitation, whom he did not intend to expel even though he was desperately longing for a place to stay: "I'm educated, I understand. . . . I'm also a human being (*binadamu*); I'm not an animal," he reasoned.

Two and a half months later, I met Joseph again on the street. Michael had kept on deceiving him, he lamented, so he had finally decided to cut his relationship with him too. He had taken his two bicycles and went with them to his mother's house. Joseph said that he had massive financial problems and did not know how to pay his monthly amortizations to AFREDA. Adding to the burden, he also had to pay the monthly water bill for Grace, Isaac, and himself. Before I could inquire into whether this meant that there had been some sort of reapproximation between him and his siblings, he said goodbye and rode away on my former bicycle into the evening sun. I did not know that this would be the last time I saw him.

One year later, after I had returned to Germany and was due to start my second field stay, I received an email from one of Joseph's nephews: Joseph's health status did not allow him to continue working as a night guard. "He spends all day sleeping because of unexpected diseases," the nephew wrote. Furthermore, Joseph no longer had a job and had sold two of his bicycles in order to pay his daughter's school fees. When the money was depleted, she was expelled from school. Joseph had finally tried to reconcile with his elder brother, but Benjamin persistently refused to forgive him "because he knows Joseph can't escape from his trouble," the short message read.

During the four months of my second field stay in Tanga, I did not meet Joseph again, because he had disappeared. At his house, I met only Grace and Zachary, another brother. Grace told me that during the first months after my departure, Joseph continued to spend only the nights at their house. Their relationship continued to be full of conflict and mutual allegations. At some point, their brother Benjamin also ceased his support for them because he had gotten into financial difficulties himself. Joseph's health deteriorated. He got wounds and fevers. And then, suddenly, he was gone without saying goodbye or telling anyone where he was going. This time, it was Grace who expressed her indignation over such a lack of solidarity. But both Grace and Zachary kept explaining that this was not so uncommon in these difficult times.

> Zachary: We are alone even though we have many relatives, but they . . .
> Grace: Everyone cares about his/her own [nuclear] family.
> Zachary: African people have changed. . . . Every day, you will find more people who only look after their own family, how they can *attain* [English expression in original Swahili quote] their future. Nowadays, you find that every family only *respects* their own [problems] and seeks for ways to survive themselves. . . .

Zachary worked as a freelancer selling mobile phone vouchers and supported Grace and her children with part of his irregular income. This was by no means sufficient for their needs. Grace had to take her children out of school in order to save on the school fees, and they could only afford one proper meal per day. The conflict between Benjamin and Irene was still not settled, and Irene supposedly intended to litigate the court decision concerning their mother's house. The animosity between the opponents and their respective allies seemed to be enormous. Grace and Zachary had no doubt that Irene would accept it with great rejoicing if the two of them suddenly fell dead.

Unable to find out anything about Joseph's whereabouts from his siblings, a few weeks later, I met with Michael, who did not have any news about him either. In fact, he had not seen him ever since the day he had removed his bicycles from the rental stand near Michael's home. In contrast to Joseph's allegations that Michael had betrayed him, Michael suspected that after he had found work as a night guard and managed to become the owner of two bicycles, Joseph must have reasoned that his situation had stabilized sufficiently to renounce their friendship and cease sharing his income with him. In the meantime, Michael had also moved out of his father's place because of the many quarrels he had had with him. He lived in a small clay hut, continued renting out his boss's bicycles, and struggled to make ends meet on his own.

"I Am Also a Human Being": The Delicate Nexus of Social Capital and Moral Recognition

Conflict, Disruption, and Reconfiguration of Social Relations

Joseph's story underscores the high degree of contingency that shaped the lives of many people living with ARVs in Tanga who "may be said to live on the margins of society, but at the same time, these 'margins' are so densely populated that we cannot talk about them as [an] exception to the rules" (Mogensen 2010, 66). In the light of increasing living expenses, mostly low levels of education, and limited job opportunities, many people face ever more difficulties in securing their livelihood, and their survival depends all the more on the help of relatives or other supportive social relationships. To put it in Bourdieuian terms, their biological existence becomes contingent on their ability to accumulate social capital that can at least partially translate into material capital (cf. Steuer 2012, 48f). The inheritance dispute among Joseph's brothers and sisters and the resulting disrupted support suggest the importance of not overestimating the moral ideal of kin-based amity (Fortes 2009). Families (and households) are not as inherently altruistic, homogenous, and cohesive as this classic axiom implies[6] (cf. Alber and Martin 2007, 161; Whyte, Mogensen, and Twebaze 2014, 106f). In Joseph's case, in fact, kinship ceased to be the principal regulator of solidarity and micro-level economic exchange in times of dire need. The social relations in his household were characterized by covered and open confrontations as well as mere indifference. The destructive dynamics of the hereditary conflict, blended with tendencies of ostracism predicated on his health status, produced a high degree of individualization among the family members, and culminated in a significant reduction (and ultimate interruption) of intrafamilial interaction and communication. This not only inflicted profound emotional pain on Joseph and gave rise to his indignation, as he expected at least his closest consanguine relatives to support him. It also complicated his struggles to continue his therapy, exacerbated his critical health situation, and constituted a threat to his very existence.

Fortunately, Joseph managed to establish new social relations that at least partway made up for this threatening loss. Spending time with the group of young men at the bicycle rental restored some joy to his life and provided him with a new sense of belonging. Through his dyadic relationship with Michael, he managed to garner moral, social, and material support at a time when he most needed it. And even the relationship with the politician whose house he was employed to guard proved to be beneficial for him, as his night shifts turned into a zone of safety and urgently needed regeneration, albeit of short duration.

In sum, the social support arrangements that Joseph managed to establish and broach were shaped by a high degree of contingency[7] and temporariness. Joseph was situated in an almost permanent process of crafting new connections with individuals or institutions that would yield material and immaterial help after other supportive relationships had been disrupted. This implied rather hard work, and the success and setbacks he experienced in this endeavor of permanent negotiation directly translated into amelioration or deterioration of his health status. The process was furthermore shaped by a continuous oscillation between agency and structural limitations. To some degree, he actively determined his path through life and made free decisions about whether to maintain or terminate particular social relationships. In so doing, he balanced, perhaps unwittingly, the advantages and disadvantages accruing from these ties. In the face of permanent uncertainty, of never knowing where the next strike might come from, he held on to his relationship with Michael, even when this itself became a source of uncertainty.

The agency Joseph displayed in his struggle to cope with the adversities of everyday life and to forge supportive social bonds was reflected in the way in which he conceptualized his future. His way of handling the subjunctivity of his own "therapeutic emplotment" (Mattingly 1994, 811) was remarkable. Notwithstanding his severe economic hardship and social uncertainty, his narrative tells of a clear teleological structure and a vanishing point of a life with his own place to stay, work, enough food—and ARVs. He decidedly resisted yielding to the existential disruptions he had experienced and put all his effort into maintaining a sense of coherent temporality instead of living in the "empty present" (Davies 1997, 568). He thus constantly made efforts to transform suffering into action, uncertainty into potentiality, and to "search for possibilities that lead in hopeful directions" (Mogensen 2009, 185).

Joseph's drive to stabilize his life situation and the progress he had made was, however, time and again determined by structural impediments and contingent upon the benevolence of influential others. For months, he did not succeed in finding work. Neither did he dispose of the financial means and material assets to become a member of the (self-)support group and microcredit initiative that promised redress in his destitute situation. Ultimately, he only managed to gain access to these support structures through the extraordinary engagement of a well-minded "gatekeeper."

Another point that becomes particularly evident in Joseph's close alliance with Michael is the need to critically interrogate the significance of kin relations in the context of HIV and ART. As discussed above, there is no doubt that enormous efforts were made mostly by patients' consanguine kin, but also their affine relatives, to provide care and support within extended family networks. However, these intrafamilial relations could be highly strained and fragile. When they collapsed, other forms of connectedness were put in place, which suggest that the crucial underlying basis of solidarity that people living with ARVs could count on was not necessarily kinship in the traditional sense but rather relatedness established through *doing* care in practice (cf. also Alber et al. 2010; Carsten 2000). This concurs with Susan Whyte and colleagues' (Whyte, Mogensen, and Twebaze 2014, 111) findings from their observation of ART patients' care relations in Uganda: "It is the actual performance of sharing and caring that realizes a relationship—that is that makes it strong or weak. Living with ART involves just such enactments of 'looking after' by feeding, supporting, accommodating, and providing money." And yet kinship apparently remained a central frame of reference for conceptualizing such other forms of enacted relatedness. After all, Joseph referred to his friend Michael using the word *jamaa*, a Swahili term of Arabic origin that means *companion/fellow*, but is first of all designated to (the members of) one's family.

Aspiring for Recognition and Belonging

One might argue that aside from the benefits of assisting each other in adhering to their therapy, Joseph and Michael's temporary close connection was predominantly based on their dire need for mutual economic support. Joseph's relationship with Benjamin and Grace, in turn, pointed to a further important variable in his decisions about which social relationships to pursue and which to disregard. The themes of dignity, being acknowledged as a morally upright person, and being bestowed with social recognition ran like a red thread through all of the longer conversations I had with him over the course of my fieldwork. His profound and frequently expressed emotional disturbance about being so vehemently "abandoned" by his own brothers and sisters pointed to the fact that he expected mutuality and recognition, both in a social and a moral sense, to be an obligatory and somewhat natural characteristic of kin relations. That he had taken this for granted exacerbated the disappointment he felt after his experiences to the contrary.

As his relationships with his consanguine brothers and sisters as well as with his *jamaa* Michael demonstrated, Joseph was quite aware of a certain limit to how much indignity he could "accept" from others in order to still maintain his self-esteem. Consequently, he seemed always to meticulously gauge the moral imbalances involved in his social relations and to be engaged in a permanent process of flexibly modifying and balancing his social proximity and distance to others accordingly. The fact that he lived with ARVs certainly had an impact on these subtle negotiations. The drugs aggravated situations in which he suffered from hunger, and the resulting higher need for financial and other assistance perhaps motivated him to occasionally hold on to "questionable" relationships longer than he would have, had he not been on treatment or HIV-positive in the first place.

It was all the more striking, however, that Joseph's most substantial concern was not about living on ARVs without hunger but about having a place in the world as someone who was respected and accepted as a person and an equal human being. At least temporarily, this longing seemed so powerful that he placed more value on his moral integrity than his biological survival, which he could have perhaps secured more easily through an apology to Benjamin.

Although he was well aware that without ARVs, he would not be able to achieve his goals in life, the drugs remarkably only figured as one theme among others in his projected future. Dignity and social recognition—both in the form of "its inscription in language" and "embod[ied] in acts of care" (Le Marcis 2012, 488)—constituted the core of his aspirations, and the question of belonging was more important to him than being a biomedically rational "pharmaceutical self" (Dumit 2002, 126), in the sense of taking every possible measure to optimize his treatment adherence. This and similar antagonistic relationships between biologically based medical requirements and patients' profound sociomoral longings, which have been reported from other settings of ART provision in sub-Saharan Africa (e.g., Meinert 2013, 129; Mogensen 2010; Steuer 2012), underscore the urgent need to pay "greater attention to the way persons, on an everyday basis, develop new ways of being and new spaces of recognition, building on the resources available" (Le Marcis 2012, 488). To what extent these new spaces of recognition are able to replace kin relations as the primary source of a sense of belonging, particularly in times of crisis and suffering, is a question in need of constant empirical validation.

Finally, Joseph's case demonstrates that the reasons for patients' longing for social recognition can vary and blend into each other in a way that makes it difficult to clearly differentiate between them. Thus, on the one hand, Joseph wished to be viewed as a morally upright person, for this conformed to his own self-image that he seemed to have developed, or at least consolidated, as an explicit refutation of his family's and others' discriminatory behavior. On the other hand, he had developed the impression that being recognized as a physically and morally flawless person was a prerequisite for being considered a potential partner in new economic projects or being incorporated into microarrangements of mutual support outside of Tanga's limited economy of institutional support for people living with HIV (cf. Frank and Rödlach 2013). HIV stigma, social and moral recognition, economic survival, and particular practices and strategies of disclosure and secrecy thus constitute an intricate nexus that is explored in greater detail in the following section.

ART and Its Impact on HIV-Related Stigma, Disclosure, and Secrecy

HIV disclosure figured as an issue of central significance to the protagonists of all of the case studies presented so far, including that of Haruna and Zahra, as discussed in the introduction. Haruna and Zahra did not tell anybody about their predicament, and Haruna decided to further conceal it after Zahra's death, even though this implied a potential danger to the health of his newborn child. Furaha (Case Study A) only disclosed her status to some of those who stemmed "from the same womb," but imagined that at some point, she would begin to selectively reveal her situation to "outsiders" whom she suspected of suffering from HIV but who had not yet tested. Issa never took the step of telling his wife about his affliction, for he worried about the psychological distress it would cause her, and perhaps because he feared blame and rejection. Fatuma, Joseph, and Michael were attentive that only a few close relatives came to know the secret of their HIV infection (in Joseph's case, these efforts were undermined by his sister Grace), because they feared gossip and discrimination. These few examples already point to the complexity of HIV disclosure and the multitude of questions that those concerned are confronted with: Should they reveal their health status to others, and if so to whom? Why would they need, want, or have to do so? What would be the right moment and way to disclose? Would the benefits of sharing the secret outweigh the possible disadvantages? Where could they find assistance in dealing with their difficulties in disclosing to others?

The number of persons to whom the protagonists voluntarily disclosed naturally differed from one case study to the other. While Haruna and Zahra followed a strict nondisclosure policy and had not even shared their condition with a single third person aside from myself, Furaha and Imani had actively informed several members of their extended family about their infection. All of the protagonists, however, were strongly preoccupied with staying in control of where and to whom the information about their infection was disseminated outside of the "protected" realms of familial networks or (self-) support groups. Issa was the only one who had disclosed his status to some of his friends, though at a later point, he seemed to regret this openness and returned to a more cautious way of sharing the information about his condition.

Concealing one's health status in the wider community had also acquired a great significance for most other people living with HIV and ARVs whom I got to know in Tanga. In fact, of the many patients I talked to, not even a handful seemed to have fully ascribed to the public health and HIV activist mantra of living openly with HIV in order to reduce stigma (cf. Moyer 2012, 2013). Forty-three-year-old Fadhila, who had been living with HIV for eight years and with ARVs for four, was the most outspoken. On World AIDS Day 2008, she appeared with a wide smile on her face in an awareness raising event, where she proudly told a crowd of several hundred people about the "normal" life she lived with ARVs despite her HIV infection, and encouraged everyone to get tested, preferably in one of the mobile VCT stations in one of the nearby erected tents. Even in the most private and intimate situations of her everyday life, she claimed to always be open and to inform a potential sexual partner about her health status. In the remainder of this section, let me shed light on why so few patients followed Fadhila's example.

On Stigma and Discrimination

People's attitudes and practices in regard to HIV disclosure were closely related to whether and how they had previously experienced and how they anticipated HIV-related stigmatization. Before exploring these experiences and anxieties in greater detail, a few words on health-related "stigma" are important, as the concept has been applied to describe such diverse phenomena in a wide variety of contexts that "it [has] suffered from a 'conceptual inflation' and a consequent lack of analytical clarity" (Deacon 2006, 419). Even with regard to the more specific context of HIV/AIDS, the body of respective literature is enormous (e.g., Bohle 2013; Castro and Farmer 2005; Deacon 2006; Deacon, Stephney, and Prosalendis 2005; Link and Phelan 2001; Ogden and Nyblade 2005; Parker and Aggleton 2002, 2003; Theilgaard et al. 2011). In these works, a great number and variety of origins, principles, types, effects, and scales of HIV-related stigmatization have been elaborated, which cannot be presented here in their entirety. But let me point out a few conceptual nuances that are relevant for the analysis of the empirical material that will follow.

In Erving Goffman's words, stigma refers to a "deeply discrediting attribute" that can be based on "abominations of the body . . . blemishes of individual character," or social categories like "race, nation, and religion" (Goffman 1963, 4). The crucial idea about stigma understood in this sense is that it emerges through a particular relationship between what is conventionally perceived to be normal by one individual or group and the deviance from these norms of another, which results in particular ways of interaction between the two. Despite referring to Goffman as their conceptual origin, many works on stigma that have been published since the 1960s have neglected this central aspect and instead feature highly individualizing and psychologizing approaches. They have focused on stigma "as though it were *a kind of thing* (in particular, a cultural or even individual value)—a relatively static characteristic or feature [that is seen] as something *in* the person stigmatized, rather than as a designation that others attach *to* that individual" (Parker and Aggleton 2003, 14f). Contrary to these works, I suggest (re-)placing emphasis on stigma as a deeply relational and social process, as this facilitates taking into consideration processes of change, which are of primary interest in an analysis of the societal effects of ART on understandings of HIV/AIDS.

A further important point concerns the distinction between stigma and discrimination. The weakness of many works on health-related stigma is their unclear differentiation between these terms, where the first has often been defined through the latter. A conflation of the two terms is, however, an analytic hindrance, inasmuch as

> defining stigma in terms of discrimination stretches the concept of stigma to accommodate both stigmatizing beliefs themselves (unjustified negative things people believe about others that involve a moral judgment) and the effects of some stigmatization processes—discrimination (what people do to disadvantage others). (Deacon 2006, 419)

For this reason, I follow Deacon (2006, 421) in defining stigma as a social process in which

> illness is constructed as preventable or controllable . . . ; immoral behaviors causing the illness are identified . . . ; these behaviors are associated with "carriers" of the illness in other groups, drawing on existing social constructions of the "other" . . . ; certain people are thus blamed for their

own infection . . . ; and status loss is projected onto the "other," which may (or may not) result in disadvantage to them.

Stigma (or stigmatization), defined in this way, and discrimination are two closely related but different phenomena. While stigmatization is a cognitive process, discrimination refers to the actual behavior of persons and groups to the disadvantage of others. Discrimination is frequently, but not always and necessarily, the consequence of stigmatization. Furthermore, there are several forms of discrimination against people living with HIV that do not involve any moral judgment and are therefore unconnected to HIV-related stigma in the strict sense of the term.

"She No Longer Deserves to Be Called a Human": *Experiences of HIV-Related Discrimination*

Many patients I talked to were confronted with a wide spectrum of discriminatory actions as a consequence of their voluntary or involuntary HIV disclosure. At times, it was difficult to distinguish legitimate differential treatment resulting from others' attempts to protect themselves from actual discrimination that would work to the patients' disadvantage. Drawing the demarcation was a highly subjective matter, as some people tolerated more "special treatment" than others without feeling excluded or discriminated against. Nonetheless, a large number of patients' narratives featured moments that had a significant psychological impact on them, and some felt compelled to take rather drastic steps in order to reorganize their lives—geographically, economically, and socially—in a way that would shield them from further harm.

Discriminatory actions were not exclusively committed by immediate relatives or restricted to the domestic sphere. However, in a similar manner as Joseph, many people living with ARVs were particularly aggrieved by the rejection, exclusion, and contempt they experienced within their own families, not least because this ran so strongly against their expectations of mutual assistance in the kin group, which constituted one of the most important elements of their identity and sense of belonging. Ismail, for instance, recounted that at the mosque where he went to pray, people avoided touching him for they suspected him of being HIV-positive. But he felt far more humiliated by the habits that his relatives developed when they learned about his infection. When he became bedridden, his mother was the only person who dared to enter his room. When she was not around, his other family members would push his plate toward his bed with a stick. Fortunately, however, with his family's increasing comprehension of the routes of HIV transmission during the months following his commencement on ART, the situation gradually improved.

Thirty-eight-year-old Ahmed, who also had an HIV-positive wife and two little daughters living with ARVs, complained bitterly about his sister, "who was born out of the same womb," who had informed a large number of people in their community about his and his family's health condition right after she had learned of it herself. From that time on, she would no longer touch her nieces, warned other people to keep their children away from them, and finally cut all contact with Ahmed and his family.

Some narratives pointed to the fact that those in the surroundings of people living with HIV and ARVs—this obviously included family members, but also people in other settings in the wider community—not only dreaded and avoided direct physical contact with them, but even shunned touching or ingesting things that they had touched. For thirty-four-year-old Zalika, this had severe economic consequences, as some of her clients would no longer buy and drink the milk she sold on the street after she had disclosed to them that she was HIV-positive. This form of "instrumental stigma," that is, "intended discrimination based on an inflated fear of contracting HIV"[8] (Deacon et al. 2005, 41), also affected many children. Ahmed, for instance, recounted what one of his daughters had told him about the way in which two of her HIV-positive classmates at primary school were being treated on a daily basis.

> There is a lot of stigmatization at school. . . . Those [two children], even when they sit with their fellow students, they are segregated. When one of them, for example, has touched a biscuit, his/her fellow is scared to eat it, because s/he believes s/he will get the infection. . . . S/he would not even touch his/her fellow's exercise book, if he/she has touched it before. (Ahmed, thirty-eight years, living with HIV for seven years, 16 August 2011)

A second form of "instrumental stigma" in the sense of "intended discrimination on the basis of resource concerns due to judgments about the likely contribution of a person living with HIV/AIDS" (Deacon et al. 2005, 41) seemed to be equally pervasive in Tanga. Despite the wide-scale availability of ARVs and the growing number of people recovering their health after treatment uptake, many patients confirmed that an HIV infection was still widely associated with a rapid death or at least the concerned person's permanent frailty and inability to partake in social and economic processes of reciprocal exchange. Joseph put it like this:

> For the people who do not have this disease, as soon as they learn that their companion has it, they think by themselves, "This one only has two or three more days to live." . . . As soon as they see that you are using these medicines [ARVs], they believe . . . he is on the journey and will necessarily go ahead [and die before me]. (Joseph, forty years, fourth year of ART, 19 January 2009)

While Joseph learned that due to such attitudes, it was hardly possible to find a business partner while being known to be HIV-positive, forty-six-year-old Alika had a similar experience of being devalued, albeit in an indirect manner. After she had been repeatedly hospitalized, several of her husband's relatives urged him to get rid of her and look for a healthy and productive wife, on the mere suspicion that she could be HIV-positive and therefore could die at any moment. On countless occasions during my interviews, the association of HIV with a premature death and the decrease or loss of an infected person's market value (cf. Frank and Rödlach 2013) were brought up. Abdallahman expressed most compellingly how closely entangled the social, economic, and moral implications of this association and corresponding social practices could be.

> Everyone who has this disease is [perceived to] be dying at any minute. . . . His/her life has already reached the end. So . . . he/she does not deserve to be part of society anymore. . . . He/she is no longer in the community of those who deserve to exist, to be called a human (*watu wanaostahili kuwepo, kuitwa watu*). (Abdallahman, forty years, third year of ART, 16 August 2011)

This form of discrimination could have severely detrimental consequences for children as well. Most of the orphaned children I worked with, in fact, reported highly emotionally straining "itineraries of care" subsequent to the death of one or both parents. Some were rejected by their surviving parent and passed on from one relative to the other, and did not find a stable place to stay for considerable stretches of time until they were finally hospitalized or through the engagement of health personnel or engaged community members were admitted to the orphanage. Eighteen-year-old Elizabeth told me that after her mother had died of AIDS, her father did not want her to live in his house any longer, and even warned his relatives not to take her in, because she "could die in their hands [and] in their house" (Elizabeth, eighteen years, sixth year of ART, 6 August 2011). Other children and adolescents were deprived of proper nutrition and care and fell victim to psychological humiliation and outright physical violence because they no longer ranked as family or community members who were deemed worthy of financial investment and humane treatment (Mattes 2014b). In some ways, these young patients were thus stripped of their "domestic citizenship" (Das and Addlakha 2001, 513) and rendered nonpersons (cf. Root 2012, 43).

While in some cases it seemed legitimate to clearly identify particular processes of discrimination as "instrumental stigma," in many others, distinguishing analytically between the different forms of discrimination that people faced over longer periods of time was difficult. This was particularly the case for forty-eight-year-old Jemima, who was in her second year of ART (see Case Study E). After the repeated hospitalizations of her ten- and nineteen-year-old sons, she decided to have them and herself tested for HIV. Shortly after the test, she found the courage to disclose to her husband that they were all HIV-positive and had been initiated on treatment. His reaction was one of strong rejection, Jemima told me with a tone that revealed how much her husband's behavior had hurt her. "He decided to throw me and the children out. He told me, 'I don't know [where you got it from], this disease is yours and that of your children. You leave now and look for another place to stay with them!'" (Interview, 2 June 2011). Suddenly without shelter, Jemima wished to return to her parental home in the countryside, but her eldest brother who had taken charge of the family affairs after their father's death did not want her and her sons to live nearby. "I felt that he was afraid that when we get back there, [our] problems will demand too much of him," Jemima said. Upon her brother's rejection, she rented two rooms in a house in Tanga. Contact with her brother largely broke off, and he never came to visit them. Soon after relocating to the new house, Jemima faced further rejection because, she suspected, someone had seen her at the CTC and had spread the word about her and her children's HIV infection.

> At that place where I rented accommodation, there was tremendous stigmatization (*kulikuwa na unyanyapaa wa ajabu*). Wherever I went, they segregated me, [saying,] "This is the sick one and her children." When the children took something, they said, "Don't touch this; you will infect us!" This situation took away all happiness from me. . . . It really bothered me, at that house . . . the flatmates, [who were supposed to be] my companions, did not want to have anything at all to do either with me or with my children. So, I decided to leave [again] with the children and to rent another house. (Interview, 2 June 2011)

Since Jemima and her husband had separated, her sons had only had sporadic contact with their father. His conduct suggests that he had thrown his family out of his house because he feared "courtesy stigma" (Deacon et al. 2005, 26), a form of secondary stigmatization that extends to the caregivers and families of stigmatized persons. His fear of being associated with HIV through his wife and children was so intense that he repeatedly pressed Jemima to stop going to the hospital and to interrupt her and their sons' ART so that no one would see them at the CTC. Jemima assumed that her husband's overly dismissive attitude and behavior mainly resulted from his apprehension about being infected with HIV himself, a disease that he viewed as highly shameful, as it has its origin in unregulated, excessive sexuality. Such interpretations were reproduced within both Christian and Muslim communities, whose leaders promoted the idea of HIV/AIDS as God's retribution for committing adultery and engaging in prostitution. Hodari told me that in her mosque's congregation, the global HIV/AIDS pandemic was viewed as an apocalypse signaling the nearing end of the world (*kiama*).

> At the beginning, there were the prophets who said that when the end of the world is near, there will be many [moral] rebellions (*maasi*). People will no longer revere the Almighty God, you understand? People will walk around uncoveredly, women walk around with their underwear sticking out, so some say that [HIV] is God's bludgeon. (Hodari, thirty-three years, first year of ART, 28 July 2011)

Some patients decidedly resisted such strongly moralistic (and often sexist) religious etiologies—at least in private conversations. Hodari herself expressed her indignation over such sweeping moral judgments, stating, "If you get [HIV], many say 'Ehee, it's her whoring around that made her catch HIV, whereas [in reality] it is your husband who has brought the disease to your home" (ibid.). Christina, by contrast, an elderly member of a local Pentecostal community, stood for many others who were less critical and did not call the moralizing discourse prevailing within their congregation into question.

> AIDS . . . comes from going against God's prescriptions. . . . If you violate those commands of God, there will be . . . things like promiscuity, adultery, and so forth. So, even in the church, they say that if someone gets the AIDS disease, it is because he/she has violated God's command. (Christina, fifty-nine years, third year of ART, 4 September 2009)

The fact that the virus was still incurable reinforced Christina's conviction that it was God's chastisement for adultery. Obviously, she reasoned, this was evidence of the Tanzanian and other societies' continuing moral decay.

In addition to the persistent conceptualizations of HIV as an indicator of impending premature death, such moralistic religious discourses doubtlessly contributed their fair share to an atmosphere that prompted the large majority of people living with HIV in Tanga's neighborhoods to meticulously gauge the range of persons to whom they would disclose their health condition. This even applied to the people who claimed that they had never been discriminated against. The permanent anticipation and expectation of being stigmatized or discriminated against after HIV disclosure could be just as taxing for those who kept their health status secret as the actual experience of discrimination. At times, in fact, it seemed that "the fear of discrimination was worse than the reality" (Iliffe 2006, 88).

Becoming the "Story of the Streets": Anticipated Stigma and the Lack of Comprehensive Knowledge about HIV and ART

People's fear of being socially and morally discredited and excluded from kin- or community-based social webs of exchange and mutual care was anything but incomprehensible. Even those who no one suspected of being HIV-positive had witnessed enough discouraging examples of how badly people living with HIV were often treated. Haruna and Zahra, for instance, were terrified by the case of an

HIV-positive woman who had lived close to their house and had recently passed away. Like Joseph, she had been given her own set of plates and cups during the months before her death, and when she became bedridden, her relatives would not care for her because they would not touch her. Apparently, the woman had eventually accepted her relatives' contemptuous behavior and internalized the HIV stigma to the point that she herself had suggested that they should not nurse her and simply let her die.

Such extreme forms of discrimination were not as exceptional as it might seem. Tanzanian newspapers frequently featured articles about HIV-positive people living in all parts of the country who were being treated in a most appalling manner by relatives and community members. Apparently, the effect of governmental and nongovernmental awareness raising campaigns for the destigmatization of HIV/AIDS that have been rolled-out across the country over the recent years still have some way to go. In fact, the Tanzania HIV/AIDS and Malaria Indicator Survey 2011–12 (THMIS) stated that there had been no increase in terms of accepting attitudes toward people living with HIV/AIDS since the last survey in 2007–2008 (TACAIDS 2013a, 64).

In the light of the rather low level of comprehensive acceptance of people living with HIV, which was statistically identified to prevail on the national level but could also be experienced in the most intimate personal relationships, it is little wonder that for the majority of my respondents, the anxiety of "being gossiped about" was often given as the main reason for nondisclosure. Many referred to "being talked about" and "being pointed at" as a profoundly damaging phenomenon that had to be avoided. Some patients, however, specified more concretely that they expected the information about their health status to spread like wildfire, which would result in increasing rejection, neglect, and exclusion. This, in turn, would have a negative effect on their health. Haruna was one of those who described such a calamitous chain of causation in explaining his and his wife's secrecy.

> There is no advantage [of disclosure] for us in view of the situation here in the neighborhood. The way we have come to know the [character of the] Swahili people, there is no advantage. To the contrary, it brings only loss. You will be excluded a lot and you will be talked about all the time. . . . You will get thin, because you always think about it. Wherever you go,

they will point their fingers at you. . . . These stories of the street (*hadithi ya mitaani*) can make you lose weight and you die quickly. (Haruna, forty years, not on ART, 3 May 2009)

In a similar way, caretakers were worried about the impact that such "stories of the street" about their own children or grandchildren could have on them. The grandmother of seventeen-year-old Latifa, who had been taking ARVs for four years, for instance, suspected that once one of Latifa's peers would learn of her disease, sooner or later, all the youngsters in the neighborhood would viciously gossip about her.

> You know, these adolescents nowadays behave badly. When they fight each other, they don't have limits and at any cost [keep fighting] until one defaces the other (*lazima watamwumbua*). [And then] they boast about it, [saying,] "You . . ." I don't know what. . . . If they will gossip about [Latifa], her self will be broken [literally: lynched—*nafsi yake itanyongeka*]. Now, once it is broken, nothing is good anymore; she won't have any joy in life anymore. And this is undesirable, according to what we've been told [at the hospital], it is undesirable to make her sad [and to confront her with] issues that make her go backward. (Bibi Latifa, sixty-four years, 21 June 2011)

Many patients who had experienced HIV-related discrimination against themselves or others ascribed this to the low level of comprehensive knowledge about HIV and ART within their communities and among the general population. Reflecting on her experiences after the involuntary disclosure of her HIV status among her family and in her neighborhood, Jemima forged this link in a particularly clear manner.

> If someone discovers that you are ill [with HIV], he/she runs away from you. Even if you have been friends, he/she excludes you, because he/she doesn't know that this is a normal disease that can be prevented or that you can live with it without infecting others if you follow the rules. . . . They believe that if they sit together with you being sick, you have already infected them. There are many who are like that. Only very few have enough education. (Jemima, forty-eight years, second year of ART, 2 June 2011)

Another peculiar phenomenon in this regard consisted of the assumed interrelation between HIV-related stigma and ethnicity, inasmuch as some patients held low levels of education and resulting HIV-related discriminatory behavior to be a specific characteristic of particular ethnic collectives whose scope varied widely. In some cases, the collective in question included the speaker; in others it did not. Haruna, for instance, affiliated the fact that in his neighborhood HIV was still considered a shameful disease and a death sentence to the lack of knowledge of "us uneducated Africans" and "the Swahili" (Interview, 15 February 2009). Others, in contrast, believed to have identified a tendency toward mutual stigmatization and discrimination as a typical trait of a specific "tribe" (*kabila*). Hodari's related judgment referred to her husband's *kabila*:

> The Wadigo, once you've disclosed that you have this problem [HIV], you are considered to be dying. . . . These people stigmatize you beyond all measure, because, most of all, many of them have not received much education. . . . Once they have finished seventh grade, they go and work on the fields. . . . Even those who have been born from one womb stigmatize each other. . . . (Hodari, thirty-three years, first year of ART, 28 July 2011)

Jemima and Hodari's complaints once more confirmed what the rumors about ARVs that were circulating in Tanga's neighborhoods suggested, namely that beyond the bounds of treatment centers and patient communities, solid information about ARVs was scarce. Several years after the initiation of the national treatment program, many people still seemed not to know that HIV could be treated, and that ARVs enable infected persons not only to extend their lives for a couple of weeks or months, but gave them the chance to survive and lead productive lives for many years, if not decades. In fact, several patients emphasized that before they had been tested and had participated in the adherence classes, they themselves had not been aware of treatment for HIV. Others had heard of it but only had a very vague idea of what it implied. Medical professionals also mentioned the unsatisfactory pervasion of information on ART in the general population. Building on her experience with ART beginners over the previous years, one nurse estimated that some fifty percent of the population knew about the existence of ARVs. Moreover, she pointed to stark differences in the availability and accessibility of information between rural and urban areas.

It was difficult to deduce from my conversations with patients and medical professionals whether, in general, the dearth of reliable comprehension of HIV and, more importantly, the limited awareness of the possibility and effectiveness of its treatment were stronger drivers of the persistent HIV-related stigmatization and discrimination than the continuous reproduction of moralistic discourses about the disease. From the patients' perspective, this certainly varied from one individual setting to the other. No matter how much these particular contexts and situations differed in terms of the frequency, intensity, and forms of stigmatization and discrimination patients were exposed to, however, their reactions to experienced or anticipated rejection, exclusion, and violence on the basis of their health status had many things in common.

Reactions to and Consequences of HIV-Related Discrimination

Providing Education

Several patients applied the strategy of actively confronting HIV-related discrimination by gradually correcting their family and community members' misconceptions and continuously providing them with factual knowledge about the disease and its treatment, until they would lose their inordinate fear of contagion and abandon their discriminatory habits. Fadhila recounted how she had successfully made such efforts:

> There were situations of being stigmatized. . . . For example, when guests come to our house—you know, there are some families like ours, we have the habit of eating from one plate. So, these people say, "Why are we served on the same plate as Fadhila? Fadhila should receive her own plate." Mama tells these guests, "You eat from your plate. I will eat together with my child." This happened sometimes. But after that, I made great efforts to provide education that it is not contagious to eat with me or to sleep together [in one place] . . . until they understood. (Fadhila, forty-three years, fifth year of ART, 28 January 2009)

Zalika reacted in an equally confrontational manner when she learned of another person rejecting the milk she sold because of her health status.

> Someone came and told me, "Eh, a certain person has bought your milk but poured it away; he/she said you have the virus." . . . And I told him/her, "It's true, it's not a lie, he/she was right: I have the virus, but my virus does not stay in the milk, and neither can I infect anyone with the milk! Tell him/her that! If he/she wants education, fine, he/she'll get it. But tell

him/her that it's true, I am taking medicine [ARVs]." Then they could not believe that someone living with AIDS would speak out. After that, they accepted it and knew that I am really living with HIV. (Zalika, thirty-four years, fourth year of ART, 22 May 2009)

In contrast to these women who started to provide education *after* they had experienced discriminatory incidents, Annan (thirty-three years, second year of ART) did so in order to *prevent* himself from having such bad experiences in the first place. Every now and then, he explained, he would inconspicuously give information material on HIV to those family members to whom he planned to disclose in the future. This way, he hoped that they would refrain from adhering to a moralistic discourse of blame and not develop an exaggerated fear of contagion that would translate into his exclusion.

Selective Disclosure

Aside from such (pro)active educatory interventions, many patients kept the danger of falling victim to discrediting and discriminatory behavior at bay by keeping the circle of people to whom they disclosed as small as possible. Many patients revealed their HIV infection solely to their spouses and a few close relatives, like their children, parents, grandparents, or siblings (Bohle 2013; Bohle, Dilger, and Groß 2014; cf. Lugalla 2008, 60). Others selectively added some members of their extended family and perhaps a few friends or housemates to the circle of people in whom they confided. While many patients preferred to disclose to close relatives living within the same household, however, social proximity was not the only or most important criterion for selecting confidants. The invisible line separating the informed from those who were left uninformed often ran between persons who had the closest contact in day-to-day life. A woman would thus not tell her husband, or, as in Issa's case, vice versa; another one would tell her husband but not his mother who lived in the same house with them; a mother would only inform one of her adolescent twin children; to mention just a few examples. Patients' reasons for providing information on their health status to particular persons and withholding it from others were multiple and often overlapping. Some of them, however, were mentioned so frequently as to suggest that they were the predominant principles guiding such decisions.

An important selection criterion consisted of the prospective confidant's discreetness, which many patients obviously felt they could expect more from close kin than from unrelated "outsiders." Similarly to how patients reasoned about others' inclination to discriminate against people living with HIV, discreetness and trustworthiness were often closely associated with higher educational attainment and a reasonable comprehension about HIV. "Many of those who do not have education, if you tell them, they will stigmatize you, and there are many of these kind where we live," explained Ahmed. After his younger sister had completely shunned him, his wife, and his children after she had learned of their predicament, he therefore turned to another, better-educated sister of his.

> I also have a sister . . . who is a schoolteacher. It is her to whom I talked about this problem because she has received education. I explained myself to her; but those other ones, I live with them, but every day we hide from them. They don't know the least bit about this issue. . . . Because the first thing they'd do is to point their fingers at the children. . . . "You see this kid over there? She has this problem. . . ." They won't stop; they don't have any brains. . . . So, we have learned that the problem is the lack of education. (Ahmed, thirty-eight years, living with HIV for seven years, 1 June 2011)

A second rather obvious criterion, which at times interfered with that of immediate social proximity, was the help—material or immaterial—that people were expected to be able and willing to provide once the information about the patient's infection was shared with them (cf. Whyte, Mogensen, and Twebaze 2014, 115). As Joseph's financial dependence on his brother Benjamin illustrates, those persons deemed trustworthy and well off enough to provide significant support were not necessarily living in patients' household or even nearby, though it is important to note that no matter how far away these people resided, the majority of them were relatives. Some patients' network of supportive kin to whom they would confide thus spanned hundreds of kilometers and was spread across the entire country.

The types of support people expected were diverse. Aside from financial and material assistance that would help them get back on their feet after prolonged periods of illness, which often entirely consumed patients' sparse reserve assets, many hoped for practical help in the daily management of their therapy and in case of medical emergencies. Others aimed to garner a more passive form of support. They hoped that through disclosure to particular significant persons, they would obtain the entitlement of special treatment out of deference to their health situation. Thirty-two-year-old and widowed Zuwena, who was enrolled on the treatment program but had not yet started ART, hoped to be spared from overly straining domestic work like washing large amounts of clothes or collecting firewood and spending much time in the smoky kitchen by telling her housemates about her HIV infection. Some parents of children living with ARVs would, in turn, inform the teachers about their children's affliction and ask them to spare them from the harsh and all too frequent corporal punishment that is used as a common instrument of coercion within schools.

On several occasions, patients reported how they directly balanced the presumed discreetness of their prospective confidant with the support that could be expected from him or her, in order to estimate whether the benefits of disclosure would outweigh the possible disadvantages. Joseph's temporary ally, Michael, had been applying this selection principle for years.

> A few of my friends know; I can't tell the others. I have told only those few who can provide help within a close relationship (*ambao wenye msaada wa karibu*). But people who have no means to help, I can't tell them. *Mzee* [honorific form of addressing elder persons, here referring to his father] knows, my sister-in-law knows, my brother knows, some of my friends know. It's only a few people, and I can't tell many others because they talk very much. (Michael, thirty-four years, fifth year of ART, 19 July 2011)

Protecting others from contracting HIV formed another motivation for patients to disclose their health status, at least to their sexual partners and other people in their closest surroundings. Mwanahamisi (thirty-seven years, third year of ART) was afraid of being rejected by her husband upon disclosing to him that she was HIV-positive. Nonetheless, she perceived taking this step as absolutely obligatory and finally, as mentioned in the previous chapter, she found a way to break the news to him through an intermediary. Remembering her helplessness during an episode of being bedridden before she had been tested, she also informed a few relatives and other household members, so that they would be able to protect themselves from the virus, should they ever have to care for her in similar situations.

The intention to protect others from possible suffering was writ large in another way too. Several patients explained that aside from selecting their confidants according to their expected confidentiality and ability to provide support, they would specifically approach persons within their surroundings whose health had repeatedly been failing and whom they suspected of also being HIV-positive. Furaha expressed this intention but had not yet started to realize it (see Case Study A), as did Salma. A few weeks after she had been tested and initiated on ART, Salma had told only her mother and her children about her health status, and she did not intend to tell any other family members, let alone her neighbors. However, she conceded that she might possibly make some exceptions:

> I am very strict about this, but when I see a companion [in a similar situation], I have to explain to her/him. I have to give her/him a class [about HIV] and tell him about the situation I was in and how I live now. (Salma, forty-two years, first year of ART, 19 June 2009)

Amir similarly told me that only his brother (in whose house he lived) and his sister-in-law knew about his HIV infection. But he also suggested that once he had gained some emotional and economic stability (*uwezo*), he would feel morally obliged to motivate presumably HIV-positive peers to take an HIV test and give them emotional support by drawing on his own positive example.

Some patients felt that it was not necessary to face the potentially negative consequences of their own HIV disclosure in order to help others overcome their anxieties of getting tested. In fact, they engaged in what could be termed "undercover counseling." Hodari, for instance, first told me about how she had recently lost a friend who, she assumed, had died of AIDS because he had opted for traditional healing rituals rather than an HIV test. She therefore made even greater efforts to motivate a severely sick housemate of hers, whom she also suspected of being HIV-positive, to get tested.

> I feared that I would lose her too. So, I advised her, "Let's go to the hospital so that you can have a big blood test [*ukapime damu kubwa*—common phrase for HIV test] and see if there is this problem [HIV]." But she does not know, she does not understand . . . that I have that problem too. . . . I took her to the hospital, and she was admitted for two weeks. I told the

doctors to test her and give her the result because there is this problem, and she does not want to, so please test her so that we don't lose her. The doctor tested her and told her, "Sister, you have that problem." And the doctor counseled her well, so that it entered her heart, and there, at home, I am with her and give her my advice too. (Hodari, thirty-three years, first year of ART, 28 July 28 2011)

Ahmed presented a slightly different version of this reasoning. While his wife and he were strongly determined not to let anyone know about their disease apart from his trustworthy sister, he could still imagine specifically approaching other relatives whom he suspected of being infected with HIV, convincing them to get tested, but only revealing to them that he was living with the virus if they did indeed turn out to be positive too.

Trajectories of Revelation: HIV Disclosure as a Long-Term and Situational Process

As has become apparent above, temporality plays an important role with regard to disclosure. Several patients who had only been living with the knowledge of being HIV-positive for a few weeks or months asserted that they could only imagine being more open about their health status once they had recovered their health and a certain degree of normalcy had been restored to their lives. Building a house, successfully establishing a business, and, most importantly, becoming the mother or father of an HIV-negative child were considered prerequisites for wider disclosure that could only be achieved with time. After the initial state of disorientation that followed their discovery of being HIV-positive, Fadhila and other patients also needed time to develop a reasonable level of understanding about the disease, its treatment, and the possibilities of living an everyday life with it before they felt ready to open up toward others. In fact, it had taken Fadhila quite some time to become the exemplarily open- and positive-minded patient that health professionals were eager to present during adherence and morning classes at the CTCs:

First, I thought, if I tell someone I have the infection, they will stigmatize me a lot, how will that be? But gradually, with the days passing, I got more and more education and I more and more shed off this fear, and I more and more understood that you don't infect someone else in this way but in that way. . . . The more education I got, the more it helped me become open. (Fadhila, forty-three years, fifth year of ART, 28 January 2009)

Disclosure, thus, is not a binary event of telling or not telling others about one's affliction at a particular point in time, but a long-term process that is closely tied to the patient's social relations and experiences they live through as time passes (see Moyer 2012, S68). Yet it is important to note that being open about one's HIV status was usually, in practice, far more complex than Fadhila's trajectory suggests. Various people described a less linear movement from strict concealment to broad revelation of their health status. Issa (Case Study B), in fact, developed a considerable *dis*inclination toward telling anyone else about his infection over time. Though he had disclosed to a number of family members, friends, and even workmates during the months immediately following his treatment initiation, some two years later, he was a lot more wary about informing others due to the potential discrimination that this implied. That he had told some of his friends and workmates but not his wife illustrates how greatly the dynamics of HIV disclosure can vary in correspondence to different categories of potential confidants.

Ismail's attitude and practice with regard to living openly with HIV serves as another case in point. For him, the passage of time also played an important role, in the sense that the symptoms through which his affliction was once exposed to others successively disappeared after treatment uptake. This increasingly gave him the chance to conceal his infection from those who had never seen him in a state of failing health. But his turn backward toward maintaining strict secrecy about his infection in his neighborhood was also contingent upon other changes in his life situation. In 2009, when I had the first two interviews with him, Ismail still lived in the house where he had lived when he had gone through the severe illness episode that preceded his HIV test a few years before. Many people in his neighborhood had witnessed how destitute he had been during that time, and rather than refuting their suspicions that he had AIDS, after returning from the hospital, he was more or less open about his infection. When I met him again in 2011, however, he gladly told me that he had gotten married to a woman who was also living with HIV. Together, they had moved to another neighborhood, and both of them took this as an opportunity for a new beginning.

The sine qua non for this, they agreed, was the strict concealment of their health status.

In spite of these concerns, Ismail still voluntarily assisted in enrolling patients on ART at one of the local treatment centers. In this context, he openly dealt with his HIV infection and, just like the peer educators involved in treatment preparation, time after time, he drew on his own example in order to cheer up and give hope to desperate patients. Through this voluntary engagement and his openness—which was nonetheless largely constricted to the hospital grounds—he had managed to gain the status of a reliable and deserving exemplary expert patient and peer educator who every now and then was invited to participate in workshops, whose per diems would at least occasionally remunerate his constant, year-long engagement.

A further intriguing example of how deeply situation- and context-related, but also performative, people's lived openness about their HIV infection could be was forty-six-year-old Alika who, like Ismail, had been living with ARVs for several years. Alika was also extraordinarily engaged as a peer educator in various treatment centers and (self-)support groups. It is reasonable to assume that, through these activities, her serostatus was known to several hundred people in Tanga. Moreover, over the course of several months in 2009, she successively told her story about living with HIV and ART as part of a radio feature that was supposed to familiarize the public with the benefits and (surmountable) difficulties of living with HIV treatment. Despite the chance that some of her relatives and friends might have learned about her infection through this radio feature, in which she used no pseudonym, in her close private surroundings, she nevertheless preferred to tell only her husband and children about her infection. Not even her husband's mother who lived in the same house knew about her ailment.

Routines of Concealment

The large majority of my interlocutors living with HIV and ARVs went to great lengths to establish and maintain an impervious wall of silence around their HIV infection. As illustrated by Joseph, Ismail, and Jemima's examples, several patients whose HIV status had become known to community members in one way or another reverted to the active disruption of social relations and geographical relocation to distant neighborhoods in order to flee into a sphere of protective secrecy.

In contrast to the patients whose HIV infection was exposed to others, whether they liked it or not, when they had been suffering from AIDS in an advanced stage, those who started ART before developing any visible AIDS symptoms had the advantage of staying in control of who learned about their affliction. They did not have to cut social ties and physically distance themselves from their neighborhoods in order to protect themselves from discrimination. Several patients expressed their relief and gratitude that they had never developed any conditions that would attract others' attention and suspicion. But like those who started a new life after moving to other places, they also had to apply particular strategies to conceal their HIV infection from others, including the secret management of its treatment.

Regular control visits and ARV refill appointments at the clinic implied the continuous risk of revealing one's health status by being seen entering one of the CTCs. Frequent visits to the hospital also raised the suspicions, for instance, of attentive housemates. In this regard, patients recounted and displayed various strategies to protect their secret. Every time Jemima had to go to the hospital in order to get a drug refill or accompany one of her sons to his control visit, she would invent excuses, saying that one of them did not feel good and needed to see a doctor. Mwanahamisi and Ahmed told me that they usually pretended to visit a hospitalized friend in order to satisfy the inquisitiveness of acquaintances they met on the way to the CTC.

On the way to the clinic, women often wore their *buibui*, a long garment common for Muslim women on the Swahili coast, and a *ninja*, a veil that covered their face excluding the eye area; and even inside the treatment centers, some would only uncover their faces upon health workers' explicit requests. Other patients who were worried about being recognized at the treatment centers would deliberately show up shortly before the closing hour in order to avoid the large number of other patients who crowded the hallways throughout the day. Although health workers strongly disapproved of this habit and often reprimanded the patients for delaying the hospital routines, most of the time, they eventually attended to these patients, who often had a higher social status than the majority of people undergoing treatment at public health facilities. Occasionally, it even happened that local officials called one of the nurses on the phone asking them to bring them their next ARV ration to a car outside the hospital grounds so that they would not have to enter the CTC. As outlined above, most of the better-situated people living with HIV, however, would enroll in treatment at one of the private health centers offering ART, which guaranteed a higher degree of confidentiality.

For some people, the fear of being associated with HIV/AIDS through regular visits by an HBC provider prompted them to deny any such offers. As one nurse explained, in some cases, it did not even help to clarify that the care providers would come by foot and in civilian clothes, as patients would counter that in their neighborhood, the care providers were widely known, and every contact with these persons would raise suspicion of them being HIV-positive. Other patients would, in turn, not join their neighborhood's (self-) support group, for this implied disclosing at least to fellow group members who might eventually—even unwittingly—reveal their secret to other community members.

In consideration of the large patient crowds at public treatment centers, it is self-evident that despite all efforts, patients could not entirely avoid meeting people they knew during their clinic visits. Many patients thus told me that, much to their surprise, they had occasionally met one of their neighbors queuing for ARVs. Interestingly, there seemed to exist a tacit agreement among those involved in such encounters to mutually respect their need for confidentiality. Off the hospital grounds, they would not let loose a single word about their common ailment. While some patients conceived of such habits as a form of mutual care and respect, others interpreted it as a sign of deplorable selfishness and mutual disinterest among persons who shared the same affliction.

Maintaining secrecy around one's HIV infection also included the concealment of taking ARVs every morning and evening. Some patients thus explained that they enter their bedroom or bathroom to swallow their pills. Others related how they would tell those present at the time of their drug intake that they were not feeling well and needed to take a tablet for their aching head, before quickly pulling a single ARV capsule out of their pocket and swallowing it.

Caretakers of HIV-positive children and adolescents also passed on the maintenance of secrecy about their health status as a crucial requirement for leading a life free of discrimination, either by way of example or by direct verbal indication. Bibi Latifa always made sure that no one saw her washing her granddaughter's clothes with rubber gloves by protecting the spot where she did her laundry from neighbors' glances with visual covers made of braided palm leaves. Sixteen-year-old Amir's sister-in-law repeatedly admonished him never to share the information that he was living with HIV with anyone else, because she was afraid that neighbors and his fellow students at school would start shunning and discriminating against him. How profoundly embodied the habit of maintaining secrecy around HIV could become, even in small children, was demonstrated by Ahmed's six-year-old daughter who, according to Ahmed, would run and hide her ARVs when she saw visitors approaching their house.

Chapter Conclusion

Kin-based networks of support were vital for people living with HIV and ARVs to successfully manage their therapy on a daily basis and maintain its positive effects in the long term. While many benefitted from the support they received from members of their extended family, particularly during the phase following ART uptake, however, kin-based solidarity could not be taken for granted. Joseph and several other patients' accounts thus featured instances of disrupted kin ties, which not only left them with the existential question of how to survive economically, but also in a state of sociomoral uprootedness, as their sense of belonging was predominantly defined through a stable social and emotional entrenchment in their extended families (cf. Dilger 2005, 339f, 2008; Whyte 2005, 156).

The disintegration of family ties (co-)induced by a family member's HIV infection has to be seen in the wider context of continuing, often-intense dynamics of HIV-related discrimination and stigmatization. Only few patients (and health workers) felt that the availability of ART over the recent years had brought about a significant change in this regard. The manifold examples of the discrimination people experienced, not only during episodes of acute bodily ailment, confirmed this perception. An HIV infection was still widely considered a death sentence (Moyer 2012, S76) and associated with norm breaking, sinful, and immoral behavior (cf. Roura et al. 2009). People living with the virus were still frequently blamed for their condition and treated with contempt, separated for fear of contagion and excluded from vital networks of economic and other kinds of support, since investing in a reciprocal relationship with them was assumed to be futile.

Consequently, most patients had an enhanced interest in hiding their infection from the wider community. In fact, their practices and strategies of concealing their ailment were so effective that several of my interlocutors asserted that, perhaps aside from other relatives or the members of their (self-)support group (if they belonged to one), they only knew one or two people living with HIV in their neighborhood—if at all. This concurs with the results of a study on HIV disclosure among women in Tanga that

> refute the expectations of a re-conceptualisation of HIV and AIDS with the implementation of universal access to ART, as raised by WHO, and underline how the "drastic breakthrough" in the struggle against the disease, that was associated with the introduction of ART in sub-Saharan Africa, has not materialized. (Bohle et al. 2014, 225)

As in other regions of sub-Saharan Africa, a correlation between the expansion and increasing accessibility of HIV treatment and a reduction of HIV-related discrimination was hardly discernible (cf. Roura et al. 2009; Wolfe et al. 2008). Even though with the help of ARVs, many people living with HIV have been able to resume a productive life, and periodic medical checkups and drug refills at treatment centers have become routine for them—"just like buying sweets at the store," as a nurse at the Bombo Regional Hospital once put it—most of these persons were well aware of the socially denormalizing effects of an HIV infection and the negative impact this could have on supportive kin ties and their daily lives in their neighborhoods (cf. Kendall and Hill 2010). ARVs were, therefore, mostly welcomed as a "technology of invisibilization" that helped them to maintain secrecy and limit rejection and ostracism (cf. Beckmann 2013; Hardon and Posel 2012). In this sense, ART indeed contributed to a certain normalization of patients' lives with HIV. Whether it induced a fundamental and wide-scale transformation of the social construction of the condition, from a heavily stigmatized ailment to a morally neutral "manageable disease like any other," remains, however, difficult to conclusively deduce from the experiences of my interlocutors.

According to the logic of public health interventions, the blame for the failure to materialize this desired larger transformation is to be found in patients' insufficient assertiveness. Those who do not manage or want to widely share the information about their HIV infection with others ultimately fail to feel "confident enough . . . to defy hegemonic norms of concealment," an act which, in keeping with the public health reasoning, is considered "an *a priori* psychological and social good, a presumed condition of psychic and social health and an ethical imperative in the concerted effort to de-stigmatize HIV/AIDS" (Hardon and Posel 2012, S2). Many of the health workers' endlessly repeated mantras vis-à-vis patients could also be read along these lines: They should not stigmatize and exclude themselves and become tense in the endeavor to hide their condition at all costs. Instead, they should confidently take their medications in public and develop a positive attitude toward their disease, which is so "normal" that there is ultimately no reason to hide it. Framing nondisclosure and practices of secrecy as a mere sign of patients' moral frailty and lack of empowerment does not, however, do justice to their life situations, as described above. In light of the persistent danger of emotional harm and social and economic discrimination resulting from the disclosure of their health status, the meticulous guarding of their secret could be seen as a highly reasonable decision that has little to do with self-contempt resulting from internalized moral stigmatization.

Considering the constant need to ponder over whom to confide in, and which negative or positive consequences this might have, life with HIV continues to be a constant balancing act in times of ART (cf. Moyer 2012, S77). Permanent "balancing work" is not only demanded of patients with regard to their decision about whom to disclose to, and the need to reappraise these decisions time and again in the light of their "social life [which] is always fluid and changing" (Manderson 2015, 4). In the context of widely shared economic precariousness, they also need to continuously balance decisions about which of their existing relationships are profitable enough to invest in, while, as demonstrated by Joseph's case, simultaneously gauging their need for financial and social support with their aspiration for social and moral recognition and a sense of belonging.

Individuals as fortunate as Furaha (Case Study A) manage to have both of these needs largely met within their familial networks.

As several examples in this chapter have shown, however, many patients' pursuits of continuity and normalcy after commencing ART are repeatedly threatened and hampered by the involuntary exposure of their HIV status, the disruption of supportive kin relations, and the collapse of economic security. In many ways, these people's lives remain affected by an undercurrent of contingency and uncertainty, which needs to be countered by a permanent alertness with regard to new, temporarily emerging sources of institutional support. Many people thus go to great lengths to permanently navigate between various social contexts that promise material and immaterial help to rebuild their lives, to enable them to make meaning of their condition beyond biomedical reasoning, and to help them maintain their hope for a promising future. Particularly important in this regard are community-based HIV (self-)support groups, which will be the concern of the following chapter.

Notes

1. Parts of this chapter have been published in Mattes 2012 and 2014a.
2. There had been a misunderstanding between us in this regard, as prior to our first interview, I had assumed that Fatuma was taking ARVs.
3. This is a common phrase for the period of time (up to three months) that it takes for the immune system to produce detectable HIV antibodies after infection with the virus.
4. The reasons for this are explained in Chapter 7.
5. That it was Fatuma and, to a lesser extent, her mother and sister Halima who were in charge of the ART and other health-related issues of Fatuma's brothers' children concurs with a general gender imbalance in relation to care provision that has been observed in sub-Saharan Africa (e.g., Kipp et al. 2006). Women are responsible for managing the domestic sphere, which includes nursing the sick and frail, while men are ascribed the role of provider of the household. My observations at the Bombo Regional Hospital's Children's Clinic confirmed this "traditional" gendered role allocation, as those accompanying the children and youths to their control visits and doctor consultations were mostly close female family members. However, it can be argued that the massive impact of HIV/AIDS on the social fabric of African societies has set in motion a process of subtle, perforce diversification and a loosening up of such rigid gender roles. I met women who had either lost their husband to the disease or had been thrown out by him after disclosing their HIV status and thus needed to take on the role of providing for their equally rejected children. On the other hand, I met several men who were enormously engaged in and felt profoundly responsible for the

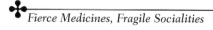

health and well-being of their children, including the practical aspects of their HIV treatment.

6. In fact, Joseph's correlation of social closeness with vulnerability and danger corresponds with equally classical research on the nexus of relatedness, social tensions, and witchcraft accusations that in some ways contradicts this axiom. Middleton and Winter (1963, 11), for instance, stated that "accusations of wizardry . . . are always made by people against others with whom they are involved in a network of social relationships and, furthermore, the relationships between the accused and the accusers are usually important to them." Such structural–functionalist interpretations may partly hold true for the situation of people with HIV in Tanga, who are expelled from solidarity networks due to their "norm transgression" that may be perceived as a danger to their social surroundings. Yet the involved people's subjective experiences and emotions largely fall outside of the margins. Joseph's narrative implies that in the face of disease and suffering, these experiential dimensions play significantly on the conceptualization of social intimacy, relatedness, and correlated notions such as dignity and belonging.

7. For an elaboration on the distinctive semantic nuances between "uncertainty," "security," and "contingency," see Whyte (2009). In Joseph's narrative, all three semantic fields were closely intertwined.

8. According to the terminological distinction between stigma and discrimination made above, what Deacon and colleagues have called "instrumental stigma" should more precisely be termed "instrumental discrimination," since it does not necessarily refer to any processes of moral blame.

Chapter 7

HIV (Self-)Support Groups

Competition, Bureaucracy, and the Limitations of Biosociality

Community-based (self-)support groups have existed in Tanzania since the early 1990s. Over the years, some developed into large professional organizations with regional branches across the country (Bujra and Mokake 2000; Dilger 2005, 184–226). As in other parts of the world, within these groups, members have received psychosocial support as well as hands-on care from their peers; gained increasing knowledge about their illness and how to deal with it; and learned to cope with stigmatization and discrimination (cf. Mundell et al. 2012, 175; Spirig 1998). In resource-poor settings like Tanzania, an additional important function of (self-)support groups has been to facilitate collective small-scale income-generating projects that provide members with some additional revenue and—in the ideal case—eventually enable them to build sustainable livelihoods. The groups thus constitute an important substitute for "failing" kin-based support networks in terms of providing both psychosocial as well as economic and material help (cf. Cassidy 2010, S1601; Moyer and Igonya 2014).

A further central concern of many groups has been to capacitate members to "live positively" with HIV, which implies a range of conceptual and practical transformations that they should perform on themselves (cf. Dilger 2005, 180ff; Marsland 2012). These include: developing a positive sense of self; achieving a self-conscious way of disclosing to others and openly dealing with the disease in public; leading a healthy lifestyle by abstaining from drugs, eating a balanced diet, and regularly engaging in physical exercise; reducing sexual activity and abstaining from unprotected intercourse; and adopting an overall optimistic attitude with regard to one's future life. As these objectives were almost identical to those pursued in the adherence classes provided at treatment centers, it is hardly surprising that patients' regular participation in a (self-)support group continues to be desirable from a public health perspective in times of ART. As discussed in Chapter 3, community-based (self-) support groups were envisioned as constituting another form of institutionalized care and support, but also ART patients' long-term surveillance. A synergistic effect was thus attained in the sense that the groups were expected to provide material and immaterial help to their members and simultaneously foster their treatment adherence, facilitate the identification of patients lost to follow-up, and thus ultimately contribute to better treatment retention rates and the greater overall success of the national treatment program.

In this chapter, I explore the extent to which (self-)support groups in Tanga met such expectations by presenting exemplary passages of (bi)weekly group meetings that I attended over the course of eleven months. On the one hand, these passages illustrate similarities between the social process of treatment enrollment at treatment centers and practices of "patient empowerment" in NGO-facilitated groups. On the other hand, they highlight the difficulties members faced in navigating the local landscape of social support.

When exploring the social dynamics and practical outcomes of Tanga's (self-)support groups, considerable differences were observable between the TALPHA groups facilitated by the well-established, internationally funded TAWG (see Chapter 1), and the majority of the so-called "neighborhood groups" (*vitundi vya mitaani*) that only sporadically received financial and practical assistance from other community- or faith-based organizations. The members of the former were privileged in various ways: they were more frequently and reliably provided with material and nutritional support; they had better access to expert information on HIV/AIDS and ART through the TAWG staff; and they had greater chances of gaining access to the temporary support initiatives that were offered by third parties.

Tanga People Living with HIV/AIDS (TALPHA)

Homework Done?

The sheets of corrugated iron above our heads emitted occasional loud cracking sounds as they heated up in the relentless, blazing summer sun. It was a morning in early December 2008, and I was participating for the first time in a group meeting at the CHICC. The center was run by the TAWG and located in the middle of Tanga's most vibrant commercial quarter, where on market days, the *daladalas* had difficulties navigating through the masses of pedestrians crisscrossing the roads from one street vendor offering her goods on the side of the dusty sidewalks to the other.

The *Umoja*[1] group that I participated in that morning was one of four groups facilitated by the TAWG. It had twenty-one participants (thirteen women, eight men[2]), all of whom lived in Tanga and, with the exception of three, were enrolled on ART at the Bombo Regional Hospital. The meeting was led by three people: forty-six-year-old Salma, who volunteered as the coordinator of all four TALPHA groups; forty-five-year-old Happiness, whose HIV diagnosis dated back fifteen years, and who was the chair of *Umoja*; and Fadhila, the widow who had been talking to the crowds about her life with ARVs on World AIDS Day only a few days earlier.

After I had been introduced and had explained the objectives of my research, Fadhila provided me with some information on the group. At each meeting, every group member was provided with 1,000 TSH as a compensation for their costs of travelling to the CHICC. They also received a cup of porridge and lunch during the meetings. Moreover, every two or three months, each member was provided with nutritional support (5 kg of rice and 4 kg of beans). The TAWG also supported small income-generating projects, like the production and sale of small snacks on the street, and covered members' transport costs to the hospital in case of emergencies. In implying that these services often outstripped the support that group members received from their relatives, Fadhila emphasized that many members felt a lot closer to their TALPHA peers than to their own families.

With regard to ART, Fadhila continued, the members assisted each other in taking their medicines and often exchanged advice on how to cope with particular side effects. Some also functioned as treatment assistants for one another. Generally, they had a very positive attitude toward ARVs, Fadhila claimed. "We get strong, we can smile," she commented on the benefits of taking the medicines, while some of the group members nodded affirmatively.

After these introductory explanations, the agenda of the actual group meeting was opened with an appraisal of a kind of "homework" that the members had apparently been assigned in the last meeting. Each member had to report on how many persons s/he had disclosed her/his HIV status to, and how many people s/he had managed to talk into taking an HIV test. Fadhila noted down the results (ranging from between two and seven persons), all the while encouraging her peers to educate other people, accompany them to get tested, and to write down small minutes of their conversations, which they could then discuss together in the next meeting.

This was followed by an end-of-year review offered by Salma, which predominantly recalled the success of awareness-raising activities at local schools, in which a few of the present group members had been involved. These activities, Salma explained, were to be enhanced in 2009, and she encouraged the members to get engaged in the theater and dance performances as well as in the dissemination of information material on HIV, stigma, and ART that were planned in further schools and villages around Tanga. While Salma compiled a list of twenty villages to be targeted, one woman spontaneously expressed her appreciation for the TAWG, emphasizing that she and other members had been rescued by the organization after their families had dismissed them. Salma thanked the woman, once more invoked the members to be open—to disclose to their relatives, friends, and neighbors—and then invited them to have lunch.

Afterward, Salma hung several sheets of paper on the wall, each of which had a long list of names. In the new year, she explained, the four current TALPHA groups needed to be divided into six, due to the large demand in the community. Every new group was to be constituted of old and new members, so that the latter could benefit from the experiences of the former.

Shortly before the group meeting terminated, the conversation turned to a nonattendant male group member. Some of the participants complained bitterly about his erratic presence at the meetings, and others vociferously alleged him of deliberately risking the health of his sexual partners, with whom he supposedly never used condoms. While I did not hear any of the group leaders' comments on this "problem case" amid the noise of everyone getting ready for departure, I did notice how efficiently the group seemed to work as a kind of social corrective (an apparatus for what could be called "benevolent denunciation") with regard to individual members' deviation from their shared rules of conduct. In a follow-up meeting, I was to gain further insight into what the group's moral norms entailed and how new members were calibrated accordingly.

Attuning the Novices

Four weeks later, I participated in a meeting of the "new" *Umoja* group, which was again led by Salma and Fadhila. Of the twenty-seven persons listed as group members, fourteen attended the meeting, only three of whom were men.

After an opening prayer, Salma turned especially to the new group members. She asked them what they had told their families about where they were going when they had left their homes in order to attend the meeting. No one seemed eager to answer the question, but Salma insisted. A few started muttering "CHICC," but when Salma asked them what the acronym stood for, they did not know. Neither could any participant explain the meaning of TALPHA. Salma finally spelled out the acronyms for the group and explained that the purpose of *Umoja* was to provide adequate education and support to its members and to let them see and feel that they were not alone with their problems.

Fadhila then took over with a long monologue, during which she read out the entire constitution of TALPHA, complemented by further explanations of the financial conditions for membership: every member had to pay an entrance fee of 10,000 TSH, which could be paid in installments, and a monthly fee of 1,000 TSH.[3] Persons who could not pay anything at all were not necessarily excluded from participating in the group meetings, but they were not allowed to receive any of the occasionally distributed food rations nor to participate in the initiatives and support projects offered by third parties that recruited their beneficiaries through TALPHA. When members were absent from group meetings without an excuse more than four times, their membership was annulled.

Before releasing the members for a short break, Fadhila further instructed the audience to guard the "secrets of the groups" (*kutunza siri ya kikundi*), especially any details of the financial support they received within the group, from the members of other (self-)support groups. During the previous year, she warned, considerable tensions had arisen when some TALPHA members disregarded this principle and told members of other groups about a onetime cash contribution that they had received at the CHICC. This, Fadhila added in a dismissive tone, had been rather "unstrategic" of them.

After a short porridge break, various long-term TAWG staff members spoke to the group. Their speeches obviously served as a first attunement of the audience to their new social and moral obligations as TALPHA members. George, a clinician and program manager, started off by repeatedly appealing to the audience that an HIV infection was no excuse to rely solely on external support instead of taking one's life into one's own hands. As if to preventatively warn the present members and motivate them to always exert themselves and work hard for their own progress, he related an unsuccessful previous attempt to provide members with economic seed capital through a microcredit initiative. Ten TALPHA members had been given a credit of 100,000 TSH, and a further ten were to be provided with the same amount as soon as the first cohort had amortized their share. Unfortunately, not even one of the ten initial beneficiaries had repaid their credit, which was why the initiative had come to an abrupt end. No one should join TALPHA with the sole or prior expectation of being helped financially, George advised, as neither the TAWG nor TALPHA itself had the means to provide the large number of members with a substantial—let alone regular—financial contribution. Instead, he encouraged the members to see the benefit of their membership first and foremost in terms of receiving education, which they could then publicly disseminate in order to provoke a change in attitude toward people living with HIV in Tanga and the entire country.

Following this, George quickly mentioned how important it was for people living with ARVs to drastically reduce their sexual activity. Frequent sexual intercourse was not only dangerous in terms of the risk it posed to sexual partners of contracting the virus, but it was also detrimental to one's own health in terms of implying a significant loss of energy.

With this, George handed over to his elderly female colleague Dr. Msangi, who reaffirmed several of his explanations by encouraging the audience to "break the silence" and get engaged in HIV peer education; advising them to abstain from sex as much as they could and to always use condoms; urging them to continue whatever economic projects they were pursuing in order to secure their own livelihood; and motivating them not to despair (*kukata tamaa*) or lose confidence in their future. Not least, a positive attitude helped to avoid depression and "stress," and this, she explained smilingly, kept their CD4 count high.

At this point, Ismail, who also belonged to the group, added for consideration that sometimes women did not want to use condoms. This aroused immediate protest among several female group members, who argued that it was *they*, women, who were in a disadvantaged position, for they had no rights to suggest to the male "breadwinner of the family" to have protected intercourse. Instead of elaborating on this controversial issue, Dr. Msangi instead broached the topic of the rights of people living with HIV being the same as those of everyone else, which included the right to education, mobility, work, public services, marriage, sex, and having children. Regarding procreation, Dr. Msangi emphasized the problem of unplanned pregnancies, which could pose a significant danger for women with low CD4 counts. She strongly urged those women present to talk to health experts about their plans to have a child in advance, so that they could assess whether their current health condition would allow for a pregnancy. Furthermore, women were advised not to breastfeed their babies for six months after birth,[4] which required additional planning and the timely diversion of financial means for the acquisition of nutritional substitutes.

With this, the provision of information to the group came to an end. After an extended lunch break, the members paid their monthly fees, were refunded their travel costs, and after some had carefully placed large boxes of condoms offered by the TAWG staff in their bags so that no one would see them when they stepped out onto the street, everyone left.

Techniques of Continuous Member Modeling

While the above-described meeting illustrates how newcomers were introduced to the formal rules of the group, as well as to the ethos and moral conduct that they were expected to display, a meeting that I attended a few weeks later was more dialogical and thus instructive of the group leaders' teaching methods and the power relations implicated in their interactions with the group members. This meeting was attended by seven women and three men, one of whom was Joseph (Case Study D), who attended as a "guest" since he was unable to pay the entrance fee.

Salma opened up the meeting by asking the participants whether they had read any information material about HIV/AIDS at home since they last had gotten together. After an initial silence, a few members said in a low voice that they had not read anything, and an elderly woman added that she could not read in the first place. Salma insisted that they all had to keep informing themselves about their condition by whatever means available, before suggesting to the elderly woman that she find a trusted person who could assist her by reading information material to her. "The virus," Salma emphasized with a warning look on her face, "changes every single day." It was therefore of utmost importance that TALPHA members knew all information by heart, in order to be prepared for every one of the virus' tricks.

Following this initial intervention, Salma asked the participants one by one what the letters HIV (in Swahili VVU = *virusi vya ukimwi*) stood for. The first three members she addressed did not remember. The fourth woman gave it a try, answering "Parasites that live inside the human body," but this did not quite satisfy Salma. Fadhila and another woman present who was also one of the TALPHA leaders grew increasingly impatient. In an enervated tone, the latter finally interrupted the exercise, saying out loud that HIV was "the name of the virus that causes AIDS," wherein she once more urged the participants to read as much as they could about the disease.

Grace then asked everyone to specify the different transmission routes of HIV. Again, the members had difficulties. The elderly illiterate woman contributed by saying "to wander around carelessly" (*kutembelea ovyo*), a common expression for having unprotected sex with a multitude of partners. She was compelled by the group leaders to rephrase her contribution again and again, until she finally used the word *kujamiiana* (to copulate). Obviously, they wanted her to use a more explicit and precise term and were only satisfied when she used one that is also commonly used in biomedical settings to refer to sexual intercourse.

Shortly afterward, it was Joseph's turn to have his terminology corrected. When, in his attempt to mention another route of HIV transmission, he referred to people living with HIV by using the term "the affected" (*waathirika*), Fadhila intervened energetically. She explained that in times of widespread prevalence of HIV/AIDS, nearly everyone in Tanzania was "affected," which deprived the term of any meaningfulness. "We are people who live with HIV!" she insisted instead, implying once more that members were expected to call things by their proper names.

An hour after the meeting had begun, a young woman entered the room. In a sharp tone, Fadhila reprimanded her that her late arrival was very inconvenient, for at this time, the attendance list had already been signed and passed on to the person who prepared the disbursement of the travel allowances. She then wrote down the woman's name and her offence of arriving late in a register. At the same time, a young mother attending the meeting began to feed her baby milk out of a used plastic bottle. Vehemently, Fadhila told her to use a cup instead and, additionally, to take her veil off so that everyone could see her face properly. The woman looked somewhat startled, but she obeyed in silence.

Fadhila then gave another monologue about the members' prior obligations to continuously improve their own knowledge about HIV, but to also carry their knowledge into their community in order to contribute to the frequently discussed theme of "education for society" (*elimu kwa jamii*). During her long and monotonous appeal, the elderly woman fell asleep. When Fadhila noticed this, she woke her up and requested her to stand up, walk across the room, shake my hand, and return to her chair. Even though the woman was unsteady on her feet, Fadhila insisted. The old woman slowly completed the exercise amid the benevolent laughter of her peers.

After the ensuing lunch break, the participants were asked to agree on a range of topics that they were going to discuss during the following meetings. Listed on the agenda were nutrition, the "truth" about HIV/AIDS, living with hope, sexually transmitted diseases, income-generating projects, and condom use. Then someone suggested "stigmatization" (*unyanyapaa*) as a topic, and Fadhila asked the group in return what this was. The youngest woman in the room, approximately twenty-two years old, asserted that she simply felt it when she was being stigmatized. John interjected that stigma was "To be separated by society" (*kutengwa na jamii*). Another woman said it was "To view yourself as different from the others." Fadhila nodded and complemented their explanations by saying that stigmatization meant "To treat someone differently than others due to his/her situation (*hali*) [of living with HIV]."

She then broached the topic of the situation at the entry gate to the Bombo Regional Hospital. Presumably in an attempt to demonstrate to the participants that being treated differently could also have its good side, she pointed out how easy it was to obtain access to the hospital grounds outside normal visiting hours by simply showing the guards one's blue CTC card as an "entry ticket." Even better than that, she added, was the fact that HIV-positive people did not have to pay a cent for any kind of treatment and medication at the hospital. Some group members, however, had had quite opposite experiences. Several of them, including Joseph, explained to their peers that on various occasions, they did have to pay for the services they received at treatment centers. Fadhila seemed surprised and, in a somewhat defenseless manner, advised them to insist more strongly on their rights.

Subsequently, the topic was abruptly switched by a man who asked: "So what about the medicines [ARVs]? Shouldn't we also receive a lesson about the medicines?" Fadhila agreed and immediately started reeling off the basic dos and don'ts of ARV use, much in the style of how patients were educated at the treatment centers: "The medicines are effective for twelve hours. If patients do not take their pills in time, the virus wakes up, sees that there are no 'guards' around, and immediately starts to breed more of its kind."

Between Empowerment and Discipline, Social Support and Social Control

As these extracts show, the processes of shaping patients' subjectivities that took place at treatment centers were carried on at the TALPHA groups (cf. Kalofonos 2008, 147). Members were continuously being reminded to act responsibly with regard to their sexuality and procreative desires, about the proper way of taking their medicines, and about the importance of adhering to a healthy lifestyle, much in the same way as patients were instructed during the adherence classes described in Chapter 4.

Another parallel between the TALPHA groups and the medical context of treatment preparation consisted of the endeavor to introduce patients/members to the scientific basics about HIV and ART. In the (self-)support groups, however, even greater emphasis was placed on the members' obligations to continuously and self-responsibly enhance their HIV-related expertise—including the acquisition of a semantically precise and scientifically sound terminology—by whatever means available to them.

There were also similarities in terms of how group leaders and health professionals established their authority vis-à-vis members/patients, as exemplified by Fadhila's occasional direct admonishments of single group members. Power did not only play out in the interaction between group leaders and ordinary members, however, but also among the members themselves, and this might be the point of prior interest from a public health perspective. Aside from the rather strict formal rules of the group, whose observance was painstakingly monitored, the main disciplinary mode of the group seemed to lie in their members' mutual social control in the context of their everyday lives. In the above case, people complained about a fellow member's irresponsible sexual practices. In other meetings, I witnessed people reporting to the group leaders on their peers' irregular ARV intake or their turn toward "traditional" ritual healing and their consequent interruption of their biomedical treatment. By identifying treatment defaulters and opening them up to the intervention of health professionals, HBC providers, or peer educators, the (self-)support groups at least occasionally seemed to function as a community-near instance of ART surveillance, as envisioned by public health and biomedical professionals.

A further obvious overlap in the interests of biomedical/public health authorities and the facilitators of the TALPHA groups consisted of the destigmatization of HIV/AIDS. In fact, the importance of actively contributing to a substantial change in attitude among the public, through disclosure and openness vis-à-vis family, friends, neighbors, and workmates, and through one's engagement in public awareness raising campaigns, was pronounced even more emphatically in the (self-)support groups than in biomedical settings. There was certainly an empowering effect to this "mission," inasmuch as it entailed the reinforcement of people's self-confidence to stand up and speak out about their life with HIV in public (best exemplified by Fadhila's performance on World AIDS Day). However, there was possibly also a considerable degree of enforcement connected to this process of openness. Apparently, only a small fraction of the TALPHA members was ready to disclose their status to large audiences at schools and other places. Furthermore, those who did participate were not necessarily convinced that this was the right thing to do, but they had a more or less diffuse feeling of being obliged to make such a contribution; or, as I would learn later, they were actually paid for this kind of engagement.

For thirty-three-year-old Chris, for instance, the main motivation for his participation in a campaign at one of Tanga's secondary schools, during which he disclosed to a large group of students, was the compensation of 2,000 TSH (for performances in villages further away in the countryside, the compensation was 5,000 TSH). At that particular event, however, there were several students from his own neighborhood, including one of his nephews, among the audience. Much to Chris's regret, these young people spread the information about his HIV status to other neighbors, which caused immense difficulties for him. In Chris's view, the TAWG facilitators would not really care about such "collateral damage," even if he told them about his problem, as they would not even define it as damage but rather as a sort of painful but necessary step forward. He therefore kept his frustrations to himself. Taking this into account, I found that some aspects of the work and dynamics of the TALPHA groups were characterized by a profound ambivalence, which made it difficult to judge whether it was the empowering or the disciplining effects that ultimately prevailed, or where the line between the two should be drawn.

Equally ambiguous was the microcredit initiative for TALPHA members that was not offered by, but was centrally mediated through, the TAWG. During my first field stay, this was the most relevant initiative regarding monetary support offered to people living with HIV in Tanga, and the only one of its kind. As alluded to briefly in the story of Joseph (Case Study D), some people did temporarily benefit greatly from this initiative. Other patients' experiences with the program, however, were more problematic. By drawing on these people's accounts, I use the initiative as a prism highlighting, first,

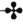

the limitations of group solidarity and loyalty among TALPHA members (and those of other groups), and, second, the intense sense of competitiveness prevalent among the many groups struggling to secure their share of the scarce material and social support being offered in the city.

Microcredits and the Limitations of Biosociality

I first heard about the microcredit program offered by AFREDA in a meeting of *Umoja*, when Fadhila made an announcement that the nationally operating Tanzanian NGO was about to recruit potential participants in Tanga. "Trusted" beneficiaries were to be selected predominantly via the TALPHA groups, Fadhila explained, and the main selection criterion was members' previous stable attendance at group meetings. On the following day, interested members would be provided with more details about the requirements of participation. Fadhila warned the audience, however, that the program's capacities were not large enough to enroll all TALPHA members.

Unfortunately, I could not attend the initial information event. But over the following months, several patients, including Joseph and Fatuma Ramadhani, as well as TAWG staff kept me informed about the progress of the initiative. Toward the end of my first field stay, I also paid a visit to the AFREDA office in Tanga, situated in one of the poorer residential areas quite far away from the city center. The house was painted bright pink, which made it seem somewhat out of place. I rang the bell and was welcomed by a woman in her early twenties who introduced herself as Nadia, the secretary, and who led me into a spacious office room. With shiny tiles on the floor and completely empty apart from one large office desk with a computer and two plastic chairs, the room had a strangely cold ambience, which did not only stem from the air conditioning that was obviously running at full blast.

Nadia explained that both the project officer and coordinator were currently in Dar es Salaam, but perhaps she could help me. She then explained that AFREDA was running microcredit initiatives specifically for people living with HIV/AIDS in four districts of Tanzania. They would soon reach the limit of seven hundred beneficiaries set for this round of the program. After three years, AFREDA would have to submit a report to the donors, and, subject to a positive evaluation, there would be a second round. The main donor to the microcredit initiative was the German Evangelical Development Service (Evangelischer Entwicklungsdienst [EED]). Nadia was not sure if there were other donors involved as well.[5]

The beneficiaries had to organize themselves into groups of ten to twenty persons. In Tanga, ten groups had been recruited via the TAWG. These groups had then received training on how to establish an income-generating project, and individuals were provided with credits of between 50,000 and 200,000 TSH. Participants had to repay one fifth of the provided credit at the beginning of each month for six months in a row. If they managed to do this, half of the overpaid amount would be returned to the beneficiary, and the other half retained as interest.

Several times during our conversation, Nadia emphasized that the aim of the program was to reinstall a sense of responsibility among the participants, who were "too used to keeping their hands open and begging for help" instead of (re)gaining control over their own lives. In her perspective, this had worked out well. Proudly, she explained that so far, only three persons had not been able to repay their dues.

The conversations I had with patients about their experiences in the initiative revealed a somewhat more ambiguous picture. A first critical issue concerned the strategy for recruiting beneficiaries, which privileged TALPHA members and excluded those of other groups that were not facilitated by the TAWG. Although, as Joseph's case suggests, it was possible to gain access to TALPHA and, in a second step, the microcredit initiative without paying the regular member fees, this was highly contingent on the particular relationship one was able to build with influential TAWG members. Moreover, the crucial issue was to receive information about the initiative in the first place, and this was spread to people living with HIV mainly through the TALPHA groups. Consequently, I met many non-TALPHA members who simply did not know about the opportunity. I even encountered a leader of one of the neighborhood groups who had participated in the AFREDA initiative but had concealed this fact from the other group members; the latter were outraged when, during a meeting I attended, they coincidentally learned that she had secretly benefitted from the program. Other (self-)support groups did receive notice of the initiative, though bitterly complained that beneficiaries were exclusively chosen through TALPHA and that they, as so often, were left empty handed.

Resentment was not only evoked by people who felt excluded from the initiative due to the situation of limited access. Tensions also arose within the microcredit groups themselves, for instance with regard to power inequalities among the members. Fatuma Ramadhani explained that some of the group leaders had set a limit of 100,000 TSH as the maximum credit amount that single group members could apply for. While this practice might have been a precautionary measure, considering that the group leaders acted as guarantors for their groups, it was met with strong objections from some participants, particularly because the leaders were said to claim larger credits for themselves. Moreover, some participants considered 100,000 TSH (and even the 200,000 TSH that was the maximum credit amount set by AFREDA) too little to really help them build up a small-scale business that might have a chance of prospering and leading to their self-sufficiency. Francis, for instance, who was a learned tailor and wished to set up a moderately small tailor shop, mentioned that the purchase of a single sewing machine would cost him 500,000 TSH. He was, nevertheless, still grateful for the credit he had received and stressed that he made great efforts to pay his monthly amortizations in time. Unfortunately, he added, most of the other members in his microcredit group did not seem to feel an equally strong moral obligation in this regard. In fact, he claimed that he and one other man out of ten group members were the only ones who reliably paid their dues. The resulting uncertainty about whether the endeavor would ultimately end in success for him caused him considerable distress.

The fact that the members of the microcredit groups had to bail for each other turned out to be a problematic issue in other groups too. Olivia explained that the inability of one woman in her group to pay her dues had sparked off considerable dissent, as the other group members were neither able nor willing to stand in for her. Ultimately, the woman had to sell some of her few belongings in order to be able to repay her credit. Several other people living with HIV in Tanga whom I talked to, who would potentially have had the chance to enroll in the initiative through TALPHA, did not do so, precisely because they anticipated being held responsible for the failure of other group members. In their view, the potential damage of putting their trust in the "wrong" people outweighed the advantages of receiving the credit. Conversely, other TALPHA members, including Fatuma Ramadhani, did not take a credit, for they anticipated that they would not be able to pay their amortizations within the agreed period. The fact that others would be held responsible for their own potential failure led to the decision not to even give it a try.

Interestingly, the component of the initiative that involved a collective income-generating group project seemed to be only a minor priority for the members of the microcredit groups. Olivia was the only one who even mentioned her group's project of growing teakwood. Unfortunately, it was not as profit yielding as the group had hoped, since half of the trees they had planted died before their wood could be sold. At the time of my interview with Olivia, the group was still in the process of "inventing" another project, as she termed it.

In light of the above-described tensions and difficulties, the microcredit initiative can be taken as an instance of the limitations of solidarity within biosocial collectives with regard to the participating groups, several of which apparently only remained in existence at the cost of "well-functioning" and "responsible" individuals, who stood in for their peers who failed to fulfill the terms and conditions, willingly or unwillingly. Power differentials within some groups further decreased people's will to contribute to the expected mutual solidarity, an idea that for others seemed so unrealistic that they did not join these collectives in the first place.

At a larger scale, the tensions AFREDA evoked among the highly fragmented HIV-positive citizenship of Tanga exemplified the intense atmosphere of competitiveness that these people were subjected to (cf. Marsland 2012). As we will see further below, accessing and securing technical and financial support to establish small-scale economic projects in this competitive field was particularly difficult for the majority of the neighborhood groups that were not facilitated by well-established NGOs like the TAWG. For the countless members of these groups, access to material help seemed to be a lot more relevant than getting engaged in the political mission of fighting for the rights of people living with HIV and transforming the societal discourse around HIV/AIDS. Through a particular event—or rather process—that took place in early 2009, I nevertheless learned that this also applied to the majority of the groups facilitated by the

TAWG, the organization that, more than any other in Tanga, could be viewed as a platform for the forging of politically conscious and active therapeutic citizens. This was the temporary closure of the organization.

Donor Dependency and the Fragility of Social Support: The Temporary Shutdown of the Tanga AIDS Working Group

In late April 2009, soon upon my return to Tanga after a six-week stay in Germany, I arrived at the CHICC again in order to attend another meeting of *Umoja*. Salma and the present TAWG staff members welcomed me with an unusual downheartedness. I did not have the chance to ask them immediately what was wrong, as they were fully occupied with compiling lists with names of TALPHA members. As they explained shortly while rushing through their piles of papers, TACAIDS was offering some help for women living with HIV, but had demanded to know the number and details of all female TALPHA members. Meanwhile, the two men and one woman, the latter of whom had a roughly one-year-old child with her, who had come to attend the meeting patiently waited in silence.

After a while, Salma took a seat next to me and almost whispered that the CHICC would possibly be closed down soon. During one of the previous group meetings, they had already informed the members that in the future, there would be neither any provision of meals during the meetings nor reimbursement of their travel costs. If the CHICC really closed its doors, Salma stressed with concern, the six TALPHA groups with more than 130 participants would not have a place to meet.

Salma finally opened the meeting by greeting the small audience and went through a comparably short agenda with significantly less passion than usual. Just twenty minutes later, she handed the meeting over to the TAWG clinician in charge of the CHICC, who provided the group members and me with further details concerning the TAWG's immediate future. In the following week, she explained, the organization would be "closed" until further notice, since major donors had entirely ceased their support. In order to at least partly mitigate the impact of this on clients, the TALPHA groups had been offered to temporarily continue their meetings at the CHICC, as long as this did not imply any consumption of water or electricity. The three participants seemed unsurprised upon hearing this, as they had been forewarned in their last meeting.

After the meeting, the clinician gave free rein to her indignation about the imminent closure of the TAWG, which she predicted would have extremely negative effects. After all, the organization was the most relevant nongovernmental actor involved in HIV prevention and care in the Tanga region. At the CHICC alone, ten to fifteen people were tested for HIV every day. The TAWG teams also distributed condoms at bars and hotels, conducted public awareness raising events, and organized large HIV testing campaigns in rural areas. A profound impact was also to be expected in the area of HBC, where hundreds of clients would be left unattended. Finally, the microcredit groups would be deprived of their TAWG supervision. Salma would be the only person maintaining contact with the groups, a task that was far too demanding for an unpaid volunteer. In short, the clinician implied that the shutdown of the TAWG would have an enormously detrimental impact on countless people living with HIV in the region.

Perturbed by this news, I went to the TAWG headquarters the next morning in order to find out more. I talked to members of the management, and over the following months, the program manager regularly provided me with brief updates on the situation. The progression of events that I was eventually able to compose on the basis of my conversations with TAWG staff, some of the clients, and a representative of one of the TAWG's main donors, was too complex to be reproduced here in detail. At the core, however, lay the allegations of two former TAWG employees, who sometime in 2008 had informed the organization's three main donors (OXFAM Ireland; African Medical and Research Foundation [AMREF], which as a principal recipient of the Global Fund channeled funding to the TAWG as a subrecipient; and the EED) that the TAWG's management had claimed funding from all three of them for the implementation of particular campaigns and activities. These allegations eventually caused OXFAM to commission an external auditor to inspect the TAWG's activities and accounting practices. His report indeed pinpointed some irregularities, which, in the view of the TAWG management, were negligible and possibly even attributable to mere slips in transferring data from the manually kept cashbooks into an electronic database. OXFAM, AMREF, and the EED, how-ever, judged the identified inconsistencies to be grave enough to suspend further disbursements until all obscurities had been solved. Since December 2008, basically all of the TAWG's vital sources of money had thus been cut off.

What followed were tedious negotiations between the TAWG and its donors, as well as discussions among the latter about the conditions for a possible continuation of funding. Donor representa-tives visited the TAWG, further audits were conducted, and reports written. The donors finally required the inclusion of nonmedical professionals, such as accountants and legal experts in the TAWG's board, the introduction and application of professional finance con-trol software, and the hiring of professional accountants who would take charge of the organization's bookkeeping in order to consider the continuation of their support. While, according to their own indications, the TAWG made every effort to meet these require-ments as quickly as possible, things still did not move forward. Month after month, the program manager kept telling me that they were still waiting for the donors' final decision.

Many details of the lengthy negotiations between the involved parties remained opaque to me, and I am not in a position to judge the extent to which the donors' allegations of mismanagement were substantiated and whether the conditions they imposed on the TAWG constituted an adequate response. In many ways, how-ever, the extensive consequences of the funding cut and the mas-sive reduction—if not interruption—of most of the organization's activities were very tangible.

After the funding had been suspended, it became increasingly difficult for the TAWG to pay staff salaries, and eventually, the contracts of nineteen of their forty-four regular employees had to be put on hold. Even though some of these people continued doing at least part of their work on a voluntary basis, in mid-May, the program manager expected that around half would soon have found other work. Indeed, I knew of two HBC providers who had already managed to find jobs at one of the local CTCs soon after they had been dismissed by the TAWG. This, the program manager lamented, was particularly regrettable, because the organization had invested considerable time and money in their advanced training, which was why they were so "marketable" in the first place.

Due to its strongly reduced workforce and the lack of money to fill its cars' gasoline tanks, the TAWG's HBC services were ceased. As the few remaining professional providers could no longer visit their clients at their homes, they focused on the provision of rudimentary medical care at the headquarters. This had particularly grave implications. Some patients, for example, refused to come to the CTCs to pick up their monthly ARV supplies, for they were too afraid of exposing their HIV status to others. The HBC providers had therefore been providing them with their drug rations at home. Faced with the interruption of this service, these patients either had to overcome their anxieties and risk being recognized as HIV-positive in public or interrupt their therapy. One provider estimated that around fifteen of her clients had chosen the latter option.

As the TAWG had no more capacities to coordinate its roughly one hundred volunteer community HBC providers and at least moderately compensate their work expenses, it was assumed that most of them had also stopped visiting their clients. The conversations I had with some of these volunteers verified that this was indeed the case, which meant the interruption of connections with hundreds of people living with HIV and ARVs in Tanga. These people were deprived of potential emergency care that was often provided by the TAWG's medical professionals upon the reports of the volunteers. Conversely, the disruption constituted a significant setback for the establishment of seamless patient surveillance from medical institutions to patients' households.

Finally, as Salma had explained, the TALPHA groups had not been interrupted per instruction of the TAWG. However, while the members were offered to continue holding their meetings at the CHICC, they were no longer provided with information materials, food, or compensation for their travel costs. As the low attendance of the *Umoja* group meeting suggested, this had a significant impact on the morale of many members, who obviously felt that there was no longer any point in participating in the meetings. During a visit I paid to Fatuma Ramadhani at the end of April, she confirmed this, relating that since March, the members of her group had not been refunded their travel costs. This had not yet inhibited the majority of the group members from attending their meetings. But after the provision of lunch during the meetings had been cancelled in early April, most members abruptly stopped showing up. "They have enough information about HIV. They simply want to eat," Fatuma stated pragmatically.

For some people, the falling apart of their group meant a loss, not only of the modest but at least regularly provided nutritional and material support, but also in a more psychological sense. Joseph, for instance, perceived this discontinuation as yet another setback in his quest for a sense of belonging and talked about it in emotionally laded language:

> It was at the CHICC where I found more support than at the Bombo Regional Hospital. . . . Since I've joined [the TALPHA group meeting at] the CHICC, I noticed that there were certain changes. . . . The CHICC helped, and it's been shut down! My soul still hurts me (*bado roho inaniuma*). I feel like we are missing a lot of things [now]. It's been different than over there at the [hospital]. When you go there, you only wait in the line, take your medicine, your weight is taken, and you return home; there's nothing else.

In a similar way, Fatuma expressed her concern about what would happen to her and the many other people who were benefitting from the TAWG's work. Her sense of being left behind emerged more subtly in an increased attachment to Edna and me. After our above-mentioned conversation at her house, for instance, she walked us all the way back to the city center, despite our repeated assurance that this was not necessary. Again and again, she pleaded with us to come by and look after her again, as we would no longer have the chance to meet at the CHICC. I could not avoid the impression that she feared being forgotten and abandoned to her fate if our regular visits should also come to an end.

By and large, the future of the TAWG remained uncertain throughout the following months. In August, OXFAM resumed the disbursement of funding, and an additional ten employees could be paid again. Yet a significant part of the funding was now tied to capacity building measures for the staff, which meant that in terms of its regular activities, the organization kept operating at a very basic level. Moreover, the TAWG's program manager explained that due to the global financial crisis, the donors themselves had to cope with budget cuts and delayed disbursements (from the Global Fund, for instance), and these problems also had an influence on their decisions with regard to the TAWG.

In early October 2009, when my first research stay came to an end, the decisions of AMREF and the EED were still pending. When I returned to Tanga in May 2011, I learned that in the intervening time, the situation had not improved. In fact, OXFAM had entirely withdrawn its funding because of an interest shift from HIV to other areas such as economic and gender justice. The EED had resumed its funding, but at a reduced level, and even this decreased support would run out at the end of 2011. With a reduced staffing level (the number of paid employees had once more decreased to twenty-two) and a budget that was far below the level prior to the crisis, the TAWG's services offered to its clients and the public were thus still being maintained only in a minimal way.[6] Heavily preoccupied with the additional task of writing funding proposals, the program manager admitted that the question of how to secure the financial basis for the organization's wide range of activities for the years to come gave him considerable headaches.

Quite apart from the fact that the TAWG's funding crisis was possibly self-induced, its near shutdown in 2009 and its severely hampered level of operation over the following years serve as yet another example of how fragile and problematic the project of public health care provision and the delegation of responsibility for providing fundamental social services to externally funded, nongovernmental actors can be (cf. Prince 2014b; Whyte 2013). Ultimately, innumerous people living with HIV and ARVs in Tanga were deprived of medical, social, and psychological support, and the continuation of their biomedical therapies was indirectly jeopardized because of the TAWG's overdependence on a small number of donor organizations and funding mechanisms whose logics of accountability prescribed the interruption of the disbursement of funds despite all of the damage that this would foreseeably bring about for the beneficiaries.

Secondly, the collapse of the TALPHA groups as a consequence of the TAWG's termination of the provision of food and compensation for travel expenses suggests that many people's participation in the groups was more profoundly based on their hopes of garnering tangible support than on their eagerness to be part of the TAWG's sociopolitical endeavor of challenging prevailing moralistic and condemning views of people living with HIV. In this regard, these former group members came to resemble the hundreds of HIV-positive people who had never enjoyed the privileges of TALPHA in the first place, and who were desperately seeking to enhance their chances of accessing whatever support was available through their participation in one of Tanga's countless neighborhood groups.

The Neighborhood Groups (*vikundi vya mitaani*)

Considering that at their peak the TALPHA groups only had some 130 members, the majority of an estimated several hundred people living with HIV in Tanga who engaged in collective struggles for support did so in so-called neighborhood groups, whose establishment was strongly encouraged and desired by AIDSRelief (see Chapter 3). In contrast to TALPHA, these groups could not draw on consistent and long-term nongovernmental, let alone governmental, support. They were, therefore, much more contingent on their members' reciprocal commitment and their ability to develop crucial capacities, such as writing funding proposals, without which it was virtually impossible to obtain any kind of assistance.

Another feature that distinguished the neighborhood groups from patient associations such as TALPHA was, as their name suggests, that their membership was usually made up of people living within the same neighborhood. Moreover, the groups' closer attachment to a particular community was often reflected in the locations where their weekly or biweekly meetings took place. These were mostly held in public buildings such as primary schools or dispensaries in the neighborhood.

During my first field stay, aside from participating in the TALPHA meetings, I attended some twenty meetings of four such neighborhood groups over a period of ten months. Drawing on the discussions that evolved during these meetings, in the following, I explore the obstacles that these groups were confronted with in their struggle to garner external support, but also to self-organize in a way that would render them platforms of sustainable mutual solidarity. Some of these discussions, furthermore, illustrate the challenges of unifying the countless small groups at the grassroots level under the roof of an umbrella network that could lend their members a more powerful voice to claim their stake vis-à-vis government authorities and nongovernmental organizations.

319

The Attritional Effect of State Bureaucracy

In mid-December 2008, I participated for the first time in a meeting of the *Amani* group, which met on the porch of a building housing a local NGO that had encouraged its foundation. Despite the fact that the group had already existed for more than half a year and had thirty-three regular members, it had not yet started any income-generating project. Instead, the first months had been consumed by discussing and agreeing upon the group's aims and basic regulations and, subsequently, a lengthy and complex odyssey through a wide range of governmental offices at different administrative levels in the quest to officially register the group as an association. This, I was told, was a sine qua non for both opening a bank account and applying for any sort of institutional funding.

The first meeting I attended was particularly instructive in terms of how time consuming and exhausting it was to navigate through this process. The chair, secretary, and treasurer of the group reported in detail on how many requirements they had been required to fulfill in order to get the right stamps from the right persons on the right documents. They had moved back and forth between the offices of local officials at their ward, the city hall, and the district administration. They had filled in registration forms, submitted photocopies of passports, transferred stamped documents and confirmation letters from one official to the other, and more than once had been dismissed to come back at a later point in time.

The biggest challenge, however, consisted of coming up with a professional, notary-certified constitution for their association. As they had no precise idea of what such a document had to include, they had borrowed the constitution of an already registered (self-) support group, copied its structure, and adapted the content according to their needs. This, again, was a long process involving many hours of discussion among the members. On the morning of the very meeting I first attended, the chair and secretary had finally managed to submit the outcome of their efforts to the local public notary. However, as they explained to the group, he had been very busy and could not tell them exactly when he would find the time to attend to their concern. The result was that they had invested an amount of 28,000 TSH in official documents, photocopies, and service fees, but still had not been able to finish the registration process and open up a bank account.

The rest of the meeting largely consisted of a detailed presentation of the group's constitution, which the secretary read aloud to the twenty-four attendant members (nineteen women, five men), many of whom had apparently missed the discussions about its contents during previous meetings. To my surprise, the financial requirements for membership were as high as those of the TALPHA groups; once the constitution became effective at the beginning of 2009, members would have to pay an entry fee of 10,000 TSH (formerly 3,000 TSH) and a monthly fee of 1,000 TSH. Indeed, this stirred up some discussion among the participants, but in the end, all objections were allayed and the group agreed. They also agreed that members' high attendance levels at the meetings were crucial for the group to move forward and therefore decided that three unexcused absences should be fined with 1,000 TSH.

During another meeting that I attended in mid-January 2009, the participants were still very preoccupied with the details of the group's formal set-up. Furthermore, another controversial debate evolved about the monthly membership fees. Several women referred to their difficult life circumstances and asked to be exempted from paying the fees for January. The group was divided. While some insisted on the punctual payment of fees in order to keep up all members' morale and eventually enable them to collectively make progress, others argued for more flexibility in this regard. Each and every member of the group, they warned, could sooner or later find themselves temporarily unable to pay. Finally, an agreement was reached that the monthly fees could at least be paid in installments. After the exhausted chair closed the meeting, all members walked away, some of them visibly irritated. I, for my part, was impressed by how grueling it was for the members to agree on the details of their formal self-organization. It was unfortunate, I thought, that they lost so much time discussing these issues instead of thinking about how they could set up some sort of small-scale economic project from which they could all benefit.

Almost four months later, I visited the group again. In the meantime they had finally managed to have their constitution certified by the public notary and to officially register as an association. However, this was apparently still not enough to apply for funding from the

Tanzania Social Action Fund (TASAF), a governmental initiative for vulnerable and marginalized groups in Tanzania,[7] which offered virtually the only opportunity for HIV (self-)support groups in Tanga to apply for governmental funding. At the local TASAF office, the group's secretary was told that the fund required a considerably more sophisticated constitution. With the help of a local NGO staff member, the constitution was therefore once more amended and improved, though it still did not meet TASAF's requirements. The group then managed to find another NGO employee who consented to help them elaborate it even further, but this appointment had been scheduled for two months later, and ever since then, the secretary had not heard anything from the woman.

In contrast to this rather unsatisfactory news, *Amani*'s chair subsequently reported that in the meantime, the NGO that had helped found the group had promised to offer them a piece of land for cultivation right next to the building where they held their meetings. This raised the mood of the present members, and they agreed to clarify the details and timeframe of this offer with the NGO as soon as possible.

Four weeks later, when I approached the building where *Amani* met in order to attend another meeting, Samuel, one of its most talkative members, saw me from afar. He rushed toward me, took me by the hand, and led me to a field of broken up soil right behind the building. He explained furiously that another NGO employee had given precisely this piece of land that they had been promised for their gardening project to another group of people that were "not even HIV-positive." These people had obviously started working the soil, but then left it unattended, which further increased Samuel's indignation.

During the subsequent group meeting, more bad news was announced. The treasurer of the group reported that at her last visit to the bank, she had noticed that 38,000 TSH of the groups 270,000 TSH was missing. This incited a long and heated discussion among the members, including fierce recriminations of the chair, the secretary, and the treasurer herself, as they were the only persons who had access to the account. All three of them vehemently denied their responsibility for any kind of loss. It took a while until all members settled their minds and lowered their voices again. They agreed first of all to inquire at the bank about the details of all recent transactions on their account in order to compare these data to the entries in their own registry books, and thus detect any potential discrepancies.

The secretary then mentioned another critical issue. Of the thirty-three members of *Amani*, she explained, only six regularly attended the meetings. Samuel replied that this was due to the fact that many members simply could no longer afford to invest their time in the group's endless and often inconclusive discussions. Another group member interjected, suggesting that they dissolve the group and divide its financial capital among those who regularly appeared at the meetings; but the others stridently rejected the man's suggestion as being unfair, irrational, and ultimately illegal. The group did not come up with a satisfactory solution to the problem other than insisting more strictly on the payment of fines for unexcused absence.

Two and a half months later, shortly before the end of my first field stay, I attended another meeting of *Amani*. It seemed as if the group had made no progress whatsoever. They had not settled the issue of the piece of land that they desired to cultivate and had received no notification of whether TASAF had accepted their revised constitution, which would allow them to submit a funding proposal. With frustration, the handful of present participants kept complaining about the large quantities of money that were being poured into the country for the fight against HIV/AIDS and care for the affected, of which so little was trickling down to the actual target groups. It seemed like the group had lost all its impetus to continue the fight for assistance in their quest for economic self-sustenance.

When I arrived in Tanga for my second field stay in May 2011, *Amani* no longer existed. An employee of the NGO that had assisted in launching the group explained that it had split up after a cash donation had allegedly landed in a group member's pocket rather than in the group's bank account. As far as I could ascertain, up to that point, *Amani* had neither managed to start any sort of income-generating activity nor secure funding through TASAF.

"They Planted the Seeds, and Then the Rain Was Stopped"

Throughout its relatively short existence, the *Amani* group faced several difficulties that ultimately led to its collapse. They struggled to navigate the extremely bureaucratic structures of public administration in their quest for formal recognition. They foundered due to the lack of the "right" connections in a clientelistic system of informal social support. Furthermore, given that the suspicions and allegations of financial misconduct turned out to be justified, they were confronted with individual members' propensity toward corruption in a context of extreme poverty that perhaps made it particularly difficult to withstand the temptation of squeezing financial profit from even slightly privileged social positions.

The *Maisha Marefu* group faced similar challenges, particularly with regard to establishing productive social ties with relevant local government authorities or NGOs that could translate into sustainable financial or informational support. *Maisha Marefu* was a neighborhood group founded in January 2008 with fifteen regular members, the majority of whom—as in the other neighborhood groups I got to know—had no formal work and lived off small-scale farming, petty trade, or the aid of relatives. The group was located in the same village as the *Uhuru* Health Center, so some 15 km from Tanga. This geographic distance from the city certainly contributed to the group members' sense of isolation. But they mainly felt neglected because, despite the fact that the group had been founded on the initiative of one of Tanga's NGOs, it had thereupon never received any support that could have enabled them to make any significant progress. Throughout 2008, PASADIT had provided the group with food rations twice, and on another occasion, the organization had made a small financial contribution to the care of two group members' orphaned children. Yet the group's chairman emphasized during one of their meetings that these initiatives were too few and far between to make a difference. "They planted the seeds, and then the rain was stopped," he commented bitterly.

The group lacked the starting capital to realize their plan to establish a small chicken farm or cultivate a piece of land. They simply did not know how to mobilize the necessary resources. Time and again, the chairman told me in frustration, they had invited the local government authorities in charge of social welfare to visit their group, but they never received a response; and up till September 2009, when I last talked to the group, no authority had ever reacted to their requests.

Maisha Marefu members also lamented that, despite all their efforts, there was no "direct communication" between the group and the Tanzania Red Cross Tanga Branch or the TAWG. Therefore, the chairman explained, the group had never received any further expert advice on how to deal with the quandaries of daily life with ARVs. He also mentioned that it was quite difficult for *Maisha Marefu* to stay updated on whatever temporary governmental or nongovernmental support initiatives were potentially accessible in Tanga and, in a second step, to meet the respective formal requirements, such as submitting project proposals, without the expertise of such organizations.

Nonetheless, the group gathered regularly, even during specific periods of the year when many of the members were particularly occupied by their farming work. They shared their experiences of being rejected, abused, and stigmatized, and provided mutual moral support. They shared advice that they had been given by medical professionals at the clinic with fellow group members suffering from similar adverse drug effects or temporary medical conditions. Members who needed help in an emergency situation were provided with a modest contribution from an "emergency fund" composed of the members' entrance fees (1,000 TSH) and the fines of 200 TSH that they had to pay when they showed up to a meeting more than twenty minutes late.

That they additionally invested their time in patiently answering the questions of a foreign anthropologist was anything but self-evident: Earlier that year, the chairman explained to me, *Maisha Marefu* had had a negative experience with another "white researcher" (*mtafiti mzungu*) who had approached the group with a request similar to mine. They had welcomed this woman to their meetings, and she had attended several times. One day, she arrived with some other people, supposedly the committee of a "donor organization" involved in AIDS work, and had pretended that she was the facilitator of *Maisha Marefu*. Thereafter, she had never shown up again, and the group suspected that she had used them to apply for research funding, of which they never saw a single Shilling themselves (for a very similar account of the abuse of a [self-]support group in Tanzania, see Marsland 2012).

Quite apart from the question of how much of the group's suspicions concerning the other researcher were true, this story not only explained *Maisha Marefu*'s members' initial reservations with respect to my research endeavor, but was also striking to me because it showed that the group members were quite aware of the "value" that their shared biological affliction could have for others. In consideration of their multiple failed attempts to forge social ties with relevant NGOs and local government officials that might be supportive in mobilizing economic resources, it must have been a particularly frustrating experience to see how someone else had capitalized on their "biovalue" in such an unscrupulous manner.

More Overwhelming Bureaucracy: The Tanzanian Social Action Fund (TASAF)

A profound sense of being disadvantaged, put off, and neglected, predominantly by government authorities, also emerged in the discussions during the meetings of the *Imara* and *Neema* groups, two further neighborhood groups in Tanga with some ten to fifteen regularly attending members.[8] A major reason for this was their highly unsatisfactory experience with TASAF. Both groups repeatedly complained about the arbitrary communication policy of the local government officials in charge concerning the funding requirements. Moreover, they felt powerless in the face of the highly bureaucratic and drawn-out processing procedures that, in their view, made it virtually impossible for them to obtain the desired support. With frustration, *Imara*'s thirty-eight-year-old chairwoman Tunaji told me during a group meeting in early September 2009 that they were still waiting for a response concerning their funding proposal, which they had submitted to TASAF more than a year earlier. Several times they had visited the office in the meantime, she explained, but they had never received any response other than that their proposal was "in progress."

As with many other groups in Tanga, *Imara* also wished to start a chicken breeding project, but the 128,000 TSH in their account would not carry them far. The longer the members discussed the seemingly deadlocked situation with regard to their TASAF proposal, the louder their voices grew. Frustration and anger broke out as they mentioned other groups of people who were *not* HIV-positive but who had supposedly received several millions of TSH from TASAF. "Where are *our* rights?!" they wondered vociferously. Then they brought up an argument that I was familiar with from my participation in the other groups: ultimately, they had been losing

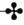

many members because it seemed so unlikely that the group would actually manage to get any funding and make even slight progress. Male members in particular, they claimed, had resigned from the group since it did not promise any material or financial gains for them. Every day, they finally remarked, they heard news on the radio about how much money was being invested in improving the care for people living with HIV in Tanzania. "These are all lies!" they concluded resentfully.

After the meeting, Tunaji invited me to her nearby house where she introduced me to her family. She pointed to a wooden construction in the backyard and explained that this was the only part of *Imara*'s planned chicken farm that existed so far. But their money did not suffice for more than a few wooden planks and some wire mesh. Since there were no chickens to go in the henhouse, in the meantime, Tunaji's family was using it as a rack to dry their laundry. Before I left, Tunaji asked me if I could possibly pass by the TASAF office and make another attempt to find out about the current status of their proposal. A white researcher, she assumed, might be more readily provided with concrete information than any other representative of their group.

When I arrived at Tanga's municipal building at nine o'clock in the morning a few days later in order to talk to the government employee in charge, a crowd of people was already waiting in front of his office. They were members of other community-based groups with queries regarding their funding applications. When it was finally my turn, I introduced myself, explained briefly about the purpose of my research, and asked the official if he could kindly provide me with a rough overview of TASAF activities in Tanga. Whether it was because he was aware of how many more people were waiting in front of his office or because he did not like the fact that an inquisitive researcher was using up his working time, he grumpily asked me who had sent me. I suddenly had the feeling that it might be detrimental to the *Imara* group if I told him that I had come upon their request, and so I told him that I had contact with several (self-)support groups in Tanga that in one way or another had had difficulties in applying for TASAF funding, which is why I wished to better understand the application process myself and get to know the perspective of the provider. "Okay, fine. Let's talk business," the official replied, even though he still did not seem quite satisfied. Quickly, he provided me with the key parameters of TASAF's operations in Tanga.

In total, there were seventeen community-based groups in Tanga District that at that particular point in time were receiving support from the fund, only one of which was a group of people living with HIV. Ten further funding proposals were currently in progress. TASAF had conducted eight "awareness meetings" in different neighborhoods of Tanga, particularly to inform the local ward councilors about the existence and purpose of the fund. These ward councilors were local government agents who officially had to confirm the neediness of the community-based groups in their ward that wished to apply for TASAF funding.

The groups themselves first needed to fill in an application form including the group's name, contact person, and planned project, have it signed by the ward councilor, and submit four copies to the TASAF office. If the application was deemed valid, a meeting was arranged with the group and their ward councilor in order to agree on the practical and financial details of the group's planned project. In a next step, the group had to submit a written proposal of the project, which was then presented to the Council Finance Committee, which was constituted of twelve to fifteen ward councilors and held meetings once a month. Once the committee had approved the proposal, the application was then sent to the TASAF headquarters in Dar es Salaam for final consideration.

The upper limit of funding per group amounted to 5 million TSH, and every group could only submit an application once. More than one hundred application forms had been submitted to his office, the official explained, pointing to piles of documents on his desk. Despite this large quantity, and the fact that the groups were required to submit a full proposal, he stated that the processing time per application should not exceed two to three months from submission of the proposal to a first funding disbursement. With this, he intimated that he now had to get back to work, and I left his office, after expressing my gratitude for his help and time.

Even though I had unfortunately not managed to find out about the precise current status of the evaluation of *Imara*'s funding proposal, this conversation was instructive to me as it showed what a highly intricate and bureaucratic process (self-) support groups had to pass through in order to have their funding proposal accepted and passed on to Dar es Salaam, which was itself still no guarantee of ultimately being granted their desired amount of money—if any at all. Furthermore, it seemed that this formal procedure was not only challenging to the applicant groups. The large number of applications that had been submitted to the TASAF office in Tanga suggested that the government officials in charge of processing these documents might have been equally overwhelmed by the enormous demand for financial support from the fund. Assuming that in other districts the number of applications were equally high, it is no wonder that none of the few neighborhood groups in Tanga that I knew of that had managed to submit a funding proposal had received any decisive response from the TASAF headquarters, even though—like the *Imara* group—they had already been waiting for many months. These groups' experiences constituted yet another example of the insufficiencies of governmental initiatives intended to provide financial and social support for people living with HIV, both in terms of their quantity and operationality.

Chapter Conclusion

It was rather challenging and cumbersome for people living with HIV in Tanga to mobilize financial, material, and social resources that could contribute to their social advancement, even if they made significant collective efforts in one of the countless (self-)support groups that mushroomed in all parts of the city. The demands of the innumerous group members, who were not only living with HIV but also below the poverty line and struggling for daily survival, by far outweighed the supply in terms of temporary governmental and nongovernmental support initiatives. The consequence was highly competitive relations between HIV (self-)support groups (cf. Cassidy and Leach 2009; Dilger 2012; Marsland 2012), but also between the various groups and other collectives of socially disadvantaged people fighting for the same few resources offered through initiatives such as TASAF.

In this highly contested field, the only ones who succeeded, firstly, were those who managed to obtain up-to-date information about specific programs offering assistance, and, secondly, those who were able to forge beneficial relationships with influential individuals or relevant institutions that could give them an advantage with regard to accessing these initiatives. In this respect, the provision of social support for people living with HIV could be viewed as a manifestation of patron–client relations that has been observed in other contexts of HIV/AIDS-related "development aid" in sub-Saharan Africa (cf. Beckmann and Bujra 2010; Cassidy 2010; Swidler 2009). For both individuals and entire (self-)support groups, it became highly relevant to become the "client" of the right "patron," in terms of a local NGO that was powerful enough to serve as a viable partner for larger national or transnational donor organizations. However, as the example of the *Maisha Marefu* group has shown, most of the self-organized neighborhood groups were not successful in forging such social links, not least because even the capacities of the larger NGOs like the TAWG were limited in relation to the large demand for their services. The lack of such ties was particularly impedimentary, because the neighborhood groups were largely made up of people with basic formal education who did not command the language to communicate with potential donor organizations at a high level and who lacked the expertise to submit funding proposals to respective initiatives without external help. There was, in short, a high degree of inequality regarding the opportunities that different groups in Tanga had in order to productively engage with the global treatment assemblage, as outlined in Chapter 2. And even though workshops were occasionally offered in which groups could learn how to set up income-generating projects, most groups simply failed to acquire sufficient starting capital to build up projects that could yield any significant profit. There was therefore a touch of bitter irony in health workers' and NGO staff members' all too frequently repeated admonitions of patient groups to take their fate into their own hands and strive for self-sustenance, without any further explanation of how to actually accomplish this.

Moreover, as evidenced by the episode of the TAWG's temporary shutdown and its subsequent limited resumption of services, even for those people who could afford to become members of a "well-nurtured" patient association like TALPHA, the sustainability of the support they received was anything but secure due to their "patron's" own vulnerable structural position in the global treatment assemblage, which rendered it highly contingent on the temporary thematic interests and agendas of transnational donor organizations.

A further problem that (self-)support groups faced were the highly bureaucratic procedures of the few available governmental support programs. The acquisition of a notary-certified constitution and the preparation of a formally acceptable funding proposal not only required the command of a particular terminology and an understanding of the logics of the respective funding institutions, which most groups lacked, it also posed enormous financial and logistical challenges. Additionally, unclear communication from the side of government officials made it hard for group leaders to fully comprehend the detailed requirements of particular application processes in the first place.

The intricate bureaucratic procedures that civil society groups were required to traverse in order to achieve governmental recognition can be viewed as the product of a particular history of the relationship between the state and civil society in Tanzania. During both the colonial and the socialist eras of the country, state authorities were keen on "keeping associations out of politics" (Marsland 2012, 479). And even though during the decades of structural adjustment in the postsocialist era "many government services were handed over to the NGO sector . . . strict government surveillance of NGOs continued in the form of tight bureaucratic procedures and restrictive definitions of the work that this sector was expected to do" (Marsland 2012, 479). On the one hand, the bureaucratic regulations that HIV (self-)support groups in Tanga were subjected to in order to receive governmental assistance reflected this history of the state's wariness vis-à-vis a politicized civil society (cf. Dilger 2013a, 184f). On the other hand, it is reasonable to assume that in the light of the limited available governmental resources for social support, the reduction of demand through the rejection of formally incomplete funding proposals constituted a secondary effect that was not entirely undesired.

Conclusions can also be drawn from the above-presented observations in Tanga's (self-)support groups with respect to the degree to which these groups could be viewed as platforms for the forging of adherent, self-responsible, politically active therapeutic citizens. In the neighborhood groups, I argue that this was the case only to a limited extent. Undoubtedly, the members of these groups contributed to each other's treatment adherence in terms of reminding one another of the correct intake of their pills, exchanging advice on how to better cope with particular side effects, and encouraging each other to endure difficult phases of the therapy. These group members nevertheless had a very marginal interest in getting engaged in political struggles for the rights of people living with HIV or actively expediting a larger change in attitude toward people living with the virus by disclosing their status and acting as role models in the wider public domain. Stemming mostly from the poorest social strata, they were instead predominantly in search of any opportunity that would help them make even slight economic progress. In fact, several members of the manifold groups that had been founded in mid-2009 on the initiative of AIDSRelief (see Chapter 3) told me that their groups had been established for the sole reason of having been promised that anytime soon, considerable amounts of funding would be made available for formally registered collectives of people living with HIV.

In the TALPHA groups, the situation differed inasmuch as the TAWG staff put greater efforts toward actively promoting their members' positive sense of self and adherence to a lifestyle in accordance with the requirements of their biomedical therapy, but also in terms of achieving their readiness to become "teachers of society" (*walimu wa jamii*). A core group of members indeed regularly offered testimonials about their life with HIV and ARVs in public events. However, this was only a small fraction of the entire body of TALPHA members. Furthermore, these members' engagement was not a form of confrontational politics vis-à-vis local government authorities, decision makers in the realm of global health policy, transnational donor organizations, or the pharmaceutical industry, as has been the case in South Africa, where the Treatment Action Campaign served as a prototype for social movements that could be conceptualized as the "production sites" of therapeutic or health citizenship (Robins 2004, 2006). The engagement of TALPHA members in Tanzania was largely in line with the government's as well as the international donor community's agendas of instilling biomedical rationality among the general public and motivating as many citizens as possible to regularly test for HIV. The lack of a spirit of or interest in politically challenging local, national, or international authorities, policies, or funding structures in relation to HIV/AIDS, in turn, is hardly surprising given the groups' financial dependency on the very actors and agencies that constitute this field (cf. Dilger 2005, 193; 2013a, 188).

Finally, the near complete breakdown of the TALPHA groups after the distribution of food and travel cost compensation had been stopped once more points to the fact that the large majority of these groups' members had most likely not joined the groups with the initial aim of gaining political clout in the fight for the rights of people living with HIV. Like most members of the neighborhood groups, they had rather done so primarily in the hope of obtaining whatever support might alleviate their dire living conditions.

The (self-)support groups unmistakably provided new members with a sense of belonging and the reassurance that life with HIV and ARVs could be manageable and perhaps even prosperous by way of the example of other members who had been living well with drugs for years. Nevertheless, the breakdown of the TALPHA groups, as well as the tensions that arose in the subgroups participating in the AFREDA initiative, suggest that biosociality—that is, a sense of commonality based on a shared biological predicament (Rabinow 1996)—was an insufficient foundation for the group members' cohesion and mutual solidarity. In the context of severe economic precariousness, many preferred to stop attending the group meetings and instead struggle for themselves alone when it became evident that no material benefits were to be expected from participation. Others perceived the act of engaging in relationships of mutual dependency with other members in equally precarious situations, in terms of joining specific subcollectives as required by AFREDA, as too risky. Ultimately, all of these people were thrown back yet again to rely on the support that they received (if any) within their kin-based networks of solidarity.

Finally, with respect to the idea of the (self-)support groups functioning as community-near platforms of patient surveillance, it can be concluded that to a certain extent, they did indeed serve this purpose. Both the members of the TALPHA and the neighborhood groups occasionally reported other members' deviance from their biomedical treatment regimes to the group, and in some cases, this information was indeed passed on to the CTC in charge. Aside from this, the TALPHA groups could be considered spaces where transnational governmentality played out at the local scale, insofar as their members were regularly provided with scientifically sound knowledge about HIV and reminded to act responsibly and in accordance with biomedical and public health reasoning. As the next—and final—chapter will show, however, the effect of these persistent "emancipatory" efforts remained limited. In fact, ideas and practices of religious healing—at times diametrically opposed to the biomedical understanding and treatment of HIV—were at least as appealing to ARV users as the advice and services they received in treatment centers and (self-)support groups; not least because they entailed the promise of being completely cured from the virus.

Notes

1. All group names are pseudonyms.
2. The generally observable gender imbalance in the groups reflects the same imbalance among people who get tested and enroll on treatment. Several reasons cause this phenomenon. Women usually have more contact with the health system through enrollment in antenatal care, which is obligatory for pregnant women in Tanzania. Moreover, women (particularly young and unmarried women and widows) have a more socially vulnerable position in society than men due to domestic gender-related power imbalances and economic marginalization, which is why they may perceive a greater incentive to join social collectives that promise support independently of familial and societal norms and obligations (cf. Dilger 2005, 189). Additionally, research in various parts of sub-Saharan Africa has shown that men exhibit a disinclination to make use of HIV services because of particular constructions of masculinity that "required men to be and act in control, to have know-how, be strong, resilient, disease free, highly sexual and economically productive" (cf. also Skovdal et al. 2011, 1; Reihling 2013). Such a notion of manhood, however, runs counter to "the 'good patient' persona who is expected to accept being HIV positive, take instructions from nurses and engage in health-enabling behaviours such as attending regular hospital visits and refraining from alcohol and unprotected extra-marital sex" (Skovdal et al. 2011, 1).
3. During the lunch break some time later, Salma explained to me that paying the membership fee and thus being listed as a regular group member was of utmost importance when approaching donors with a request for support. Donors were always keen to know exactly how many members the groups had, and this needed to be proved with the membership lists. Moreover, she added, the registration as a nonprofit association alone cost 50,000 TSH per year.
4. This contradicted the instructions provided to mothers of newborns at health institutions, which advised them to breastfeed their children exclusively during the first six months after birth.
5. According to its website (www.afredatanzania.org), AFREDA engages in a wide range of activities aimed at the empowerment and support not only of HIV-positive people but also of other groups of disadvantaged women,

men, children, and youth. It is funded by a multitude of governmental and nongovernmental organizations, as well as individual persons.

6. Some of the TAWG's HBC clients had been transferred to the Tanzania Red Cross Tanga Branch, but the latter's capacities could not come close to filling the gap left by the TAWG's service disruption.

7. See www.tasaf.org. Last accessed 4 September 2015.

8. As was the case with many (self-)support groups, including *Amani* and *Maisha Marefu*, their membership was mainly constituted of women, and the majority of the members had no formal employment.

Chapter 8
The Blood of Jesus, Witchcraft, and CD4 Counts
HIV/AIDS and ART in the Context of Traditional and Religious Healing

It was in early March 2011 that Tanzanian newspapers first featured reports on "the Wonder of Loliondo," a "miracle cure" for HIV/AIDS and other major chronic diseases provided by Ambilikile Mwasapile, a seventy-six-year-old retired pastor of the Evangelical Lutheran Church of Tanzania (ELCT), one of the country's largest mainline churches.[1] Over the following months, hundreds of thousands of people flocked to Mwasapile's home in Samunge (Loliondo Division), a remote village in the Sonjo plains way up north close to the Kenyan border. Day after day, Mwasapile—widely referred to as "Babu wa Loliondo" (Grandfather from Loliondo)—sedulously distributed his "magic cups" filled with an herbal concoction that he claimed to produce according to godly instruction. Subsequently, countless people suffering from chronic diseases, including HIV/AIDS, ceased to take their biomedical medications on the assumption that they had been cured.

The close entanglement of religious faith and a scientifically verifiable therapeutic substance in the form of Mwasapile's herbal elixir incited a highly informative and increasingly heated public controversy among government officials, medical professionals, scientists, religious leaders, traditional healers, and ordinary citizens. While some argued over the legitimacy of Mwasapile's performance as a traditional or faith healer and the possibility or degree of his medicine's therapeutic efficacy, others problematized the government's failure to provide adequate health care and protect its citizens from

Mwasapile and similar figures whom they held to be "quacks." The sick and suffering, in turn, struggled to make sense of the phenomenon in relation to their own religious faith and their profound longing for relief from chronic pain and illness.

The Wonder of Loliondo, the complex discourses that emerged about the phenomenon, and the enormous impact it had on the treatment itineraries of a large number of ART patients in and beyond Tanzania clearly point to the relevance of attending to religious discourses around HIV/AIDS in the endeavor to gain a more profound understanding of how people make sense of and practically deal with the disease and its biomedical response. The phenomenon itself, in turn, can only be understood in the context of religious approaches to healing, including "Christian, Islamic, and African ritual and 'traditional' practices"[2] (Dilger, Burchardt, and Van Dijk 2010, 374), which, since the establishment of biomedicine during the colonial era, have continued to exert great influence on the ways in which people in East Africa respond to ill health and misfortune (Bruchhausen 2006, 2010; Feierman 1985; Parkin 2014; Vaughan 1991).

HIV/AIDS and ART in Articulation with Religious Thought and Practice

There is by now a considerable body of social science literature exploring the entanglement of HIV/AIDS with religion in sub-Saharan Africa. From the very beginning of the epidemic, affected people embedded the disease in religious understandings of health, affliction, and healing in order to give meaning to the unknown threat. The disease was interpreted, for instance, as a consequence of an increasing nonadherence to preexisting social and moral regulations intended to sustain coherence within social collectives (Dilger 2005; Mogensen 1995; Wolf 2001). This seemed all the more logical as the onset of the epidemic unfolded simultaneously with processes of substantial social transformation and increasing economic hardship in societies that were heavily affected by SAPs and increasing privatization (cf. Dilger 2010; Ferguson 2006). In this context, HIV/AIDS became a powerful metaphor for the negative consequences of "modernity." Deeply restructuring processes of change were phrased in narratives of decline (Beckmann 2009; Dilger 2003; Setel 1999) that ascribed increasing social disorder, including changing gender relations and loosening sexual mores, to an ever more pervasive nonobservance of "traditional" moral norms.

Within the framework of African traditional religion, HIV/AIDS was often seen as a result of malevolent witchcraft (Behrend 2009; Mshana et al. 2006; Rödlach 2006; Yamba 1997), an idea that gave infected people the opportunity to blame others for their condition, to achieve agency in the form of engaging in a counterattack against the evildoer, and thus to sustain hope for a cure. The concept of spirit possession, which prevails in traditional, Islamic, and Christian healing practices, equally provided the possibility of being cured through the ritual deliverance of spirits, as well as through individual and collective prayers. Moreover, these interpretations functioned "as a secondary rationalization by addressing the question 'Why me and not another?'" (Behrend 2009, 34), which was of primary importance even for those who, in the biomedical sense, considered AIDS to be caused by a virus.

The discourse of Christian and Muslim denominations that construed HIV/AIDS as a divine punishment for illicit sexual behavior (e.g., Beckmann 2009; Svensson 2009; Togarasei 2010; see also Chapter 6) also constituted a framework within which this fundamental question could be answered. However, this way of reasoning put the blame solely on the immorality of the concerned persons and thus contributed significantly to their stigmatization. For proponents of this logic, the seeming answer to the problem lay in the reestablishment of conservative moral values and rigid behavioral prescriptions that regulated people's sexual relationships according to "the scriptures." This has been observed, for instance, in neo-Pentecostal churches (Dilger 2007), among neo-Traditionalists (Prince 2009), and within reformist Muslim circles in Tanzania (Becker 2009). While in the Pentecostal context this reestablishment was found to be marked by "the creation of [church members'] rupture with the past, traditions, social relations and nation-state projects" (Van Dijk 2009, 283), such fundamentalist and disruptive tendencies were juxtaposed by the material, social, and moral support that individual religious communities provided for their members, who were thus facilitated to better navigate their increasingly uncertain life worlds (cf. Dilger 2007, 78).

The former Christian mission churches also played an important role in the care for infected and affected people throughout Africa.

338

Some of these churches only began attending to people suffering from HIV/AIDS in a serious and uncondemnatory manner relatively late in the epidemic (Kalipeni, Muula, and Liveve 2009, 7)—and the official line of the Roman Catholic Church toward condom use has obstructed HIV prevention efforts for decades. They were found not only to have introduced "Manichean morality and according behavioral prescriptions, enforced by racial and economic segregation, into the African religious imagination" (Becker and Geissler 2009, 8), but just as other religious institutions, they also enabled "*communitas* and transgression of boundaries" (Becker and Geissler 2009, 8), an aspect of particular relevance to their HIV-positive followers (cf. Klaits 2010).

While these few examples show that over the last decade or so the interrelations between HIV/AIDS and religious practice have gained heightened attention, most of the studies in this area refer to the era before the large-scale rollout of ART in Africa or do not specifically address the interrelation between ART and religious practice. Yet, as argued above, in times of ART, the embedding of HIV/AIDS within wider religious conceptual frameworks continues to be of significant analytical importance. Indeed, the longer wide-scale public treatment programs have been running, the clearer it has become that the corresponding biomedicalization of people's ideas about HIV/AIDS, suffering, and death has not materialized to the expected extent. Evidently, many patients' understanding of "healing" cannot be narrowed down to rising CD4 counts and increased body weight, and the repeated warnings of health workers that ART does not terminate the HI-virus but only "puts it to sleep" could be understood as an outright invitation to look for therapeutic alternatives that promise a "real cure."

Among the still relatively few studies on the mutual impact of expanding ART and religious practice in Africa, similarities in the fashioning of selves through Christian and biomedical techniques of counseling have raised scholarly interest (Becker 2014; Burchardt 2009; Nguyen 2009b). Other works have explored theological understandings of ART among religious leaders. Kalipeni and colleagues interviewed "a number of influential [Christian] clergy in Malawi" in order to get a preliminary sense of the "attitude of the Church with regard to ARVs and what directions are religious and practices taking [sic]" (Kalipeni et al. 2009, 8). By citing two clergy members' responses to the same questions about the use of ART in detail, the authors demonstrate significantly opposing attitudes toward ART across Christian denominations in Malawi.[3] On the one hand, they cite a representative of what they call a "compassionate" church who fully supported the provision of ART and called for the active cooperation of his church with biomedical institutions and organizations based on the conviction that "discoveries that promote life within the confinements of moral laws are permitted by God" (Kalipeni et al. 2009, 6). On the other hand, they cite the clergyman of a "not so compassionate church" who contended that "HIV/AIDS is due to immorality and the prevalence of ARVs does not cancel out this immoral basis, but simply covers it up and can only encourage the behavior" (Kalipeni et al. 2009, 10).

Based on a study of the understandings of life, death, and healing in the context of Pentecostal and African Independent Churches in Botswana, Lovemore Togarasei (2010) has pointed equally to the detrimental influence of pastors who argue that "the ability of ARVs to prolong life is challenging God who is the source of life and healing" (Togarasei 2010, 429). In opposition to this stance, and similar to the above-cited "compassionate" Malawian church leader, Togarasei calls for a new theology "that accommodates ARVs in the realm of God," a "theology of ARVs" based on the principles of "the sanctity of life" and the notion "that scientific discoveries that enhance human life should be seen as God sanctioned" (Togarasei 2010, 433).

According to Amusa Balogun (2010), such a theological argumentation in favor of ART is also fully compatible with the Qu'ran and the prophet Muhammad's *ahadith*.[4] Provided that ARVs do not contain any ingredients that, according to Islamic prescriptions, are considered unlawful, Balogun argues that "the use of ARVs should not be seen as contrary to Muslims' reliance on Allah for cures and healing, but represents compliance with the prophetic tradition that every servant of Allah must seek treatment for his diseases" (Balogun 2010, 464). Jack Ume Tocco's (2014) study of Islamic prophetic medicine in Northern Nigeria, however, shows that such a theoretical legitimization of ART according to Islamic principles by no means translates into an unconditional embrace of the treatment by all fractions that constitute a country's usually highly heterogeneous Muslim community.

As these studies suggest, several years after the introduction of large-scale biomedical treatment programs in sub-Saharan Africa, "bodies and people were not disciplined by the available biomedical treatment regimes in the ways envisaged (or at least hoped for) by national and international policymakers as well as local healthcare providers" (Dilger et al. 2010, 380). Let me now turn to the Wonder of Loliondo, which serves as a particularly vivid example of this observation.

"Relief for Troubled Mankind": The Wonder of Loliondo

It was not long before the middle-aged lady sitting next to me on the plane inquired about my opinion concerning Mwasapile. It was early May 2011, I was about to start my second field stay, and I had already gained a rough idea of what was going on in Samunge through respective online coverage of Tanzanian newspapers. Before I could answer, the lady readily explained that she was from Dar es Salaam but had worked as a nurse in Europe for decades. After expressing her professional doubts about the hygienic conditions of Mwasapile's medicinal cups, she slowly argued her way toward its potential efficacy. The skin disease of her sister's neighbor, which he had suffered from for years, had supposedly been cured by Mwasapile's medicine. Elaborating on her own indecisiveness, the lady finally concluded that she had to see for herself: "Seeing is believing!"

This woman's ambiguity was emblematic of the state of the Tanzanian public at the time, which was engaged in a multilayered and intense debate about scientificity and efficacy; religious faith; medical and religious authority; governmental, civic, and media responsibility; and economic and political development, which had been sparked by Mwasapile's magic cup.

When the Wonder of Loliondo first appeared in Tanzanian media, the sick had already been flocking to Samunge in their thousands to see Mwasapile, who claimed that God had revealed to him in a dream how to prepare a concoction from a particular tree's roots in order to cure major chronic diseases, including HIV/AIDS. In the dream, Mwasapile was also instructed that the healing concoction should be handed out exclusively by him at the modest cost of 500 TSH per cup—the price of a regular cup of tea.

Mwasapile initially provided his medicine to a few fellow villagers. Some indeed felt their afflictions improving and the word spread like bush fire. By March 2011, people were coming from all parts of Tanzania, the cars and buses queuing for kilometers on the rough dirt roads crossing the Ngorongoro Conservation Area. The public imagination was incited, and biblically inspired narratives of the lame walking and the blind seeing circulated. The first testimonial of a thirty-year-old, HIV-positive widow living in Samunge featured in a Tanzanian national newspaper in mid-March. Since drinking what Mwasapile had supposedly called "God's miracle cure for the ailing nation" (Mosoba 2011), the woman, who had been on ART for several years, claimed that her CD4 levels had started rising until, to the amazement of her clinicians, she had tested HIV-negative. A clinician at the woman's health facility confirmed the miraculous cure and instructed her to stop ART (*Mwananchi*, 14 March 2011). Certainly, this story fuelled people's hope and increased the influx to the village—and the infrastructural chaos this created in the entire region. At the height of its popularity, approximately six thousand people were provided with the cup on a daily basis. Sick people, many of whom had traveled hundreds of kilometers, had to wait days for their turn. Hygienic conditions became increasingly worse, accommodation was unavailable, and food and drinking water became scarce and expensive, a situation that seriously endangered the survival of patients who had been removed from hospitals by relatives and had already struggled with the exhausting journey on rough dirt roads.

The Minister of Health and Social Welfare, Dr. Haji Mponda, issued his first official statement on 10 March, prohibiting further distribution of the medicine until the hygienic conditions were addressed, Mwasapile had "registered his services in line with laid down procedures," and an expert task force had assured that the medicine was safe for human consumption (*The Guardian*, 10 March 2011). His orders remained without effect. Regional health authorities claimed that they had never received any written directive from the health minister and Babu continued to distribute his concoction as usual (*The Citizen*, 10 March 2011). Bishop Laizer of the Evangelical Lutheran Church reacted to the health minister's criticism with a rebuke: "It is not right to halt the service, which has spiritual elements and it is also not right to take such action without involving stakeholders who are *wananchi* [citizens]," he reprimanded, and requested that the government actively support Mwasapile's services for the benefit of citizens. On the following day, the Minister of State in the Prime Minister's Office, Mr. William Lukuvi, mitigated the health minister's directive, saying, "The government cannot interfere with religious beliefs because it is not in its policy to do so" (*Daily News*, 11 March 2011). He further explained that arrangements would be made to "ensure peace and security for the 6,000 patients already camped in the area to get the medicine before allowing more people in" and "to improve the environment by engaging more health workers, first aid teams and ambulances to make life in the otherwise surrounding bush area become 'habitable'" (*Daily News*, 11 March 2011).

The dispensing of Mwasapile's medicine was never officially stopped. On the contrary, more and more high-level politicians, including the former prime minister and several current ministers, arrived in Samunge in order to drink a cup of the concoction. One member of parliament, Beatrice Shelukindo, "the first high profile opinion leader in the country to come out in the open testifying the potency of the 'miracle drug,'" encouraged all Tanzanians to "fully exploit the golden chance" (Luhwago 2011). Claiming that relatives of hers had been cured of cancer, HIV/AIDS, and diabetes, she reasoned that "not everything is politics," that this was a matter of "divine power," and—alluding to the government's notice of ongoing scientific research on the concoction—that "God is unresearchable" (Luhwago 2011).

Two logics of healing and efficacy were entangled in Mwasapile's concoction: scientifically verifiable *materia medica* in the form of medicinal plant extracts on the one hand, and faith in God and her/his servant Mwasapile on the other. This combination rendered the magic cup a polysemantic symbol that provided ample contact surface for both proponents and critics of natural science and religiously informed concepts of illness and healing. While some traditional healers were scandalized that Mwasapile had not initially been obliged to register according to Tanzania's Traditional and Alternative Medicines Act (The United Republic of Tanzania 2002)—a procedure that was usually painstakingly followed and whose breach could be heavily fined[5] (*Mwananchi*, 26 March 2011)—Mwasapile himself did not tire of insisting that he was no traditional healer in the first place. He had, he argued, no expert knowledge of medicinal plants but simply functioned as an instrument of God; the efficacy of his medicine, he claimed, rested solely in his and others' unconditional belief in the healing powers of the Almighty (see Mbonea 2011a). "This medicine . . . has the power of the blood of Jesus Christ, the son of God, so even if the bugs [viruses] are still there, they will not be able to fight with the blood of Jesus," he explained (*An-Nuur*, 3–9 June 2011a).[6]

More than Mwasapile himself, who displayed rather modest behavior, it was his circle of close confidants and guards who, with their public sermons, started a process of mystification. The crowds were repeatedly reminded of the holiness of the pastor and urged to refrain from any sinful and antisocial behavior on his compound (see, e.g., *An-Nuur*, 3–9 June 2011b). Upon receiving complaints, Mwasapile once admonished high level society members to follow the regular procedure and wait for their turn as everyone else, otherwise the medicines would not prove effective for them (*Nipashe*, 21 March 2011). Reacting to reports of middle-aged men who, after taking the concoction, thought themselves safe to indulge in unprotected sexual activities (Figure 8.1), he also made clear that

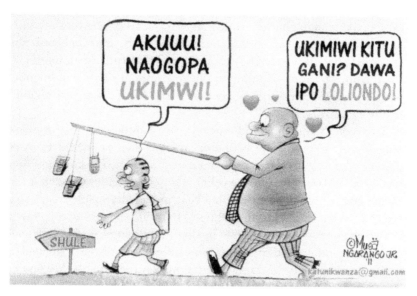

Figure 8.1. "I am afraid of AIDS!"—"AIDS, what's that? There's medicine in Loliondo!" Source: *Tanzania Daima*, 6 May 2011 © Musa Ngarango Jr., used with permission.

his medicine was only curative and should not be mistaken for a vaccine against HIV/AIDS and other diseases.

Mwasapile claimed to have communicated with God several times. God had told him to start treating the nation's orphans and inmates, whereupon he requested the government to support the organization of respective transports and initiatives (Mvungi 2011). On other occasions, God had issued concrete instructions concerning the price of the medicine and had finally allowed Mwasapile to accept donations from the cured, which he had vigorously refused before (*An-Nuur*, 3–9 June 2011b). Mwasapile also refused to have his medicine processed into pills—a recommendation made by an expert delegation from the WHO concerned about hygienic issues—arguing that God had not allowed him to do so (Juma 2011b).

The Tanzanian Christian community was divided concerning Mwasapile's alleged close ties with God. While the leaders of some mainline churches encouraged their followers "that it was alright Biblically for them to drink the Loliondo medicine" (*Daily News*, 11 March 2011) and moreover publicly ingested it themselves (Silla and Juma 2011), other—predominantly Pentecostal—leaders issued warnings against engaging in Mwasapile's "satanic work" in that way. Bishop Kakobe, founder of the Full Gospel Bible Fellowship Church and actively engaged in individual and collective faith healing ceremonies himself (see Dilger 2007), sharply attacked Mwasapile for applying the "power of darkness" (*nguvu za giza*) (Juma 2011a), precluding the possibility that God would collaborate with somebody who was not "saved."[7] Another Pentecostal pastor claimed that Mwasapile was not enlightened by God but by evil spirits (*majini*) and admonished his followers not to consult him because, rather than through the intake of herbal medicine, healing was only possible through the Word of God and prayers (Mwachali 2011).

Muslim leaders issued hardly any comments in public. The sheikh of Samunge's small Muslim community, however, explained that the inhabitants of the Sonjo Plains had been using the *mugariga* tree, the vernacular term for the plant that formed the base of Mwasapile's concoction, for centuries, long before the pastor had had his revelation. Without generally denying the plant's therapeutic efficacy, he clarified that it could not cure serious afflictions, let alone diseases like HIV/AIDS or diabetes. He rather assumed that expanding the influence of Christianity among "irreligious" locals was Mwasapile's main intention (*An-Nuur*, 1–7 July 2011). Among some of Mwasapile's proponents, the sheikh's allegations apparently incited considerable anger. A few weeks after they featured in the press, his house was set on fire and completely burned down, fortunately without causing harm to him or anyone else (*An-Nuur*, 1–7 July 2011).

These publicly staged disputes and critiques had no significant effect on the pilgrims' faith in the miracle potion. By mid-May, Mwasapile had dispensed some three million cups (Frank 2011). The continued massive influx of patients affected an immense boost of entrepreneurship in Samunge and along the main entryways leading to the village (e.g., Mikaili 2011). Government authorities issued obligatory licenses (5,000–10,000 TSH) for every car heading toward Samunge. Countless safari companies in Arusha, the closest large city to Samunge (400 km away) and the main starting point for the touristic circuits in the national parks of northern Tanzania, were quick to adjust their portfolios. Return tickets to Samunge were sold for up to 150,000 TSH, a sum easily equivalent to three or four months' salary for the poorer pilgrims. Restaurants, small shops, tent hotels, and sanitary services sprang up along the routes, providing their owners with considerable income. Even large companies jumped at the chance of capitalizing on Mwasapile's popularity. Major mobile communication companies expanded their coverage to Loliondo and gave Mwasapile cell phones as gifts. A solar energy enterprise bestowed him with a medal for his "selfless service" and a donation of technological equipment worth some four million Tanzanian Shillings (Mhala 2011).

The government authorities struggled to contain the chaos in and on the way to Loliondo. Three official points of entry to the area were established, where every car had to be registered. Upon Babu's request, Prime Minister Pinda called for the public not to set out for Loliondo for seven days, and further cars were prohibited from continuing their journey (Kisembo 2011). This caused considerable protest among travelers who held the government responsible for casualties among the waiting sick (*Nipashe*, 11 April 2011). At this point in time there were about twenty-four thousand people queuing for Babu's cup. On the other hand, the government tried to "create a conducive environment for [the] pastor's services" (Kisembo 2011). It ordered the authorities of Ngorongoro District to install water pipes at Mwasapile's house, set up tents and toilets for the waiting, improve the conditions of the roads and the local dispensary, and provide sufficient space for burying the dead (*Nipashe*, 29 March 2011). Despite such efforts, the government hardly managed to tackle even the most pressing infrastructural challenges of the mass pilgrimage to Samunge. Paradoxically, however, it did not even temporarily disrupt the run on Mwasapile's medicine by enacting the national policy on HIV/AIDS that determines that "all public claims of cures for HIV/AIDS by traditional and faith healers or other care providers shall be discouraged until such claims are authenticated and approved by government agencies" (The United Republic of Tanzania 2001, 33).

Scientific Claims and Religious Appeals

In contrast to his initially skeptical position, a few weeks after his ineffective orders to halt Mwasapile's services, Health Minister Mponda stepped into the breach *for* him. Since Mwasapile attracted equally high numbers of pilgrims among both Tanzanian and Kenyan citizens, Kenyan Public Health Minister Beth Mugo had vigorously requested that Mwasapile be immediately arrested and stopped from misleading the public. Mponda, however, dismissed this suggestion as "unfair," saying that his Kenyan colleague "had no sufficient evidence to prove her statement," and rather referred to ongoing scientific research about the safety of Mwasapile's medicine for human consumption (Philemon 2011).

Indeed, on the following day, the results of a first scientific report were published. Two researchers from the NIMR and the Muhimbili University of Health and Allied Sciences in Dar es Salaam had identified Mwasapile's miraculous tree as *Canissa Spinarum*, parts of which were commonly used for therapeutic purposes and as a nutritional supplement by various Tanzanian pastoralist ethnic groups (Malebo and Mbwambo 2011, 10f). Drawing on a meta-analysis of preexisting scientific studies on the plant's chemical properties, the researchers concluded that Mwasapile's concoction was fit for human consumption and may in fact have therapeutic effects (Malebo and Mbwambo 2011, 11ff). However, they strongly recommended further investigation "on optimum dosage, dosing schedule and duration of treatment per ailment" (Malebo and Mbwambo 2011, 21). On the basis of this report, Mponda and a representative of the Tanzania Food and Drugs Authority publicly stated that the consumption of Mwasapile's medicine was not harmful for humans. Nevertheless, they also made clear that its actual levels of efficacy were still being investigated and that the results could not be expected any time soon (*Nipashe*, 29 March 2011).

Meanwhile, the COSTECH had begun verifying the possibility of patenting Mwasapile's concoction, and, to this purpose, had tried to establish the medicine's unique characteristics (Shekighenda 2011). The possibility that—contrary to the NIMR report—the medicine could still contain an undiscovered active ingredient was equally considered in a report of the Tanzania Medicinal Plant Foundation, which claimed to have verified that the concoction either consisted of a combination of *Canissa Spinarum* and another plant, or was made from a completely different plant altogether (Katulanda 2011). The concoction's efficacy was further investigated by researchers of the NIMR, COSTECH, and WHO, who explained that they were involved in the close observation of two hundred persons who had drunk Mwasapile's potion, and, furthermore, that trials with diabetic laboratory rats were being conducted (Juma and Mshana 2011).

The absence of scientific evaluation of precisely what effects Mwasapile's medicine had on diverse physical afflictions seemed not to have any impact on the mass of pilgrims travelling to Loliondo. Incomplete and misleading media reporting further fuelled the run on the miracle cure. "Experts: Babu's cup is fantastic protection" (*Wataalamu: Kikombe cha "Babu" ni kinga bomba*) headlined the Tanzanian news source *Habari Leo* (Tesha 2011), citing the results of the preliminary NIMR report, while *Business Week* quoted a representative of the Tanzanian Medicinal Plant Foundation who said that "though not all, people are getting cured of HIV and other incurable diseases after getting Loliondo treatment" (Chiwambo 2011).

While on the one hand the government's position was informed by scientific rationality, the actions and public statements of some high-level politicians illustrated an incongruous stance and a general reservation about interfering in matters of faith. Despite affirming her intention to take strict disciplinary measures against any type of self-proclaimed healer advertising cures for chronic diseases similar to Mwasapile's (Justice 2011)—and indeed several copycats were barred from dispensing their herbal brews—Deputy Minister of

Health, Dr. Lucy Nkya, explained that the government was unable to intervene in Mwasapile's case "because his work involves faith" (*Daily News*, 1 July 2011). Reports of members of the political elite who travelled to Samunge and had a cup of the pastor's potion did not stop.

As inconsistent as the government's reactions were, Mwasapile's impact on the treatment itineraries of people living with HIV/AIDS was quite tangible. "I repeat again, those suffering from HIV/AIDS need just one cup of my medicine and they don't have to continue taking hospital medication," read his most explicit statement in this respect (Nkwame 2011). Indeed, many ART patients throughout the country and abroad gratefully acknowledged his encouraging instructions and stopped taking their medication after supposedly being cured. The numbers of patients lost-to-follow-up were reported to increase significantly at various treatment centers (e.g., *Majira*, 9 June 2011), and rising HIV-test rates in certain regions were attributed to Loliondo pilgrims inquiring about their serostatus after they had received Mwasapile's medicine (*The Citizen*, 6 August 2011).

As time elapsed, however, testimonials of people who had waited in vain for their miraculous cure to set in increased. Infuriated relatives of those who had succumbed to relapses of their afflictions after the discontinuation of their biomedical therapies raised their voices. "Medically verifiable stories of cures are totally absent in the media. Whose interests are being served, only the profiteers'?" asked a critical columnist with regard to the government officials and private entrepreneurs for whom the mass of pilgrims constituted an enormously lucrative source of income (Patten 2011). By mid-July, the "Mseto[8] of faith" (*mseto wa kiimani*) had lost much of its credibility and the increasing death reports exerted a significant impact. The number of cars passing through Samunge each day decreased to 100–150, and Samunge's "new economy" started collapsing (Mbonea 2011b).

In late July, the first threats of taking Mwasapile to court were made by Reverend Christopher Mtikila, the highly controversial leader of the anti-Islamic nationalist Tanzania Democratic Party, who claimed to act on behalf of relatives of deceased Loliondo pilgrims. He also intended to call those politicians to account who had publicly taken the pastor's potion and thus fueled the run on Loliondo (*Sani*, 20–22 July 2011). In August, the chair of TANOPHA issued similar threats (Going 2011), and the vice president of the Medical Association of Tanzania (MAT) once more called for the government to clearly communicate to its citizens how dangerous Mwasapile's healing promise was (Mlekani 2011). Health Minister Mponda, however, simply called for patience and declared that he would issue an official statement once the scientific evaluations of Mwasapile's concoction had yielded results (Makore 2011).

Mwasapile continued dispensing his medicine without hindrance, and when the tuberculosis ward at a nearby hospital was closed in mid-September due to a lack of new admissions (*The Citizen*, 17 September 2011), he took this as proof of God's healing powers and a further legitimization to continue his services: "I don't cure people, but the Almighty God does it. It is illogical to blame the one who brings relief to the troubled mankind" (*The Citizen*, 17 September 2011). However, over the following months fewer and fewer people descended on his home seeking "the cup," and with the thinning stream of pilgrims, the pastor's media attention waned.

In February 2012, Mwasapile was reported to have claimed that "God has shown him other 'new miracles,' which are beyond the current 'magic cure'" (Philemon 2012), and which presaged another, even greater wave of millions of pilgrims that would flood his village. He and his assistants thus cleared the area and prepared for the construction of several buildings to house the expected masses of patients, while he once more demanded that "the government authorities improve the main road from Arusha and other destinations to the village in order to ease transport" (Philemon 2012).

The government, however, finally announced preliminary results of the ongoing scientific study of his miracle cure's efficacy: a randomized, controlled trial with a cohort of more than two hundred patients who had ingested the concoction. Dr. Mponda's successor, Minister of Health and Social Welfare Dr. Hussein Mwinyi, informed the public that Mwasapile's medicine, which he claimed could cure chronic diseases including HIV/AIDS, "had no such effects on the virus nor on diabetes" (Shekighenda 2012).

Initially, Mwasapile was apparently little impressed by the scientists' verdict. After all, he had always clarified that the efficacy of the cup was based exclusively on the individual receiver's faith. Yet a few months later, he struck out against all opponents of his medicine. He ascribed the low demand for his medicine to "propaganda and smear campaigns waged on him by medical doctors and NGOs, and a supposed witch-hunt by Pentecostal churches, combined to frustrate him and instill fear in would-be pilgrims" (Mosoba 2012). Ever since, Mwasapile has continued announcing a soon-to-come Wonder of Loliondo, whose scope would be even bigger than its predecessor (Ayo 2015; Mwilolezi 2016).

Ambilikile Mwasapile: An Uncharismatic Semi-Prophet? A Socio-Political Interpretation

In some newspaper articles, Mwasapile was addressed as *nabii*, an Akkadian term of the Old Testament designating "one who is either called by God or announces the message of God" (Anderson and Johnson 1995, 8), which found its way into Swahili through Arabic influence. As Gerhardus Oosthuizen explains in reference to the Old Testament, "The prophet was conscious of the fact that the revelation he received came from God and that it had not origi-nated from his own consciousness" (1992, 3). In this literal sense, it seems appropriate to designate Mwasapile as a prophet. As has been argued in a considerable body of historical literature, however, the crucial aspect of what makes a prophet is his/her role as a leader in times of crisis and as an instigator of social change (cf. Wallace 1956). Throughout the nineteenth and twentieth centuries, African prophetic movements have emerged as a response to destructive external influences in the form of colonial conquest and its related epidemics, and to a community's or society's perceived inner moral decay, with all three phenomena often being closely interconnected (Ranger 1992). Indeed, David Anderson and Douglas Johnson extend the definition of prophet beyond a mere divinely informed leader of social and political protest:

> The utterances of prophets need not always be directly predictive: they will also encompass commentary upon the past, and may be interpreted as offering guidance on the regulation of social and political practice in the present. This more pervasive relation sustaining the moral community places the prophet in a social context that is much broader than mere reaction to crisis: the prophet is also a barometer of social and political behaviour. (Anderson and Johnson 1995, 19)

In order to explain the enormous momentum of the Wonder of Loliondo, I suggest examining the phenomenon in the context of prophetic movements in Africa, particularly in comparison to a similar case in Malawi where, in the early 1990s, one Billy Chisupe equally attracted hundreds of thousands with an herbal cure for HIV/AIDS. The case of Chisupe has largely been interpreted along the lines of Anderson and Johnson above (Probst 1999; Schoffeleers 1999). As with Mwasapile, he had revelational dreams, in which his grandfather and an unknown man showed him a plant that could cure HIV/AIDS. After his story had been broadcast on a national radio channel, thousands started pouring into his remote village demanding his freely dispensed concoction, known as *mchape*. The whole phenomenon was reminiscent of the witch cleansing movement that swept Malawi in the 1930s, which was referred to by the same name.

The mass influx to Chisupe's village caused infrastructural and sanitary chaos similar to the situation in Loliondo, and the Malawian government equally struggled (or hesitated) to counter Chisupe's attractiveness with scientific evidence of his concoction's inefficacy (Probst 1999, 121).

All this happened at a time of

> all-pervasive . . . crisis caused concretely by the AIDS pandemic, a severe famine triggered by a succession of poor rainy seasons, a drastic devaluation of the Malawian Kwacha and, more generally, a widely shared disappointment in the way things had been developing after the elections of 1994. (Schoffeleers 1999, 411)

Chisupe responded to this multilayered crisis by not only providing a cure that the government and scientific community had not been able to come up with, but also accompanying it with an explicitly articulated social and political protest, which induced Probst to reflect "that just as the old *mchape* was a local comment on the effects of the colonial intervention and the global economic recession, the recent *mchape* was a new and timely comment on just another feature of 'modernity's malcontents' (Comaroff and Comaroff 1993), this time in the form of AIDS" (Probst 1999, 121). The second *mchape* cult was considered a "counter-institution" to "the hegemony of the post-Banda state" (Probst 1999, 125), with Chisupe as its leader bestowed with personal charisma in the Weberian sense, implying a "break with the established order" (Ter Haar 1992, 239).

There are striking similarities between the Wonder of Loliondo and Chisupe's *mchape* '95 cult. Similar to Malawi in the mid-1990s, Tanzania's political and socioeconomic situation in the early 2010s has been widely perceived as a multilevel crisis, especially due to the large number of poor and low-educated people without formal employment or any form of social security. Disappointment was often expressed by Tanzanians who on a daily basis were confronted with large-scale corruption cases among the country's political, business, and religious leadership, as well as the government's inability to provide the most basic conditions for "development," such as a stable power supply. The complaint of "those up there" not caring about "us down here" was a persistent comment on the seemingly ruthless national elite.

Negative experiences with the national health care infrastructure were equally frustrating. Even in Tanga, a city where hospitals and health centers were in reach, basic equipment and medicines were often unavailable and had to be purchased in private pharmacies. Health centers were overcrowded; health professionals often insufficiently trained, overwhelmed, and sometimes corrupt; and treatment for serious injuries or diseases hardly available. Searching for treatment for relatively minor physical afflictions could become a painstaking odyssey through health facilities and pharmacies with an uncertain outcome, and could easily consume a family's entire financial reserves. In the light of such experiences, associating the Wonder of Loliondo with the desolate situation of national health care delivery seemed natural:

> Some say the Loliondo rush is an indication of a failed health system, which over the fifty-year independence period hasn't responded to the health demands of millions of people in the country. With an underfunded budget, Tanzania's healthcare system has in some cases become a "death trap," condemning some people to death, not because they are severely sick, but as a consequence of poor medical services. (Mgamba 2011)

There was, in short, a "serious crisis of expectation" similar to the one in Malawi during the mid-1990s, where "people had become disillusioned with politics and everything that had to do with the common good" (Schoffeleers 1999, 410). At this moment, Mwasapile emerged as an almost Messianic figure offering hope to the entire "ailing nation" (Mosoba 2011). Connections were made to Tanzania's highly venerated "father of the nation," Julius Nyerere, respectfully called *mwalimu* (teacher), who fifty years earlier had redeemed this same nation from the ailment of colonial subjugation:

> The number of women and newly born dying in delivery is among the highest in the world, and real reform is rejected in all quarters of political society, and many are preparing to destroy the peace in the country if certain preconditions of policy are not met. The Loliondo priest looks eerily like the late Mwalimu, his name Ambilikile is close to Mwalimu's teasing name of "Haambiliki," the potion he administers is the restoration of the Arusha Declaration that many wish for. (Jozen 2011)

The entanglement of longings for both spiritual and political leadership became even more apparent in an article referring to Mwasapile as the "grandfather of the nation" who, through his God-sanctioned miracle cure, was engaged in fighting disease—one of humankind's fiercest enemies (Nyenyembe 2011). Furthermore, just as Chisupe's cult was read along the lines of historic protest movements against colonialism, the Loliondo narrative carried an anti-imperialist undertone conceptualizing Mwasapile and his miracle cure as a challenge to neocolonial capitalist exploitation in the form of the Western HIV/AIDS industry alleged to capitalize on the African AIDS sufferer (Hiza 2011).

While these readings of the Wonder of Loliondo suggest a remarkable similarity with the prophetic movement of Malawi's *mchape* '95, there is a significant difference between the two phenomena. Chisupe formulated open and fierce critique against the political establishment and at the same time actively coconstructed his role as a leader in the process of Malawian society's moral renewal. Mwasapile, by contrast, was an "economically modest, socially humble, publicity-shy Loliondo senior citizen who has shot to virtual international stardom, obviously against his will" (Kaigarula 2011). Apart from his warning that his concoction should not be mistaken for an invitation to engage in "immoral sexual behavior" and his socially leveling appeal to the "rich and mighty" to queue like anyone else, Mwasapile hardly ever issued statements that could be read as judgments on society's moral state, a political protest against its fraudulent leadership, or a grab for political power. On the contrary, he repeatedly emphasized his own ordinariness and reminded the crowds to praise God instead of himself (see, e.g., Mbonea 2011b). Rather than positioning himself contra the state "as the cult's 'ritual other'" (Baumann in Probst 1999, 118), he personally welcomed every politician to Samunge, and he even politely posed in pictures wearing the VODACOM or AIRTEL T-shirts that he was given by these multinationals, who epitomize more than anything else "neo-imperialistic" capitalism.

Due to his political reticence and modest appearance, which rendered him a sort of uncharismatic semiprophet, Mwasapile was possibly perceived as not powerful enough to incite a politically motivated protest movement and was thus spared from governmental regulation and interference to a greater extent than Chisupe in Malawi. Rather than being a prophet in his own right, Mwasapile seemed to have become a projection surface for the disillusioned masses watching out for one—a state of affairs that nevertheless makes him an interesting "barometer of social and political behaviour" (Anderson and Johnson 1995, 19).

Another remarkable point is the enormous economic boost that Mwasapile's concoction brought to an entire region that is far off Tanzania's economic hubs. The masses of pilgrims constituted more than just a considerable source of income for private entrepreneurs along the pilgrimage routes. They also flushed enormous amounts of money into the registers of government authorities who, through taxing all incoming cars and helicopters, made millions of Shillings over the months. This, in turn, induced the protest of local villagers, who complained that—as so often—nothing of these revenues was trickling down to those who actually had to cope with the ecological and social damage caused by the stampede of pilgrims. By the end of March 2011, Mwasapile himself was reported to have made some 50 million TSH through dispensing his cups, of which the ELCT and Mwasapile's group of assistants were given 20 million, and Mwasapile remained with 10 million (*Nipashe*, 31 March 2011).

Aside from the economic aspects and the question of whether or not Mwasapile can be considered a prophet, the Wonder of Loliondo undeniably sparked a fierce discussion among the Tanzanian public between the proponents of biomedical science and those defending a religiously informed concept of faith healing. In practice, however, these factions were not so discrete. The government's hesitance and ambivalence, the considerable number of high-level politicians queuing up for the cup, and the masses of pilgrims for whom scientific evidence was of minor importance, suggested that large parts of the population running through all social strata did not adhere exclusively to biomedical logic but at least considered the *possibility* of there being a cure for their ailments beyond insulin, antihypertensive pills, and ARVs.

As will be outlined in the following section, the basis for such considerations is not only to be found in the influence of nationally renowned faith healers and religious authorities like Mwasapile or his fierce opponent Bishop Kakobe. Healers and religious leaders at the grassroots level also contributed a significant part to the sustenance of powerful discourses about HIV/AIDS that interpreted the disease in nonbiomedical terms and fuelled people's hope for a cure.

Staking Claims and Seeking Redemption: Religious Leaders, Traditional Healers, and ART Patients' Navigations in a Contested Field of Healing

"This Is Not What Our Religion Teaches Us": Local Religious Authorities' Opinions of the Wonder of Loliondo

All three of the religious leaders (one Pentecostal pastor and two Muslim sheikhs) that I interviewed in Tanga after the onset of the mass pilgrimage to Samunge (July/August 2011) expressed a decidedly oppositional attitude with regard to Mwasapile and his miracle cure.[9] Pastor Mary, the forty-two-year-old leader of a local neo-Pentecostal church, predominantly objected to Mwasapile's claim that his medicine had to be poured into the cup by himself. If the proclaimed cure was really the work of God, she reasoned, s/he would ensure that it would reach the greatest number of people possible instead of restricting its scope by tying its efficacy to the hands of a single person residing in an extremely remote area.

Mary was also skeptical of Mwasapile's one-dose-for-all logic. Contrasting his potion to biomedical pharmaceuticals that usually have to be administered in different dosages to children and adults, she wondered how it could be that children, adults, and old people could all be cured by a single intake of the same dosage of his concoction. The fact that Mwasapile claimed faith to be the decisive aspect of his medicine's efficacy, however, remained completely uncommented upon by Mary. Perhaps she would not formulate any critique in this regard because, as will be shown further below, she herself was engaged in faith healing of people living with HIV/AIDS.

Sheikh Hussein, the leader of a small, independent, reformist-oriented Islamic institution, did address the issue of faith in a critical way. Conceding that the cup might have at least minor therapeutic potential, he strongly opposed what he held to be Mwasapile's position with regard to his clients' religious confession. He assumed that the pastor made clients' affiliation to Christianity a sine qua non for his concoction's efficacy (this was in fact not the case). This, he reasoned, was a direct offence to Muslims, who should therefore refrain from seeking Mwasapile's cure.

Sheikh Suleiman, the leader of Tanga's largest revivalist Muslim congregation, provided the most detailed and theologically founded critique of Mwasapile's healing cult. He accused the pastor of lying, for, according to Islamic doctrine, God does not communicate with common human beings. "God will not give any instructions to ordinary people (*watu wa kawaida*)," he explained.

> [Our scriptures] say that only the prophets who were already announced and whose writings are well known talked to God, and that this will not happen again. . . . Therefore, we reject people like [Mwasapile]. If he treats people with his medicine, so be it; but he must not tell lies that he talked to God . . . and that the medicine won't have any effect if you do not receive it there [at Mwasapile's place]. . . . In Islam, medicine is *worldwide* [English expression in original Swahili quote]. If it heals, it heals [anywhere]. (Sheikh Suleiman, fifty-five years, 3 August 2011)

Despite their profound skepticism and denial of Mwasapile's miracle cure, none of the three religious leaders generally precluded the idea that HIV/AIDS is curable. In the following section, I examine the differing ideas about disease causation in relation to HIV/AIDS, which such assumptions were based on.

From God's Mercy to Divine Retribution: Christian and Muslim Discourses on HIV/AIDS and ART

Despite disparate levels of knowledge about HIV/AIDS among the Muslim and Christian leaders whom I interviewed, there was a striking similarity with regard to their conception of the ultimate cause underlying the disease. As has been observed in other African contexts, they predominantly understood HIV/AIDS as divine retribution for adultery (*zinaa*) and general moral decay. In the case of Sheikh Suleiman, such a moralistic etiological conception led to a strongly judgmental attitude toward "the sinners" whom he held culpable for their infection and incapable of performing moral catharsis. However, he insisted that "dirty" and "innocent" HIV-positive persons had to be distinguished from one another.

> We are able to know that this one was infected because he/she is a dirty person (*mtu mchafu*) and that one was infected innocently. . . . If someone has dirty and promiscuous behavior, he/she is known. If he is a man, he will all the time meet those [female] profligates who wear short clothes, he sits with them in privacy. . . . And we also recognize the one who innocently got HIV: it is [for example] . . . a person who prays and is religious, but [then] she is married to a worthless person (*mtu mbovu*). Now, we cannot segregate (*kubagua*) or . . . stigmatize this innocent one, while she has been poor, does not carry any sins. . . . Or the child who was born out of wedlock, for instance, we cannot put the blame on him/her because he/she is not the reason. (Sheikh Suleiman, fifty-five years, 3 August 2011)

According to several of the Muslim ART patients who participated in my research, mosque leaders frequently verbalized similar contemplations during Friday prayers. At the same time, they reported that there were no formalized networks of care or endeavors to foster (self-)support groups within their religious communities.[10] This, it seemed, resulted in the profound reserve of Muslims living with HIV vis-à-vis their religious authorities. Neither Sheikh Suleiman nor Sheikh Hussein had ever encountered an HIV-positive person disclosing his/her status to them during the many years that they had been leading their communities (Sheikh Hussein had been in office for twenty years). Nonetheless, both affirmed their general interest in supportive initiatives for people living with HIV/AIDS in their communities, while accentuating the fact that, in contrast to Christian churches, Muslim organizations in Tanga were largely neglected by governmental bodies when it came to financial support or technical assistance in the field of HIV/AIDS.

As moralistic as all of the interviewed religious leaders' (including the Pentecostal pastors') interpretations of HIV/AIDS were, a crucial aspect of their etiological conceptions was that they allowed for the idea of healing. Their perspectives on what exactly healing meant in the context of HIV and how it was to materialize, however, differed considerably. The Muslim leaders emphasized the element of collective expiation and comprehensive moral reorientation as the way forward. Healing, in their view, was thus first and foremost understood in terms of healing society through moral transformation, one of the benefits of which would be future generations' relief from HIV. The idea of scientific progress leading to a biomedical remedy was seamlessly incorporated into this logic. After all, as the secretary of the more liberal, government-near Muslim organization explained, the elimination of "sinful behavior" was the indispensable precondition for God to reveal the cure for HIV to biomedical scientists (cf. Balogun 2010). Furthermore, a sheikh from the same institution added, an HIV infection should be viewed as evidence of God's mercy: by becoming infected, one is given the chance to expiate one's sins and give evidence of one's faith by accepting the disease as a trial to be mastered by intensified adherence to Islamic moral canons. This idea also served as an explanation for the infection of "innocent" newborns. Like adults who may have become infected through caring for a sick relative, these children, it was reasoned, were not paying for their parents' or anyone else's sins.

While the Muslim leaders thus discussed the matter of healing in the context of HIV/AIDS in a fairly abstract and collective-oriented way, the Pentecostal leaders' conceptions and related practices were of immediate practical relevance to individual HIV-positive members of their church. Both pastors actively engaged in healing prayers and services for people living with HIV/AIDS and vividly advocated for the possibility of their cure. In their view, patients' profound devotion to a religious life and their faith in the Word of God were the preconditions for the cure, which in turn was conceived of as a testimony of divine benevolence. Pastor Mary recounted that, to date, two of her parishioners had been cured of HIV after participating in prayer meetings over a long period of time. Even those who had not yet been cured had benefitted from the prayers, she added, drawing on the evidence of their rising CD4 counts. Forty-nine-year-old Pastor Michael likewise reported having cured several of his congregants of HIV through his prayers. Though he conceded that he had never been presented with one of these persons' negative HIV test results after his intervention, this was quite irrelevant, since curing HIV did not necessarily go hand in hand with a complete elimination of the virus. As long as the cured patients adhered to the church's moral regime and abstained from sinful behavior, they could live without any negative impact, despite the virus's continuing presence in their body.

Both pastors also held spirit possession to be a possible explanation for an HIV infection. Pastor Michael regularly conducted individual exorcism ceremonies, which culminated in the withdrawal of malevolent spirits causing all kinds of diseases, among them malaria and HIV.

> There are two forms of HIV. I remember a case of conducting healing prayers. When I said, "Spirit of HIV, I rebuke you! In the name of Jesus Christ, come out right now!" And you can see, when I mention "spirit of HIV" . . . he/she is terrified. I have done this exercise very often. . . . And while this person suffered from diarrhea and had to vomit before, once you've said this, you'll find that . . . he/she expresses his/her astonishment: "I feel like eating." So everything is all right for the persons of this kind. (Pastor Michael, forty-nine years, 18 August 2009)

Both pastors as well as the Muslim leaders did not object to their parishioners undergoing ART and, with the exception of Pastor Michael, they all held a biomedical HIV test to be the ultimate measure with which to verify the effect of any religious intervention intended to cure the virus. There was also consensus among the representatives of both faiths that God was the ultimate source of scientific innovation, which is why ART did not constitute a challenge to divine power over the beginning and end of human life. A crucial difference to scientific reasoning, however, lay in the Pentecostal pastors' conviction that in case of successful religious intervention, HIV-positive persons could stop their biomedical therapy without expecting any negative consequences. This certainly explained their appeal to ART patients who were troubled with the daily drug intake and related side effects.

The question may arise, however, of why so many people preferred to go to considerable lengths to get to Samunge and seek the cup, while faith healers such as Pastor Michael, who also promised a cure, were much more easy to access. The local religious leaders' moralistic, derogatory, and often publicly announced view of people who contracted HIV through sexual intercourse was, I suggest, one reason among others why this was the case. Mwasapile, in contrast, has to my knowledge never made any statement in which he associated HIV/AIDS in particular with an immoral lifestyle or sinful behavior. In fact, he has never expressed any opinion concerning the origin of this and other diseases. Additionally, he usually referred to HIV/AIDS in precisely the same nonjudgmental manner as other chronic and noninfectious conditions like diabetes and cancer. It is reasonable to assume that this nonmoralistic way of speaking about HIV and of treating those infected with the virus significantly attributed to his enormous attraction. Moreover, despite all of the financial and practical efforts that a journey to Samunge implied, for many people, the barrier to undertake this trip once was presumably lower than to partake in prayer sessions with a local pastor over a prolonged period of time, which implied the incalculable risk that, sooner or later, other church members might learn about their health status.

"Religion Is Not the Solution": Traditional Healers' Opinions of the Wonder of Loliondo

In a similar vein as the religious leaders, the traditional healers questioned Mwasapile's—as well as his medicine's—therapeutic potential. They all lay stress upon the differences between the pastor's healing practice and their own. Perhaps even more than the religious leaders, their efforts to distance themselves from the Wonder of Loliondo could be viewed as a form of what Harry West and Tracy Luedke have referred to as "therapeutic border work" (2006, 1). "Successful healers," they argue, "must act not only as cross-border travelers but also as border guards, regulating and restricting the flow of the resources in which they traffic as well as the flow of potential competitors and the clients for whom they compete" (West and Luedke 2006, 7).

The healer who criticized Mwasapile most outspokenly was fifty-year-old Tendaji, whose therapeutic practice was mostly based on the use of herbal medicines (*dawa ya asili*). For Tendaji, the most problematic aspect of Mwasapile consisted of the pastor's insistence that rather than active herbal ingredients, patients' faith in God was what made his concoction effective. Tendaji, in turn, drew a clear-cut line between religion and the art of healing (*uganga*), which he defined to be primarily based on herbal medicine:

361

The domain of [Babu] is faith, not medicine. But what we want is medicine, not faith. This medicine is for malaria, this one is for cancer . . .
you understand? That's what we want. It's not like I had to do a particular
thing [like a ritual or prayer] in order to heal [for example] your ailing
head. This does not work. It will only heal with the right medicine. . . .
Religion is not the solution. What we need is the right (herbal) treatment.
(Tendaji, fifty years, 6 August 2011)

He further explained that there were Muslim and Christian healers in Tanga who cooperated very well, which was only possible
because they subordinated their confession to their practice as traditional healers. Tendaji himself was even a member of his mosque's
leading committee. But he claimed that this in no way intervened
with his work as a traditional healer, since every time he returned
from the mosque to his home, he left the domain of religion behind
and "simply treat[ed] patients. That's all." Tendaji took Mwasapile's
claim that God had shown him the *mugariga* tree in his dreams
as another proof that he was not truly a healing expert. Indeed,
"real" healers were often instructed about the existence of particular
officinal plants in their dreams, Tendaji conceded, but rather than
God, the instructors in such kinds of dreams were always spirits
(*majini*) (cf. Mackenrodt 2011). Finally, Tendaji referred to several
people he knew who had sought Mwasapile's medicine in the hope
that it would cure their affliction. Upon returning from Samunge,
their health had deteriorated significantly, and one person had even
died. This, Tendaji reasoned, was the ultimate proof that faith alone
was insufficient for any healing process to manifest itself—and that
Mwasapile was a quack.

Mohamedi, a healer who lived and practiced just a few hundred meters away from Tendaji's house, struggled equally with
Mwasapile's conceptual combination of religious faith and herbal
substances:

I haven't come to grips with it yet. . . . He uses medicine, a tree of which
he claims God had shown him in his dreams. But . . . he is also standing
on the side of religious faith, so I feel like he has put two entirely different
things together in one. As for the side of religion, there have been other
pastors like . . . Kakobe . . . and here in Tanga there are also such persons
who pray for people but they don't use plants. They don't take any tree in
order to make a medicine out of it. . . . Sometimes, they perhaps use [holy
water] upon which they pray and then you can drink it, but they don't

use [herbal] medicine, but [Mwasapile] distributes medicine! Now that is something that I can't fully comprehend (*kitu ambacho hakikuniingia akilini kikakaa vizuri*). . . . I personally believe that [Mwasapile's claims to cure chronic diseases] are not true. (Mohamedi, fifty-seven years, 25 June 2011)

The thirty-year-old healer Haji also argued that the matter of healing was in no way associated to religion. "We take a look at your [health] problem; we don't enter the field of religion," he explained with regard to his own healing practice, while he emphasized that his clients' confession had no influence on his treatments' effectiveness. Additionally, Haji contested Mwasapile's miracle cure in a way that resonated with Pastor Mary's argument about the medicine's lack of specificity. "Each and every medicine has healing capacities (*inatibu*), but it has its particular procedure (*utaratibu*)," he explained.

> Every medicine—you first need to find out what exactly it is good for, before people can be treated with it. But when this Babu discovered his medicine, he gave it to anyone and claimed that they all were cured. That's not true; it cannot be that it is effective for all people. Not even we ourselves [referring to traditional healers] claim such a thing! (Haji, thirty years, 22 July 2011)

Nonetheless, Haji did not call into question the fact that the health state of some Samunge pilgrims might indeed have improved after taking the cup. He viewed this, however, as a matter of mere luck and coincidence, while he himself was able to systematically and reliably treat many chronic diseases.

While healers thus showed a remarkable consensus about the ineffectiveness of combating HIV/AIDS (and disease in general) by way of Christian faith healing, they were nonetheless convinced that there were other ways to successfully respond to the disease. In fact, the treatment of HIV-positive patients formed an inherent part of their therapeutic practice, and the conceptual framework within which these healing activities were embedded were by no means as science-oriented and secular as Haji's and Tendaji's judgments of the Wonder of Loliondo, including their emphasis on the efficacy of herbal therapeutic substances, would suggest.

"God's AIDS" vs. "African AIDS": Epistemological Divides and Therapeutic Options

In consideration of the diverse nonbiomedical theories of disease causation that are prevalent in Tanzania as elsewhere in Africa, healers in Tanga had to determine whether and how to integrate HIV/AIDS into preexisting etiological classifications. According to Mohamedi, there exist four essential classes of reasons for why illness and affliction are inflicted on human beings:

> The first one consists of the things that are simply caused by the mercy of God, but other issues are caused by witchcraft. Another one, thirdly, is *mapepo* (spirits). The fourth one, which does not occur very often, is not to perform the *matambiko* (ritual offerings) for the ancestors. (Mohamedi, fifty-seven years, 25 June 2011)

The specific way in which healers incorporated HIV/AIDS into such categorizations, and how they responded to their patients' respective imaginaries, varied. Halfani—a widely known healer approximately sixty years old who introduced himself as a "traditional healer," "practitioner of alternative medicine," and "spiritualist"—claimed to adhere exclusively to the biomedical understanding of HIV/AIDS as an "immunodeficiency" (*upungufu wa kinga*) that is entirely unrelated to any immaterial or super-natural forces. But of course, he said, he was aware of the other etiological logics with which his HIV-positive patients might explain their condition. In fact, he explained that some ninety-five percent of his patients, including the HIV-positive ones, came to see him with the conviction that they had been bewitched or were being possessed by spirits, and he tried to proceed pragmatically during their consultations.

> I'm not dealing with spirits . . . but in an HIV case, you have to relieve [the patient] of whatever he's coming with. [If] he is coming with that way African [sic in originally English quote] . . . he is possessed by spirits or bewitched . . . you have to help him psychologically first. . . . If you've seen the symptoms of HIV and this one has come here and wants a service of the spirits or anything else, you should not let him down. [Otherwise,] he'll go to consult somebody else and will be lost. . . . When you tell the Africans that they have not been bewitched, they will say okay, thanks very much [and leave]. (Halfani, ca. sixty years, 1 September 2009)

Mohamedi, in contrast, claimed that there were two kinds of HIV/AIDS. The first was "a disease of God," which did not imply any human agency and in this respect coincided with the bio-medical explanation for the disease. But HIV/AIDS could also be the effect of witchcraft. Those affected by this latter form of the disease, Mohamedi explained, presented at the hospital with AIDS symptoms, but their health would not improve by any biomedical treatment. "If there is someone [a healer] who takes a look and detects *tego* [effect of witchcraft]," in contrast, "as soon as [the patient] will have been given medicine for *tego*, he will be relieved; and when he returns [to the hospital] and gets tested, there will be no more HIV."

While Mohamedi insinuated that, with the right expertise, it was not exceedingly difficult to cure this second kind of HIV/AIDS, finding the right herbal remedy for those who were suffering from the God-sent version constituted, in his view, a great challenge. He assumed that so far, he had only been successful in two such cases, and referred to his ongoing "research" (*utafiti*), which for some years he had been conducting together with another healer. The setting of their research somewhat resembled that of a biomedical pharma-ceutical trial, including treatment-naive research participants and a randomized control group. Both of the patients whom Mohamedi believed he had cured, he explained, had stopped taking their ARVs after their health had considerably improved as a result of his treat-ment. Yet they had done so in disregard of his advice to continue taking their pills until a negative HIV test at the hospital supplied the ultimate evidence of his work's success.

Haji's considerations about HIV/AIDS partly coincided with those of Mohamedi. He believed that the main cause of HIV/AIDS was fornication (*uasherati*), but he also reported having ample evidence of the existence of a strain of the disease that was caused by human intervention.

> A lot of people have already come here and said they had AIDS. . . . They were treated and went there [to the hospital] and were tested and found to not have AIDS [anymore]. So, there is really another type of AIDS: somebody bewitches you, he throws something bad on you (*anakutupia kitu kibaya*). So when you get to the hospital, you're found to have AIDS . . . but it's not AIDS, it's "African AIDS" (*UKIMWI wa kiafrika*). (Haji, thirty years, 22 July 2011)

Haji estimated that about 30 percent of all HIV infections in Tanzania were cases of "African AIDS" caused by hostile human agency, and this type could be cured completely by specific rituals. The treatment of "AIDS from God," by contrast, required further research into effective herbal cures.

Tendaji did not consider HIV/AIDS to be caused by malevolent human beings. Like Halfani, he explained the disease more or less in biomedical terms as a sexually transmitted disease. Nonetheless, like Mohamedi, he was convinced that, sooner or later, he would find a medicine that would reliably cure the disease. He too told me about a "research project" he was currently running, whereby he estimated his herbal remedies' efficacy according to biomedical indicators like rising CD4 counts. He lamented, however, that these were difficult to obtain due to many of his research participants' "lack of coopera-tion." "I'm still investigating," Tendaji recounted.

The healers' stances toward ART were significantly shaped by their stance toward biomedicine in general and their personal expe-riences with biomedical professionals. The spectrum of positions ranged from functional cooperation and regular referrals from healers to hospitals to resistance and profound critique of bio-medicine's self-asserted epistemological superiority and respective administrative regulation.

"Dr. Kiboko" was a fifty-two-year-old healer who referred to him-self as an expert of spirits (*mganga wa majini/mizimu*), but he also had long-term experience in treating people with herbal medicines and claimed to know a plant that had cured some of his HIV-positive patients. Nonetheless, he conceded that sometimes it could take some time until his herbal medicine eliminated the virus, which is why he usually told patients to simultaneously seek ART, about whose effectiveness he was quite impressed.

"Dr. Mberesero," in contrast, offered fierce criticism of the biomedical HIV treatment program. He articulated insurmountable differences between the epistemological foundations of biomedical scientists and health professionals and his own. In a tone that was both derogatory and resentful, he elaborated on "the professors" who were always eager to know the properties of each tree and would note everything in their books. "But science— ... one is born with it, then one writes it down and other people read it and understand 'you can do this and this and this.' But the one who was born with science is different from the one who reads [it]," he explained, implying the superiority of his innate and immediate knowledge over the mediated knowledge of biomedical science. In relation to this, he bitterly complained about the legal discrimination that healers faced when one of their patients died as a result of failed treatment for HIV/AIDS. Healers were strongly restricted when it came to claiming to cure HIV/AIDS, he continued, and in case of a patient dying during therapy, they were immediately taken to court. "*You* have warehouses full of medicines, but people die right there [in the hospital]. [And then you go] to 'Dr. Mberesero' and tell him, 'You're not allowed to say you treat AIDS.' Why do *you* treat it, and then the people die right there?" he reproached, apparently taking me to be a representative of the scientific community (all quotes taken from an interview conducted on 10 August 2011). In fact, he reasoned, biomedical professionals were responsible for exacerbating the spread of HIV/AIDS by providing medicines that prolonged the lives of individuals who nonetheless remained carriers of the still transmittable virus. He and the members of his healing cult, by contrast, could bring HIV/AIDS to a "real halt."

Boundary Work in a Historical Perspective

A look at the history of the relationship between biomedicine, the state, and traditional medicine helps contextualize such confrontational positions of local healers vis-à-vis biomedical science. As Rebecca Marsland argues, during the period of German and British colonial rule in Tanzania, "the organization of space and time in mission and hospital medicine were designed to instill 'modernist' values in their users, and encourage rationality over superstition" (Marsland 2007, 758; cf. also Vaughan 1991). Colonial authorities constructed a clear-cut boundary between "Western" scientific medical practice and "its other"; that is, indigenous approaches to healing based on the premise that illness and other forms of misfortune have their origin in impaired social relationships and are caused by mischievous ancestors, spirits, or witches. This boundary "between biomedicine and so-called traditional medicine emerged as a way to establish certain forms of expertise and authority that were critical to the disciplinary civilizing of colonial modernization" (Langwick 2006, 143; see also Comaroff 1993).

During the period of German colonial rule, indigenous medicine was predominantly affected by German missionaries' attempts to discourage local people from adhering to what they considered pagan and "primitive" beliefs. During the 1920s, in turn, particular traits of traditional medicine were subjected to the legal regulation of the British government. The authorities were particularly keen on making any engagement in the exercise of occult power legally prosecutable through a legal antiwitchcraft ordinance (Bruchhausen 2006, 197ff), for they had increasingly experienced how large-scale witchcraft finding movements caused social unrest and threatened public order (cf. Beck 1981, 61ff). In contrast, there have never been any attempts to legally prohibit local healers' practices that were based on the use of medicinal plants. On the contrary, since the German colonial period, herbalists' knowledge was considered to be potentially useful and governmental authorities actively fostered respective research (Bruchhausen 2006, 155–59).

This dichotomous stance with regard to indigenous healing practices continued to prevail in the postcolonial era under the rule of Julius Nyerere. The statement issued in 1968 by "a research officer in the Tanzanian Ministry of Agricultures and Cooperative Development," as cited by Stacey Langwick (2011, 58), is illustrative of the socialist government's focus on the institutionalization and standardization of herbal medicine, the only component of traditional medicine that it deemed justified due to its potential scientific verifiability. Returning from the first Symposium on African Medicinal Plants in Senegal, the officer "claimed for scientists the role of transforming 'the old or indigenous ways of curing disease' into 'new' forms of modern treatment"; that is, "transforming 'primitive medicaments' through scientific investigation" (Langwick 2011, 58). Following this call, the government "strove to delineate a national body of healing practices by systematically collecting accounts of treatments and samples of *materia medica*" and asked "all regional medical officers on the mainland . . . to collect information on the therapies of herbalists in the area, including the drugs they dispensed" (Langwick 2011, 62). At the same time, it enhanced its efforts to subject all traditional healers practicing in the country to governmental control and regulation. In this way, the application of any form of herbal therapy, as well as any attempts to discover new therapeutically exploitable substances, were to be brought under governmental surveillance.

The "ontological privileging" of science over spirit, knowledge over belief, material over immaterial (Langwick 2011, 82) that has characterized the government's position toward traditional medicine since colonial days is reflected to this day in the Tanzanian Institute of Traditional Medicine's initiatives to "integrate" traditional healers in the fight against HIV/AIDS. On the one hand, these initiatives aim to "impart the appropriate knowledge in the identified deficient areas to enable [traditional healers] to understand HIV/AIDS better" (Uiso et al. 2007, 99). On the other hand, they entail a search for herbal substances effective in the treatment of opportunistic infections (cf. Kayombo et al. 2007). While the first aspect clearly points to biomedicine's claims to exclusive knowledge with regard to HIV/AIDS, the second aspect equally implies a power imbalance between traditional healers and their biomedical counterparts, for it is the latter who determine how evidence of a specific compound's efficacy is to be established according to scientific standards. This situation indeed is not so different from how traditional medicine was dealt with during the British Mandate, when "revisions of the witchcraft ordinance and companion policies concerning native medicine divided African therapeutics into practices to be disciplined by law and those to be disciplined by science" (Langwick 2011, 40).

In light of the long history of unequal power relations between representatives of scientific medicine and traditional healers and the disciplinary measures that local healers had to expect when challenging it by way of their therapeutic practice, "Dr. Mberesero's" profound discontent about public health officials' attempts to prohibit his quest for a cure for HIV/AIDS is rather comprehensible. And in consideration of the fact that, as he quite rightly criticized, biomedical experts themselves are unable to offer a remedy, it seems even more justified. The other above-quoted healers' assertions that there is a particular form of the condition that is caused by witchcraft, which thus requires an entirely different response, in turn demonstrate how far the government was from its aim of standardizing traditional medicine through a decontextualization of material healing substances from immaterial therapeutic actants, such as malevolent spells, spirits, ancestral relations, and the personal capacities of the healer.

In this regard, the government's ambivalent response to the Wonder of Loliondo suggested that it actually constituted quite a challenge for governmental authorities to assume a consistent position with respect to religious aspects of healing. Ultimately, this resulted in the fact that, besides its attempts to improve the infrastructural conditions in Samunge and the surrounding area, the government solely focused its actions on the scientific evaluation of Mwasapile's herbal concoction, while the matter of religious faith that, according to the pastor, constituted the decisive part of the miracle cure was mostly left unattended, let alone officially contested. As the following case study shows, this omission had a direct impact on how people living with HIV/AIDS judged and involved themselves with the Wonder of Loliondo.

Case Study E: Jemima and Samuel

How to Measure Faith—Jemima

Fourty-eight-year-old Jemima was a teacher and had two sons who were ten and nineteen years old. As mentioned previously, after all three of them had been tested HIV-positive, her husband accused her of "having brought this disease" and drove them all out of his house. When I got to know Jemima and her sons in 2011, they were living in a house on the outskirts of Tanga with two tenants, from whom they concealed their illness. If the tenants were at home when it was time to take their medication, they secretly swallowed their pills in their bedrooms. Jemima had suffered from various side effects when she began taking ARVs in 2010, and still complained about disproportionate accumulations of body fat, even though "she did exercise as usual." Her sons, by contrast, were not faring badly with the medicines.

Taking ARVs every day, Jemima complained, was very exhausting, and she constantly kept looking for a medicine that might cure her sons' and her condition. Her two sisters actively supported her search by informing her about every possible remedy they came across. Jemima had already tried numerous products, but none had brought the desired effect; and at times, she felt tired of the seemingly endless procedure of trial and error. Her most serious problem, however, was the lack of financial resources. Once her sister had informed her about a promising compound from South Africa, but the price of 500,000 TSH (approximately two and a half times Jemima's monthly salary as a primary school teacher) for a single dose far exceeded her means.

Jemima would not have been able to afford the journey to Loliondo, either, had her sister not insisted and paid for her and her sons' bus tickets. They all drank Mwasapile's medicine, but even this time, Jemima remained skeptical.

> [ARVs] and faith are two different things. It's not like I was running towards the side of faith. I haven't seen anyone who said "I stopped taking the medicine [ARVs], and I was cured," [so] I'm not in a hurry. I'm going slowly. First we asked Babu, "Should we continue taking ARVs?" And he said, "If your faith is strong, leave it! But if your faith is not strong, continue taking your medicines, because my medicine works slowly." When I heard this, I did not stop and my children are still given their medicine.

Jemima had difficulties evaluating her religious commitment and assumed that it would not suffice for a manifestation of a cure.

> I don't have too much confidence. Because I am a human being and maybe I have failed God in many ways that I'm not aware of. And I don't even know why I got this problem in the first place. . . . Maybe God is trying me, saying, "You have failed me," and he wants to bring me back this way. I don't understand. . . . I don't believe that you can leave the medicines aside directly and God will cure you. . . . I don't know the amount of mistakes I have committed on [God's] account. So, there is faith, and I also believe that there is [scientific] expertise (*utaalamu*). I haven't decided yet which direction I should take.

Ultimately, Jemima considered that biomedical judgment should have the last word regarding her therapy. Unless the doctors at her treatment center told her to stop taking ARVs, she would not do so, she claimed. However, she did not put much effort into pursuing a biomedical evaluation of Babu's medicine's efficacy; several months after she and her sons had taken the cup, none of them had undergone a new HIV test. Jemima apparently preferred to continue living with her doubts—but also with the hope for the unexpected cure to manifest itself in the future.

You Need to Fish with Two Things!—Samuel

In 2008, forty-six-year-old Samuel was admitted to the hospital with cerebral malaria. Fortunately, he recovered; but from then on, he was semiparalyzed and had to begin taking ARVs, since he was also discovered to be HIV-positive. When he first started taking the drugs, he remembered being tired all the time and his legs feeling so numb that he could barely walk. Slowly, these negative effects had vanished, at least to some extent.

Three years later, in spring 2011, his younger brother who lived in England and had learned of Mwasapile through the media, proposed for Samuel to go to Loliondo and contributed 70,000 TSH for the travel expenses. Samuel had already heard several stories of sick people being cured and readily embarked on the six-day journey that would cost around 350,000 TSH. In Samunge, he managed to shake hands with Mwasapile. "If you've drunk this cup of mine, you'll already be cured," the pastor assured him. Even if the "bugs" were still visible, they had been reduced for sure, and Babu's medicine was still at work, Samuel confidently concluded.

In an interview with him (1 August 2011), he reported feeling a lot better since he had drunk the medicine—and since he had stopped taking his ARVs three months before. He regularly talked to one of Mwasapile's assistants via telephone. "If your progress is good, that's it. Just go on like that; don't use your medicines [ARVs]," the assistant had told Samuel during their last conversation. Samuel seemed to ascribe his felt improvement in equal measure to Babu's concoction and to the discontinuance of his biomedical therapy. After starting ART, his health had improved to a certain extent, he admitted. "But right now, I'm improving a lot more than at the beginning. . . . Since I stopped taking [ARVs], I feel a certain lightness." Nonetheless, he was still in a "wait-and-see mode" and was by no means averse to continuing his biomedical therapy should his improvements be limited.

> I got faith from going to Babu's. He told me not to stop believing. So I thought by myself, wait and let the [antiretroviral] medicines rest for a little bit until you see how *these* things [improvement through Babu's medicine] are developing. If there will be no changes . . . I'll continue taking [ARVs]. You have to try everything. If you see certain changes, you stop the other thing, but you have to try everything. . . . But if you don't

372

> have faith, you can't be healed. . . . Faith comes before medicine (*imani inafuatana na dawa*). If you have faith, this medicine will also help you. . . . You need to fish with two things: faith and medicine.

Similar to Jemima, Samuel could not tell where the fish would bite. After a few weeks, he intended to undergo an HIV test in order "to know what to do." "If the 'bugs' are all gone, I'll thank God. If they're still there, I'll go back to the hospital and continue with the drugs. I'll know that Babu's medicine will have decreased [the bugs'] strength, but that it didn't cure completely." Samuel knew about the risks of developing resistant virus strains when interrupting ART, but even the constant insistence of an HBC provider could not motivate him to resume therapy earlier.

When I inquired about Samuel's opinion about other healers claiming to cure HIV/AIDS, he elaborated on the government's public stance toward Mwasapile in a way that affirmed the voices of those who strongly criticized the government for not informing its citizens properly about the Loliondo cure:

> These others are liars. . . . If Babu was a liar, the government wouldn't care about him. Instead, it organizes a good procedure (*inaweka ule utaratibu vizuri*), good resting places, good transportation, permits. . . . Until today they keep putting good regulations in place for him (*wanamfuatilia sheria zake nzuri*).

Unfortunately, during my second field stay, I was unable to get in touch with Samuel and thus I do not know how his health situation further developed and whether he ever resumed his biomedical therapy.

Calculations, Pragmatism, and Hope

Both Jemima and Samuel experienced a positive impact of ART on their health, and they were grateful for being provided with the treatment. At the same time, however, their accounts underlined how ARVs had effected new hardships in their lives. Severe and persistent side effects had to be coped with and could provoke treatment fatigue throughout the course of the lifelong therapy. Experiences of discrimination, and the consequent creation of secrecy surrounding their serostatus further complicated their therapy. After all, a life with ARVs by no means equaled a life without HIV, and Jemima's and Samuel's quests for a cure—their desire to "try out everything"—raise the question of how much "redemption" there actually is in "the redemptive moment" (Dilger et al. 2010, 377) induced by the growing availability of ART in resource-poor settings.

In both Jemima's and Samuel's cases, close relatives materially and immaterially supported their quests for a cure. They also helped to estimate Mwasapile's spiritual legitimacy, though the evaluation of Jemima's and Samuel's own spiritual aptness was left to themselves. These calculations and estimations leave ample space for uncertainty, which was experienced as deeply demoralizing doubt in one moment and overwhelming confidence in the next. In both cases, however, the efficacy of the Wonder of Loliondo was undoubtedly thought to be a matter of faith. In fact, Jemima did not even mention the herbal brew in her reflections on a possible cure; and for Samuel, having faith was the indispensable condition for the medicine's efficacy. Despite this attribution of therapeutic power to faith rather than to the concoction's herbal ingredients, Mwasapile, in his role as a healer or a godly medium, seemed to be of minor relevance. While Samuel at least once mentioned him to be "a man of God," Jemima did not refer to any of his personal characteristics or statements that would point to the importance of topics such as an expiation of sins. Her speculations about religious integrity were not triggered by a "moralizing prophet" but were the result of her own reflections. Moreover, Jemima's account resembled those of others who had received the cup without even getting out of their car, and who then immediately embarked on their return trip. God's healing power, condensed in the cup, had become a commodity largely detached from the exigencies of inner catharsis or from the prioritization of profound commitment to Jesus, as issued by the leaders of Pentecostal healing churches (cf. Van Dijk 2009). In this respect, Bishop Kakobe's anxiety about losing followers to this commoditized, more easily accessible form of faith healing may not have been entirely groundless.

Finally, Jemima's and Samuel's accounts once more demonstrate that "uncertainty is intrinsically tied up with the maintenance of hope" and that people "will do whatever it takes to restore their health and status" (Kwansa 2010, 456). No matter how much effort healers and religious leaders put into establishing boundaries between different therapeutic resources in a contested field of healing, these boundaries—be they of a denominational or epistemological nature—are transgressed in a highly pragmatic and flexible way.

Chapter Conclusion

The exponential expansion of ART in Tanzania can indeed be seen as a "redemptive moment" after decades without effective treatment. Nevertheless, the biomedically declared incurability of HIV/AIDS left ample space for a polyphonic concert of healing promises from religious leaders and traditional healers—and patients readily embarked on the search for a cure in terrains other than the biomedical. The Wonder of Loliondo and the cases of Jemima and Samuel (as well as those of countless other people who interrupted their therapy after getting involved in religious and traditional healing), once again show that when it comes to the matter of health, illness, and healing, "scientific truth" remains anything but unchallenged.

More specifically, despite the government's attempts (as random as they may have been) to prevent healers from claiming to be able to cure HIV/AIDS, even the small sample of healers in Tanga whom I interviewed suggested that discourses about therapeutic options for eliminating the virus were widely prevalent. It is reasonable to assume that it was precisely the etiological ideas behind concepts such as "African AIDS" resulting from witchcraft that made these alternative discourses so attractive for patients, as they addressed their social and moral concerns and provided the hope for a cure that biomedical reasoning did not allow for.

Furthermore, the government's "mixed messaging" (cf. Doran 2007, 404) in the context of the Loliondo phenomenon suggests that while the official discourse of governmental bodies may have been the separation of *materia medica* from its religious contexts of meaning and the personal powers of healing figures (cf. Langwick 2011, 80), individual personnel did not necessarily translate this policy into their personal practice. Instead, they resorted to the very same nonscientific healing methods in the search for relief from their own afflictions. Epistemological divides, in this case, remained restricted to theory.

Aside from politicians' individual religious convictions, there is reason to assume that calculations about the extent to which Mwasapile posed a threat to governmental authority, as well as economic aspects equally influenced the authorities' decisions about whether and how to interfere in the mass healing phenomenon. For most people living with HIV/AIDS, in turn, the complex entanglements of politicians' and other actors' interests in the Wonder of Loliondo were as untransparent as their strategies to secure interpretational and therapeutic authority. Scientific evidence of certain healing practices was often unavailable, while for many it was also not fully comprehensible or was simply irrelevant. Not least, as much as patients decided where to seek remedy for their ailing body in a highly pragmatic fashion, they sought for meaning and more profound redemption in a situation of permanent—not only medical—crisis. Healers, religious leaders, and prophets—be they self- or externally constructed—will remain important figures and avenues for troubled persons in such troubled times.

Notes

1. Parts of this chapter have been published in Mattes 2014c.
2. It is important to note that similar to the use of "traditional" in relation to medical practices, the notion of "traditional" African religion needs to be critically interrogated. As Becker and Geissler point out, the term "in itself is intricately connected to missionaries' efforts to identify and manipulate what they had made out to be their indigenous 'competition,' and that the appropriation of Christian concepts in Africa has long born traces of the initial relationship between Christian masters and 'pagan' servants" (Becker and Geissler 2009, 4).
3. Unfortunately, the authors do not provide the exact denomination of the respective churches.
4. Singular: *hadith*. Written collections of supposedly verbatim quotes of the Prophet Muhammad.
5. The official registration as a "practitioner of traditional or alternative medicine" includes the payment of registration fees, the presentation of testimonials of the applicant's healing competence, and the provision of "a written statement from the local government authority within which he is practising" (The United Republic of Tanzania 2002, 12). Satisfaction of these requirements grants a certificate valid for three years.
6. The quotes taken from interviews or newspaper articles written in Swahili have been translated to English by myself.
7. The idea of being "saved" or "born again" through the complete commitment of one's life to Jesus and making a break with any "sinful" practices of one's old life is a central element of Pentecostal thought and practice (cf. Dilger 2005, 254).

8. "Mseto" is an acronym for a common artemisinin-based antimalarial pharmaceutical drug.

9. The remainder of this chapter is drawing on interviews with six traditional healers, two neo-Pentecostal pastors, two sheikhs of different reformist Muslim organizations, and a focus group discussion with several leaders of a third, more liberal Muslim congregation in Tanga.

10. In this regard, the Muslim communities differed considerably from their Pentecostal counterparts. Both pastors reported that people living with HIV frequently revealed their status to them. Certainly, their readiness to disclose was enhanced by the prospect of participating in individual healing prayer sessions, but also by the expectation of receiving social and moral support (cf. Dilger 2007). Pastor Mary, for instance, explained that every week, a group of HIV-positive congregants met in her church. They received some material support in the form of clothes and food supplements donated by their fellow parishioners. However, the individual members' health status was kept secret from other church members and they presented themselves as needy only in an economic and material sense.

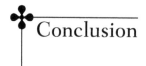
Conclusion

The global HIV treatment apparatus constitutes an exemplar of transnational "therapeutic sovereignty" (Nguyen 2010, 6), which is a novel "form of power over life [that] is exercised today in the context of international emergencies" (Nguyen 2010, 6). Transnationally operating entities of global health governance such as WHO, PEPFAR, the Global Fund, and large-scale philanthropic foundations determine which parts of the world will benefit from life-prolonging drugs for the treatment of HIV/AIDS and under which conditions. These entities define the technical and medical standards of ART delivery and regulate the continuation of funding flows according to their evaluations of the extent to which "local" treatment programs meet these standards. Moreover, they engage in practices of subject formation that aim to foster patients who subscribe fully to biomedical rationalities and who realign their bodies and lifestyles accordingly. Finally, these entities of global health governance and finance shape and help solidify the discourse of "the normalization" and not least "the end of HIV/AIDS," which ultimately legitimates their own successive divestment from respective health interventions—notwithstanding affected people's continuous experiences of disruption—which suggest that this discourse is, at best, precipitous (cf. Sangaramoorthy 2018).

I subsume the forms of political–economic domination, bureaucratic regulation, discursive dominance, and ethical subject formation enacted by these entities of global health governance and finance under the notion of HIV-related transnational governmentality (Ferguson 2006; Ferguson and Gupta 2002). In this book, I have pointed to the limitations of this particular manifestation of governmentality. More specifically, I have highlighted the frictions arising from the attempt to roll out globally standardized ART in Tanga—which in some ways may be taken as a proxy for many other politically and economically underprivileged localities in sub-Saharan Africa—by paying close attention to the (infra)structural set-up and social fabric of specific HIV treatment centers, as well as the local moral worlds in which patients strive to make ends meet and lead meaningful lives with their daily medications. By closely accompanying medical professionals in their struggles to provide quality care and by conversing with patients and family members for innumerous hours in their homes, work environments, and (self-) support groups, I gained insights that I hold to be crucial for deepening our understanding of the manifold challenges of successfully and sustainably installing "global" HIV treatment in a specific locale. Such insights constitute an essential complement to the progress and implementation reports that are being published, for instance, by many recipient countries' ministries of health as well as by major development organizations and funding initiatives, whose metrics are, to a large extent, based on numeric indicators and thus on data that are "purified" from the specificities of local treatment sites (cf. Adams 2016; Rottenburg et al. 2015).

In the following, I will summarize what I see as the most important findings of this study in relation to the major ethnographic contexts of the research—the institutional settings of the CTCs and patients' local moral worlds—before I end with some comments on its political implications and the role of anthropology in future HIV/AIDS research and interventions.

Concerning the routines of treatment enrollment and surveillance, there was a stark contrast between the nonhierarchical professional–patient relationship and patient empowerment, as stipulated in international and national policy documents, and medical professionals' conduct in practice, which was highly authoritative vis-à-vis patients during treatment preparation and throughout the course of their therapy. The health workers carried and felt a great responsibility to improve treatment adherence rates among rapidly increasing numbers of patients and to sustain these over the course of many years. In the face of this responsibility, it would seem that they trusted more in the establishment of their own unquestioned authority and the application of disciplining educational measures than in nourishing patients' sense of self-responsibility that would lead them to adhere to their treatment regimen and adopt a "healthy" and "biomedically rational" lifestyle with all its implications.

This suggests that Tanga's public treatment centers, most of whose patients had a low socioeconomic status and education level, were not generating therapeutic and "responsibilized" citizens as envisioned during the pioneering phase of ART provision in Africa. Instead, the health workers' often rather dominant ways of communicating and interacting with patients seemed to promote a disempowering process of medicalization, during which patients were transformed into docile bodies who fully surrendered to biomedical rationality and authority.

The fact that health workers failed to establish more equitable relationships with their patients should, however, by no means be blamed on their denial of the medical professional ethos. To the contrary, they often went to great lengths to provide the best possible service they could. Furthermore, most of them were well aware of how conducive a friendly and affective way of dealing with patients was for their psychological well being, the formation of trusting relationships, and, ultimately, for achieving high treatment retention rates. Nevertheless, they routinely struggled to manage the large numbers of patients who were crowding the clinics' hallways every single day of the week, at times under significant (infra)structural constraints and enormous time pressure. There was hardly ever the time or room to conduct appropriately extensive clinical examinations and unhurried individual counseling sessions that would possibly have provided the CTC staff with a sense of patients' problems beyond their most pressing physiological dysfunctions. Furthermore, the structural conditions were not conducive for patients to open up to the clinic staff and frankly discuss their concerns and attitudes with regard to their therapy, much less so if these concerns and attitudes contradicted the biomedical tenets authoritatively conveyed during treatment preparation.

Intrainstitutional organizational deficits, insufficient supervision and personnel management, and a strongly hierarchical staff structure additionally impeded efficient work routines, thwarted individual health workers' self-initiative, and inhibited constructive mutual critique and learning among the clinics' workforce. These at times rather subtle microsocial undercurrents went largely unnoticed and unattended by the AIDSRelief supervisors, who "parachuted" into the clinics for a few days per quarter. The health staff, in turn, either had no motivation or did not feel authorized to even discuss the less complex obstacles to their work routine with the AIDSRelief special-ists in order not to unnecessarily dampen their hoped-for positive impressions of their work. For, ultimately, AIDSRelief functioned not only as a cooperation partner in the endeavor to increase the quality of care provision, but they also represented a major donor, whose continuous funding—upon favorable evaluation—was abso-lutely essential for the clinics.

These institutional power dynamics constitute one example of how the effects of the presumably well-oiled machine of transna-tional governmentality in the field of HIV/AIDS may be distorted in the process of transforming global standardized policies into local clinical practice. Shifting the ethnographic focus from the insti-tutional settings of ART provision to patients' local moral worlds revealed numerous further such distortions.

I have shown that many patients did not implement health pro-fessionals' instructions on how to live their lives with ARVs to the expected extent. The disciplinary practices applied during treatment preparation and their long-term monitoring did not always bear the desired fruits, because "no matter how effective, [ARVs] take on different tenors and trajectories as they relocate from the logics of the clinical space to the 'complex calculus' of everyday lives" (Persson et al. 2016, 370). Living a life with ARVs demanded much more than timely drug intake, eating a balanced diet, and abstaining from sex or using condoms. Patients had to make careful decisions in a context of competing moral economies. Their HIV disclosure might effect the disruption of mostly kin-based solidarity networks that were essential not only for their biological survival but also for their "moral well-being." The latter can be understood in terms of feelings of social recognition, emotional connectedness, and a sense of belonging. As Joseph's case (Case Study D) has shown, a patient's will and capability to take the ARVs as prescribed could be deeply enmeshed with these existential human longings. For Joseph, maintaining his moral self-esteem and achieving social recognition, even if only temporarily, seemed to have an even higher priority than his mere physical survival.

That the disclosure or exposure of one's HIV status—possibly through the daily intake of ARVs—endangered patients' solidarity ties with relatives, neighbors, and friends followed from the fact that despite the increasing availability of ARVs and for varying reasons, HIV remained a highly stigmatized disease. Be it due to fear of contagion, moral contempt and blaming, or because of their expected premature death (implying that they thus lacked "value" in reciprocity-based forms of informal economic exchange), people living with HIV and ARVs experienced a wide range of exclusion and discrimination practices. Husbands expelled their wives after they disclosed their serostatus, pushing them into economic and social insecurity. Entire families were compelled to move and shift the center of their lives to distant neighborhoods, because they had been socially marginalized in their own. Children who had lost their parents to AIDS were rejected and abused by their relatives (Mattes 2014b).

How, one wonders, could ARVs ever heal the emotional wounds that such disruptive experiences have inflicted upon people? It is hardly surprising that both anticipated and enacted HIV stigma and experiences of discrimination compelled the large majority of my HIV-positive interlocutors to continue to conceal their health status from everyone except a very small circle of mostly close relatives, whose emotional, social, or material assistance they would or could not go without. Having experienced or heard about others' instances of massive social and moral disruption due to the exposure of their seropositivity to others, many people were painfully aware of the risks of being open about their health status and their daily ingestion of ARVs; an openness that was encouraged time and again within clinics and NGO-facilitated (self-)support groups.

In consideration of these continuing denormalizing effects of HIV that people in Tanga experienced in their daily lives, and their resulting practices of concealment and secrecy, I argue that ARVs mostly assumed the role of what could be called a "technology of invisibilization" (cf. Hardon and Posel 2012; Moyer 2012; Steuer 2012). Consequently, ARVs paradoxically did not function as the instigator of a profound conceptual and discursive transformation of HIV into a nonmoralized disease to the extent expected by public health specialists, even though ever more people were enrolled on treatment and became acquainted with the benefits of the drugs through their own or a close person's experience. The "social and moral normalization" of HIV thus lagged behind the pharmaceutically induced "biological normalization" brought about by the rollout of ART, which enabled ever more people to remain silent and to hide their HIV-positive status.

However, the "biological normalization" of HIV had its limits too. On the one hand, in spite of undergoing treatment, people living with HIV remained infectious and posed a risk for caring relatives, sexual partners, and even their unborn children. For many, this implied an ultimately irresolvable moral dilemma, inasmuch as when they decided to have unprotected sexual intercourse and/or to get pregnant, they always had to accept the risk of passing on the virus. Moreover, living with ARVs meant a life full of new biological contingencies and afflictions. Patients experienced the medicines' fierceness in the form of side effects, which, to the detriment of the many who were struggling to make ends meet, were exacerbated by their lack of sufficient nutrition (cf. Hardon et al. 2007; Kalofonos 2010).

In the face of the often-extreme ART-induced bodily impairments, it exacted quite some perseverance from patients to adhere to their strict treatment schedule of uninterrupted daily drug intake. It was thus anything but surprising that—notwithstanding their awareness of the possible consequences—some did adjust the ingestion of their pills to the momentary availability of food to go along with them, even if this implied deviating from the most emphatically transferred biomedical instruction to never skip or delay a dose. In clinical settings, such manifestations of "nonadherence" were often blamed on individual patients' insufficient understanding of the "biomedical facts" about the treatment and their lack of a sense of responsibility (cf. Beckmann 2013). This assessment fell short, however, of appreciating the structural and political–economic contexts that prevented large parts of the population from earning an income high enough to secure their livelihood and ensure regular and sufficient access to food. In some ways, it perhaps also reflected medical professionals' awareness of their own inability to do anything about large-scale factors such as unemployment and poverty, which prevented their patients from adhering to and thriving on their medication.

Acknowledging the fact that despite the indubitably positive effects of ART, the treatment also introduced new inflictions and uncertainties into affected people's lives, favors the comprehension of their widely prevailing recourse to traditional and religious healing practices, which implied the possibility of being entirely cured from HIV. As shown in Chapter 8, patients pragmatically crossed epistemological boundaries between "scientific truth" and traditional and religious discourses on HIV in their quest for conclusive redemption from their affliction. At times, they placed more importance on adhering to the "rules" of traditional healers and religious leaders and their respective therapeutic practices than those of their bio-medical therapies. Particularly when this deviance from scientific rationality occurred on such a large scale as in the context of the Wonder of Loliondo, these dynamics can be seen to reflect a significant form of friction in relation to the transnational governmentality of HIV, which most vividly materialized in the massive number of patients who interrupted their biomedical treatment in health centers all over Tanzania to receive Mwasapile's "miracle cure." This case also suggests that the implicitly expected globe-spanning biomedicalization of HIV through the rollout of ART has not yet manifested itself—and most likely will not any time soon—because nonbiomedical rationalities not only allow for the possibility of the existence of a cure, but also for providing concerned people with an explanation for and meaning of being infected with the virus, be it within the conceptual framework of witchcraft or religious discourses on HIV as a divine ordeal. Beyond this, the mass healing phenomenon of Loliondo also indicated that people's stance toward religious and traditional healing is strongly influenced by media discourses and politicians' statements and actions, the latter of which, presumably not least for economic reasons, were highly ambiguous and inconsistent.

The most important implication of these briefly summarized ethnographic findings, I believe, consists in the critical interrogation of the current global health rhetoric of the "normalization" of HIV/AIDS. This invokes the transition of HIV/AIDS from an acute and ultimately lethal disease to a well controllable and manageable chronic condition "like any other" (Moyer and Hardon 2014). The close observation of health professionals' and medical institutions' challenges in implementing national and international standards, and the in-depth insight into ARV users' day-to-day lives and social relationships, has revealed that this transition was intricate, anything but linear, and often enough failed to materialize altogether.

For many people, it was difficult to "normalize" their health condition after ART initiation and to successfully establish physical and social continuity, steadiness, and certainty. This resonates with two anthropological studies on the first generation of AIDS survivors in

Uganda, which concluded that ARVs "gave people a second chance at life that was still full of problems and pain and the specter of death" (Whyte 2014, Mogensen, and Meinert, 278) and that these people were "thinking in terms of how to return to normalcy, while slowly realizing that they might never quite achieve it" (Mogensen 2010, 76). Despite the increasing availability of ARVs, people who resumed their lives with the help of the drugs were still suffering from largely persistent dynamics of stigmatization in addition to severe economic hardship. They were also struggling to negotiate disruptions to and the reestablishment of social relations and the simultaneous endeavor to rebuild and maintain their standing in their local moral worlds.

In many respects, one could say that these people were caught in a paradoxical state of "permanent transition." They had left behind their suffering from "biological AIDS" and at times literally risen from their deathbeds with the help of ARVs. Yet despite their physical resurrection, it was impossible for them to achieve the sense of "normalcy" that they had prior to becoming infected with HIV, not least because they could never attain real "reproductive normalcy" (cf. McGrath et al. 2014).

The problem with the discourse on the normalization of HIV is that it disregards the unpredictability, social fragility, and moral struggles and dilemmas that can become dominant and constraining features in the lives of people living with ARVs over the course of many years—if not decades—of treatment. More than that, it implies the risk of falsely putting the blame for patients' inability—or reluctance—to conceptually and practically realize the "normalization" of their illness on them, rather than acknowledging the economic, social, and biological factors by which this process is inherently limited.

In order to better account for the long-term biological and social contingencies of life with HIV that persist, not only despite but also because of HIV treatment, I suggest that more attention needs to be paid to patients' lived experiences with their illness and medications. This includes their aspirations as well as their anxieties, doubts, and moral concerns. What is needed is a deeper understanding of the complex intertwining of long-term ART as a biomedical technology with the relational nature of social life. Evidently, the sites in which such an understanding can be generated include HIV clinics. By providing more room in the treatment centers for patients to discuss their persistent difficulties of living with ARVs in a nonjudgmental context, where the priority is not solely about injecting patients with a sense of biomedical rationality and making them "buy into" the idea of the "normalcy" of HIV, this will foster a more frank and constructive dialogue between health workers and patients. The potential for more profound appreciation of the factors that hinder patients from staying on treatment might provide a more fertile ground for thinking about how to tackle these problems. In the long term, I contend, this might translate into better treatment adherence and lower attrition rates.

As has become clear, however, merely providing ever more people living with HIV in resource-limited settings with drugs to reverse the suppression of their immune systems—an approach that originates in the strong contemporary tendency toward the pharmaceuticaliza-tion of public health and global health politics (Biehl 2007)—falls significantly short of the manifold needs of those targeted. Many people living with ARVs in Tanga had a hard time getting by from one day to the next. Furthermore, in the face of very limited govern-mental and nongovernmental social assistance for HIV (self-)sup-port groups, becoming a part of these biosocial collectives usually did not provide a solution for patients' economic precariousness. At the risk of repeating too often the well-rehearsed argument about the close interrelationship of both individuals' vulnerability and their resilience to HIV on the one hand, and the larger political–economic forces impinging on their lives on the other (Farmer 2006; Poku and Whiteside 2004; Schoepf 2001), I propose that patients' dire living conditions and their resulting difficulties in adhering to their ART regimen obviously point to two main interrelated issues. These consist in the government's as well as the international communi-ty's responsibility to not only provide pharmaceuticals, but also to address the socioeconomic inequalities that prevent patients from obtaining adequate formal education and an occupation that would enable them to "stand on their own feet" and successfully engage in their (newly planned) life projects.

In offering an experience-near ethnography of the inscription of ART in local moral worlds, and by linking individual and collective struggles to live a "normal" life with HIV to national and global political–economic processes, I hope to have indicated the critical implications of the increasing removal of HIV/AIDS from the global political agenda. This turn has manifested itself not least as a consequence of the thriving rhetoric of the disease's "normalization." Undoubtedly, there are numerous convincing arguments for the global donor community's shift from vertical, disease-specific health initiatives to broader, horizontal interventions such as health system strengthening and the delivery of primary care (see Marten 2014; Yang, Farmer, and McGahan 2010). And yet, particularly in the context of increasingly transnationalized, privatized, and projectified health care provision in Africa, this shift—as well as the often correlated reorientation toward merely calculating efficiency and cost reduction—has to be viewed in a critical light. As exemplified by the funding constraints of the TAWG—part of which was owed to the fact that one of its donors changed its thematic priorities away from HIV/AIDS—and the resulting disruption of important and long-standing components of service provision, the proliferating rhetoric of the dawning "end of AIDS" (Havlir and Beyrer 2012; Kenworthy et al. 2017; UNAIDS 2014) could have rather concrete and destructive implications for HIV/AIDS interventions "on the ground." This was particularly observable in Tanzania, whose entire HIV/AIDS response, including the national treatment program, was—as in many other countries—highly contingent on developments in the global economy and the closely correlated fluctuations in the volume of donor funding. As shown in Chapter 3, the Tanzanian government has had enormous difficulties in filling the gradually increasing void in health care provision that the successive withdrawal of financial and technical donor assistance has left behind.

Moreover, the rhetoric of the normalization of HIV and the nearing eradication of AIDS strikes as almost sarcastic in consideration of the fact that many people across the globe "still do not live in the age of treatment [which is] bounded less by time than it is by economics and geopolitics" (Moyer 2015, 261). The survival of the 16 million—out of the 36.9 million people living with HIV across the globe (UNAIDS 2017c, 1)—who still do not have access to life saving medicines thus essentially depends on keeping HIV/AIDS high on the agenda of decision makers in global health and trade policy, and on maintaining public pressure on pharmaceutical companies to make current and future ARV compounds—including second- and third-line regimens—affordable, and not only for governments, health insurance companies, and people in need of treatment in the Global North.

I shall end by suggesting what I hold to be the most essential contributions that anthropology can and should make to future research in the field of HIV/AIDS, and ART in particular. The first consists in what Anita Hardon and Eileen Moyer have designated as "subaltern alignment, a research strategy in which medical anthropologists reveal what really matters for people who have little power to influence global health efforts" (2014, 256). Gaining a fine-grained picture of the divergences between affected people's experiences and dominant global health narratives will hopefully result in more effective forms of intervention and assistance through closer attunement to local institutional configurations of ART provision, as well as to the cultural, social, and moral specificities of individual patients' lifeworlds.

Furthermore, anthropologists should maintain their critical engagement with wider political and economic forces, such as the neoliberal-informed downsizing and restructuring of public service provision in Africa, which aggravate existing social inequalities and can significantly enhance affected people's vulnerability and response to HIV. But aside from making transparent the constraining effects of such forces—and these may include the HIV-related transnational governmentality as described in this book—I also hold it to be a central task of anthropologists to point out the ways in which these effects are coped with, resisted, disregarded, or appropriated by particular people in their day-to-day lives. Thorough ethnographic exploration of these processes, their limitations, and the social domains in which they take place—be they intimate forms of friendship, extended families, HIV (self-)support groups, or religious communities—will inevitably demonstrate that as much as HIV/AIDS is a biological condition, it is also highly social. This is by no means a new insight, but one that is crucial to continually recollect in times of the increasing constriction of the global HIV response to biomedical technological quick fixes.

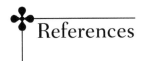

References

Adams, V., ed. 2016. *Metrics: What Counts in Global Health*. Durham, NC: Duke University Press.

Adams, V., N. J. Burke, and I. Whitmarsh. 2014. "Slow Research: Thoughts for a Movement in Global Health." *Medical Anthropology* 33, no. 3: 179–97.

Alber, E., B. Beer, J. Pauli, and M. Schnegg, eds. 2010. *Verwandtschaft heute: Positionen, Ergebnisse und Perspektiven*. Berlin: Reimer.

Alber, E., and J. Martin. 2007. "Einleitung Zum Themenschwerpunkt 'Familienwandel in Afrika.'" *Africa Spectrum* 42, no. 2: 151–66.

Alber, E., J. Martin, and C. Notermans, eds. 2013. *Child Fostering in West Africa: New Perspectives on Theory and Practices*. Leiden: Brill.

Alcorn, K. 2007. "Brazil Issues Compulsory License on Efavirenz." Retrieved 20 August 2014 from http://www.aidsmap.com/Brazil-issues-compulsory-license-on-efavirenz/page/1427206.

Anderson, D., and D. Johnson. 1995. *Revealing Prophets: Prophecy in Eastern African History*. London: Currey.

Appadurai, A. 1988. *The Social Life of Things: Commodities in Cultural Perspective*. Cambridge, UK: Cambridge University Press.

AVERT. 2014. "Antiretroviral Drug Prices." Retrieved 13 June 2014 from http://www.avert.org/antiretroviral-drug-prices.htm.

Ayo, Millard. 2015. "Babu wa Loliondo kaongea . . . tarajia hili kutoka kwake time hii!" Retrieved 15 August 2016 from http://millardayo.com/135585bll/.

Balogun, A. 2010. "Islamic Perspectives on HIV/AIDS and Antiretroviral Treatment: The Case of Nigeria." *African Journal of AIDS Research* 9, no. 4: 459–66.

Bartsch, S. 2007. "The Global Fund to Fight AIDS, Tuberculosis and Malaria." In *Global Health Governance and the Fight against HIV/AIDS*. Edited by W. Hein, S. Bartsch, and L. Kohlmorgen, 146–71. New York: Palgrave Macmillan.

Beaudin, C. L., and S. M. Chambre. 1996. "HIV/AIDS as a Chronic Disease: Emergence from the Plague Model." *American Behavioral Scientist* 39, no. 6: 684–706.

Becher, J. 1997. *Dar es Salaam, Tanga und Tabora: Stadtentwicklung in Tansania unter deutscher Kolonialherrschaft, 1885–1914*. Stuttgart: Steiner.

Beck, A. 1977. "Medicine and Society in Tanganyika, 1890–1930: A Historical Inquiry." *Transactions of the American Philosophical Society* 67, no. 3: 1–59.

———. 1981. *Medicine, Tradition, and Development in Kenya and Tanzania, 1920–1970*. Waltham, MA: Crossroads.

Becker, F. 2007. "The Virus and the Scriptures: Muslims and AIDS in Tanzania." *Journal of Religion in Africa* 37, no. 1: 16–40.

———. 2009. "Competing Explanations and Treatment Choices: Muslims, AIDS and ARVs in Tanzania." In *AIDS and Religious Practice in Africa*. Edited by F. Becker and P. W. Geissler, 155–89. Leiden: Brill.

———. 2014. "Fashioning Selves and Fashioning Styles: Negotiating the Personal and the Rhetorical in the Experience of African Recipients of ARV Treatment." In *Religion and AIDS Treatment in Africa. Saving Souls, Prolonging Lives*. Edited by R. van Dijk, H. Dilger, M. Burchardt, and T. Rasing, 27–47. Burlington, VT: Ashgate.

Becker, F., and P. W. Geissler. 2009. "Introduction: Searching for Pathways in a Landscape of Death: Religion and AIDS in Africa." In *AIDS and Religious Practice in Africa*. Edited by F. Becker and P. W. Geissler, 1–25. Leiden: Brill.

Becker, G. 1997. *Disrupted Lives: How People Create Meaning in a Chaotic World*. Berkeley: University of California Press.

Beckmann, N. 2009. "AIDS and the Power of God: Narratives of Decline and Coping Strategies in Zanzibar." In *AIDS and Religious Practice in Africa*. Edited by F. Becker and P. W. Geissler, 119–54. Leiden: Brill.

———. 2013. "Responding to Medical Crises: AIDS Treatment, Responsibilisation and the Logic of Choice." *Anthropology & Medicine* 20, no. 2: 160–74.

Beckmann, N., and J. Bujra. 2010. "The 'Politics of the Queue': The Politicization of People Living with HIV/AIDS in Tanzania." *Development and Change* 41, no. 6: 1041–64.

Behrend, H. 2009. "The Rise of Occult Powers, AIDS and the Roman Catholic Church in Western Uganda." In *AIDS and Religious Practice in Africa*. Edited by F. Becker and P. W. Geissler, 29–47. Leiden: Brill.

Behrend, H., and U. Luig, eds. 1999. *Spirit Possession, Modernity and Power in Africa*. Madison: The University of Wisconsin Press.

Benson, J. 2001. "The Impact of Privatization on Access in Tanzania." *Social Science & Medicine* 52, no. 12: 1903–15.

Bernays, S., T. Rhodes, and T. Barnett. 2007. "Hope: A New Way to Look at the HIV Epidemic." *AIDS* 21, suppl. 5: S5–11.

Biehl, J. 2004. "The Activist State: Global Pharmaceuticals, AIDS, and Citizenship in Brazil." *Social Text* 22, no. 3: 105–32.

———. 2007. "Pharmaceuticalization: AIDS Treatment and Global Health Politics." *Anthropological Quarterly* 80, no. 4: 1083–126.

———. 2010. "'Medication Is Me Now' Human Values and Political Life in the Wake of Global AIDS Treatment." In *In the Name of Humanity: The Government of Threat and Care*. Edited by I. Feldman and M. Ticktin, 151–89. Durham, NC: Duke University Press.

————. 2011. "When People Come First: Beyond Technical and Theoretical Quick-Fixes in Global Health." in *Global Political Ecology*. Edited by R. Peet, P. Robbins, and M. Watts, 100–30. London: Routledge.

Biehl, J., and A. Kleinman. 2007. "Introduction: Rethinking Subjectivity." In *Subjectivity: Ethnographic Investigations*. Edited by J. Biehl, B. Good, and A. Kleinman, 1–23. Berkeley: University of California Press.

Biehl, J., and A. Petryna, eds. 2013. *When People Come First: Critical Studies in Global Health*. Princeton, NJ: Princeton University Press.

Blower, S., and P. Farmer. 2003. "Predicting the Public Health Impact of Antiretrovirals: Preventing HIV in Developing Countries." *AIDScience* 3, no. 11. http://aidscience.org/Articles/aidscience033.asp.

Boelaert, M., W. Van Damme, B. Meessen, and P. Van der Stuyft. 2002. "Editorial: The AIDS Crisis, Cost-Effectiveness and Academic Activism." *Tropical Medicine & International Health* 7, no. 12: 1001–2.

Bohle, L. 2013. *Stigmatization, Discrimination and Illness: Experiences among HIV-Seropositive Women in Tanga, Tanzania*. Göttingen: Universitätsverlag.

Bohle, L., H. Dilger, and U. Groß. 2014. "HIV-Serostatus Disclosure in the Context of Free Antiretroviral Therapy and Socio-Economic Dependency: Experiences among Women Living with HIV in Tanzania." *African Journal of AIDS Research* 13, no. 3: 215–27.

Booth, K. 2004. *Local Women, Global Science: Fighting AIDS in Kenya*. Bloomington: Indiana University Press.

Bruchhausen, W. 2006. *Medizin zwischen den Welten: Geschichte und Gegenwart des medizinischen Pluralismus im südöstlichen Tansania*. Göttingen: V&R Unipress.

————. 2010. "Heiltraditionen oder 'Traditionelle Medizin'? Von Förderung und Verweigerung des biomedizinischen Paradigmas in Tansania." In *Medizin im Kontext. Krankheit und Gesundheit in einer vernetzten Welt*. Edited by H. Dilger and B. Hadolt, 245–65. Frankfurt: Peter Lang.

Buguzi, S., and J. Namkwahe. 2016. "Govt Needs Sh830bn for Ambitious HIV Plan." *The Citizen*. 1 December.

Bujra, J., and S. Mokake. 2000. "AIDS Activism in Dar Es Salaam: Many Struggles; a Single Goal." In *AIDS, Sexuality and Gender in Africa: Collective Strategies and Struggles in Tanzania and Zambia*. Edited by C. Baylies and J. Bujra, 153–74. London: Routledge.

Bunton, R., and A. Petersen. 2002. *Foucault, Health and Medicine*. London: Taylor & Francis.

Burawoy, M. 1998. "The Extended Case Method." *Sociological Theory* 16, no. 1: 4–33.

Burchardt, M. 2009. "Subjects of Counseling: Religion, HIV/AIDS and the Management of Everyday Life in South Africa." In *AIDS and Religious Practice in Africa*. Edited by F. Becker and P. W. Geissler, 333–58. Leiden: Brill.

Caplan, P. 2004. "Introduction." In *Swahili Modernities. Culture, Politics, and Identity on the East Coast of Africa*. Edited by P. Caplan and F. Topan, 1–18. Trenton, NJ: Africa World Press.

Carsten, J. 2000. *Cultures of Relatedness: New Approaches to the Study of Kinship*. Cambridge, UK: Cambridge University Press.

Cassidy, R. 2010. "Global Expectations and Local Practices: HIV Support Groups in the Gambia." *AIDS Care* 22, suppl. 2: S1598–605.

Cassidy, R., and M. Leach. 2009. "AIDS, Citizenship and Global Funding: A Gambian Case Study." University of Sussex, Institute of Development Studies, Working Paper no. 325.

Castro, A., and P. Farmer. 2005. "Understanding and Addressing AIDS-Related Stigma: From Anthropological Theory to Clinical Practice in Haiti." *American Journal of Public Health* 95, no. 1: 53–9.

Charmaz, K. 1983. "Loss of Self: A Fundamental Form of Suffering in the Chronically Ill." *Sociology of Health & Illness* 5, no. 2: 168–95.

———. 1995. "The Body, Identity, and Self: Adapting to Impairment." *The Sociological Quarterly* 36, no. 4: 657–80.

Chiwambo, Y. 2011. "HIV/AIDS Cure: Where Is the Truth?" *Business Week.* 13–19 May.

Coetzee, D., and H. Schneider. "Strengthening the Health System and Ensuring Equity in the Widescale Implementation of an Antiretroviral Therapy Programme in South Africa: Editorial." *South African Medical Journal* 93, no. 10: 772–3.

Comaroff, J. 1993. "The Diseased Heart of Africa: Medicine, Colonialism, and the Black Body." In *Knowledge, Power, and Practice. The Anthropology of Medicine and Everyday Life*. Edited by S. Lindenbaum and M. Lock, 305–29. Berkeley: University of California Press.

Comaroff, J., and J. Comaroff. 1993. *Modernity and Its Malcontents: Ritual and Power in Postcolonial Africa*. Chicago: University of Chicago Press.

Conrad, P. 1992. "Medicalization and Social Control." *Annual Review of Sociology* 18: 209–32.

Cooper, D., J. Harris, L. Myer, P. Orner, and H. Bracken. 2007. "'Life Is Still Going on': Reproductive Intentions among HIV-Positive Women and Men in South Africa." *Social Science & Medicine* 65, no. 2: 274–83.

Crane, J. 2013. *Scrambling for Africa: AIDS, Expertise, and the Rise of American Global Health Science*. Ithaca, NY: Cornell University Press.

Crapanzano, V. 2010. "'At the Heart of the Discipline': Critical Reflections on Fieldwork." In *Emotions in the Field: The Psychology and Anthropology of Fieldwork Experience*. Edited by J. Davies and D. Spencer, 55–78. Stanford, CA: Stanford University Press.

Csordas, T. 2008. "Intersubjectivity and Intercorporeality." *Subjectivity* 22, no. 1: 110–21.

D'Andrade, R. 1995. "Moral Models in Anthropology." *Current Anthropology* 36, no. 3: 399–408.

Das, V., and R. Addlakha. 2001. "Disability and Domestic Citizenship: Voice, Gender, and the Making of the Subject." *Public Culture* 13, no. 3: 511–31.

Davies, J. 2010. "Disorientation, Dissonance, and Altered Perception in the Field." in *Emotions in the Field: The Psychology and Anthropology of*

Fieldwork Experience. Edited by J. Davies and D. Spencer, 79–98. Stanford, CA: Stanford University Press.

Davies, M. 1997. "Shattered Assumptions: Time and the Experience of Long-Term HIV Positivity." *Social Science & Medicine* 44, no. 5: 561–71.

Deacon, H. 2006. "Towards a Sustainable Theory of Health-Related Stigma: Lessons from the HIV/AIDS Literature." *Journal of Community & Applied Social Psychology* 16, no. 6: 418–25.

Deacon, H., I. Stephney, and S. Prosalendis. 2005. *Understanding HIV/AIDS Stigma: A Theoretical and Methodological Analysis*. Cape Town: Human Sciences Research Council Press.

De Klerk, J. 2012. "The Compassion of Concealment: Silence between Older Caregivers and Dying Patients in the AIDS Era, Northwest Tanzania." *Culture, Health & Sexuality* 14, suppl. 1: S27–38.

Dilger, H. 2001. "'Living PositHIVely in Tanzania': The Global Dynamics of AIDS and the Meaning of Religion for International and Local AIDS Work." *Africa Spectrum* 36, no. 1: 73–90.

———. 2003. "Sexuality, AIDS, and the Lures of Modernity: Reflexivity and Morality among Young People in Rural Tanzania." *Medical Anthropology* 22, no. 1: 23–52.

———. 2005. *Leben mit AIDS: Krankheit, Tod und soziale Beziehungen in Afrika*. Frankfurt: Campus.

———. 2007. "Healing the Wounds of Modernity: Salvation, Community and Care in a Neo-Pentecostal Church in Dar Es Salaam, Tanzania." *Journal of Religion in Africa* 37, no. 1: 59–83.

———. 2008. "'We Are All Going to Die': Kinship, Belonging, and the Morality of HIV/AIDS-Related Illnesses and Deaths in Rural Tanzania." *Anthropological Quarterly* 81, no. 1: 207–32.

———. 2009. "Doing Better? Religion, the Virtue-Ethics of Development, and the Fragmentation of Health Politics in Tanzania." *Africa Today* 56, no. 1: 89–110.

———. 2010. "'My Relatives Are Running Away from Me!' Kinship and Care in the Wake of Structural Adjustment, Privatisation and HIV/AIDS in Tanzania." In *Morality, Hope and Grief: Anthropologies of AIDS in Africa*. Edited by H. Dilger and U. Luig, 102–24. New York: Berghahn Books.

———. 2012. "Targeting the Empowered Individual: Transnational Policy Making, the Global Economy of Aid, and the Limitations of Biopower in Tanzania." In *Medicine, Mobility, and Power in Global Africa: Transnational Health and Healing*. Edited by H. Dilger, A. Kane, and S. Langwick, 60–91. Bloomington: Indiana University Press.

———. 2013a. "No Public? Class Dynamics, the Politics of Extraversion, and the Non-Formation of Political Publics and (Religious) AIDS Activism in Urban Tanzania." In *Transnationalität und Öffentlichkeit*. Edited by C. Schmitt and A. Vonderau, 175–205. Bielefeld: transcript.

———. 2013b. "Securing Wealth, Ordering Social Relations: Kinship, Morality, and the Configuration of Subjectivity and Belonging across the Rural-Urban

Divide." In *African Migrations: Patterns and Perspectives*. Edited by A. Kane and T. Leedy, 113–32. Bloomington: Indiana University Press.

———. 2014. "Claiming Territory: Medical Mission, Interreligious Revivalism, and the Spatialization of Health Interventions in Urban Tanzania." *Medical Anthropology* 33, no. 1: 52–67.

Dilger, H., M. Burchardt, and R. Van Dijk. 2010. "Introduction: The Redemptive Moment: HIV Treatments and the Production of New Religious Spaces." *African Journal of AIDS Research* 9, no. 4: 373–83.

Doran, M. 2007. "Reconstructing Mchape '95: AIDS, Billy Chisupe, and the Politics of Persuasion." *Journal of Eastern African Studies* 1, no. 3: 397–416.

Dumit, J. 2002. "Drugs for Life." *Molecular Interventions* 2, no. 3: 124–27.

Eibl, M. 2010. "PEPFAR, Politics, and Patients. Antiretroviral Treatment in Tanzania." PhD diss., Michigan State University.

Englund, H. 1996. "Witchcraft, Modernity and the Person: The Morality of Accumulation in Central Malawi." *Critique of Anthropology* 16, no. 3: 257–79.

Estroff, S. 1989. "Self, Identity, and Subjective Experiences of Schizophrenia: In Search of the Subject." *Schizophrenia Bulletin* 15, no. 2: 189–96.

Evans, R. 2005. "Social Networks, Migration, and Care in Tanzania: Caregivers' and Children's Resilience to Coping with HIV/AIDS." *Journal of Children and Poverty* 11, no. 2: 111–29.

Evans-Pritchard, E. 1987. *Witchcraft, Oracles, and Magic among the Azande.* Oxford: Clarendon.

Farmer, P. 2006. *AIDS and Accusation: Haiti and the Geography of Blame.* Berkeley: University of California Press.

Fassin, D. 2007. *When Bodies Remember: Experiences and Politics of AIDS in South Africa.* Berkeley: University of California Press.

Feierman, S. 1985. "Struggles for Control: The Social Roots of Health and Healing in Modern Africa." *African Studies Review* 28, no. 2/3: 73–147.

Feierman, S., and J. Janzen. 1992. *The Social Basis of Health and Healing in Africa.* Berkeley: University of California Press.

Ferguson, J. 2006. *Global Shadows: Africa in the Neoliberal World Order.* Durham, NC: Duke University Press.

Ferguson, J., and A. Gupta. 2002. "Spatializing States: Toward an Ethnography of Neoliberal Governmentality." *American Ethnologist* 29, no. 4: 981–1002.

Fortes, M. 2009. *Kinship and the Social Order: The Legacy of Lewis Henry Morgan.* Brunswick, NJ: Transaction Publishers.

Foucault, M. 1977. *Discipline and Punish.* London: Penguin.

———. 1982. "The Subject and Power." In *Michel Foucault: Beyond Structuralism and Hermeneutics.* Edited by H. Dreyfus and P. Rabinow, 208–26. Brighton: Harvester.

———. 1988. *Technologies of the Self: A Seminar with Michel Foucault.* Edited by L. Martin, H. Gutman, and P. Hutton. Amherst, MA: University of Massachusetts Press.

———. 1991. "Governmentality." In *The Foucault Effect: Studies in Governmentality.* Edited by G. Burchell, C. Gordon, and P. Miller, 87–104. London: Harvester Wheatsheaf.

Frank, D. 2011. "Milioni 3 wanywa kikombe Loliondo." *Tanzania Daima.* 9 May.

Frank, E., and A. Rödlach. 2013. "To Disclose or Not to Disclose, That Is the Question! Antiretroviral Therapy, Access to Resources and Stigma in Southern Africa." *Journal of Southern African Studies* 39, no. 1: 119–33.

Galvão, J. 2005. "Brazil and Access to HIV/AIDS Drugs: A Question of Human Rights and Public Health." *American Journal of Public Health* 95, no. 7: 1110–16.

Garrett, L. 2007. "The Challenge of Global Health." *Foreign Affairs* 86, no. 1: 14–38.

Geffen, N. 2010. *Debunking Delusions: The Inside Story of the Treatment Action Campaign.* Auckland Park, South Africa: Jacana Media.

Geissler, P. W. 2015. "Introduction: A Life Science in Its African Para-State." In *Para-States and Medical Science: Making African Global Health.* Edited by P. W. Geissler, 1–44. Durham, NC: Duke University Press.

Geissler, P. W., R. Rottenburg, and J. Zenker. 2012. "21st Century African Biopolitics: Fuzzy Fringes, Cracks and Undersides, Neglected Backwaters, and Returning Politics." In *Rethinking Biomedicine and Governance in Africa: Contributions from Anthropology.* Edited by P. W. Geissler, R. Rottenburg, and J. Zenker, 7–19. Bielefeld: Transcript.

Geschiere, P., and J. Roitman. 1997. *The Modernity of Witchcraft: Politics and the Occult in Postcolonial Africa.* Charlottesville: University of Virginia Press.

Gessler, M., D. Msyua, M. Nkunya, A. Schär, M. Heinrich, and M. Tanner 1995. "Traditional Healers in Tanzania: Sociocultural Profile and Three Short Portraits." *Journal of Ethnopharmacology* 48, no. 3: 145–60.

GFATM (The Global Fund to Fight AIDS, Tuberculosis and Malaria). 2013. *Program Scorecard Tanzania HIV/AIDS.* Geneva: GFATM.

Giles, L. 1987. "Possession Cults on the Swahili Coast: A Re-Examination of Theories of Marginality." *Africa: Journal of the International African Institute* 57, no. 2: 234–58.

———. 1995. "Sociocultural Change and Spirit Possession on the Swahili Coast of East Africa." *Anthropological Quarterly* 68, no. 2: 89–106.

Goffman, E. 1963. *Stigma: Notes on the Management of Spoiled Identity.* New York: Simon & Schuster.

Going, M. 2011. "Babu kortini." *Ukweli na Uwazi.* 16–22 July.

Green, M., and S. Mesaki. 2005. "The Birth of the 'Salon': Poverty, 'Modernization,' and Dealing with Witchcraft in Southern Tanzania." *American Ethnologist* 32, no. 3: 371–88.

Grube, N. 2008. *Die indische Diaspora in Tansania zwischen Transnationalismus und Lokalität: "We are Indians even though we are not born in India."* Hamburg: Kovač.

Hardon, A. 2012. "Biomedical Hype and Hopes: AIDS Medicines in Africa." In *Rethinking Biomedicine and Governance in Africa: Contributions from*

Anthropology. Edited by P. W. Geissler, R. Rottenburg, and J. Zenker, 77–96. Bielefeld: Transcript.

Hardon, A., D. Akurut, C. Comoro, C. Ekezie, H. Irunde, T. Gerrits, J. Kglatwane, J. Kinsman, R. Kwasa, J. Maridadi, T.M. Moroka, S. Moyo, A. Nakiyemba, S. Nsimba, R. Ogenyi, T. Oyabba, F. Temu, and R. Laing. 2007. "Hunger, Waiting Time and Transport Costs: Time to Confront Challenges to ART Adherence in Africa." *AIDS Care* 19, no. 5: 658–65.

Hardon, A., and H. Dilger. 2011. "Global AIDS Medicines in East African Health Institutions." *Medical Anthropology* 30, no. 2: 136–57.

Hardon, A., and E. Moyer. 2014. "Anthropology of AIDS: Modes of Engagement." *Medical Anthropology* 33, no. 4: 255–62.

Hardon, A., and D. Posel. 2012. "Secrecy as Embodied Practice: Beyond the Confessional Imperative." *Culture, Health & Sexuality* 14, suppl. 1: S1–13.

Hardon, A., and E. Sanabria. 2017. "Fluid Drugs: Revisiting the Anthropology of Pharmaceuticals." *Annual Review of Anthropology* 46: 117–32.

Hartemink, A., and J. Wienk. 1995. "Sisal Production and Soil Fertility Decline in Tanzania." *Outlook on Agriculture* 24, no. 2: 92–96.

Havlir, D., and C. Beyrer. 2012. "The Beginning of the End of AIDS?" *The New England Journal of Medicine* 367, no. 8: 685–87.

Hearn, J. 1998. "The 'NGO-isation' of Kenyan Society: USAID & the Restructuring of Health Care." *Review of African Political Economy* 25, no. 75: 89–100.

Hegelund, A. 2005. "Objectivity and Subjectivity in the Ethnographic Method." *Qualitative Health Research* 15, no. 5: 647–68.

Hein, W. 2007. "Global Health Governance and WTO/TRIPS: Conflicts between 'Global Market-Creation' and 'Global Social Rights.'" In *Global Health Governance and the Fight against HIV/AIDS*. Edited by W. Hein, S. Bartsch, and L. Kohlmorgen, 38–66. New York: Palgrave Macmillan.

Hiza, Gazpar. 2011. "Needed: Protection to Pastor Ambilikile." *The African*. 11 May.

Hoen, E. 't. 2009. *The Global Politics of Pharmaceutical Monopoly Power: Drug Patents, Access, Innovation and the Application of the WTO Doha Declaration on TRIPS and Public Health*. Diemen, Netherlands: AMB Publishers.

Horton, M., and J. Middleton. 2000. *The Swahili: The Social Landscape of a Mercantile Society*. Oxford: Blackwell.

Iliffe, J. 1969. *Tanganyika under German Rule, 1905–1912*. London: Cambridge University Press.

———. 1979. *A Modern History of Tanganyika*. Cambridge, UK: Cambridge University Press.

———. 1998. *East African Doctors: A History of the Modern Profession*. Cambridge, UK: Cambridge University Press.

———. 2006. *The African AIDS Epidemic: A History*. Athens: Ohio University Press.

Inda, J. X. 2005. *Anthropologies of Modernity: Foucault, Governmentality, and Life Politics*. Malden, MA: Wiley.

Ingram, A. 2009. "Biosecurity and the International Response to HIV/AIDS: Governmentality, Globalisation and Security." *Area* 42, no. 3: 293–301.

———. 2013. "After the Exception: HIV/AIDS Beyond Salvation and Scarcity." *Antipode* 45, no. 2: 436–54.

International HIV/AIDS Alliance. 2012. *Don't Stop Now: How Underfunding the Global Fund to Fight AIDS, Tuberculosis and Malaria Impacts the HIV Response.* Hove, UK: International HIV/AIDS Alliance.

IRIN News. 2014. "Analysis: HIV Generics under Threat from Tighter Patenting Rules." *IRINnews*. Retrieved 13 June 2014 from http://www.irinnews.org/Report/90041/Analysis-HIV-generics-under-threat-from-tighter-patenting-rules.

Jackson, M. 1989. *Paths Toward a Clearing: Radical Empiricism and Ethnographic Inquiry*. Bloomington: Indiana University Press.

———. 1998. *Minima Ethnographica: Intersubjectivity and the Anthropological Project*. Chicago: University of Chicago Press.

Janzen, J. 1987. "Therapy Management: Concept, Reality, Process." *Medical Anthropology Quarterly* 1, no. 1: 68–84.

———. 1992. *Ngoma: Discourses of Healing in Central and Southern Africa*. Berkeley: University of California Press.

Jones, P. 2004. "When 'Development' Devastates: Donor Discourses, Access to HIV/AIDS Treatment in Africa and Rethinking the Landscape of Development." *Third World Quarterly* 25, no. 2: 385–404.

Jozen, A. 2011. "Loliondo Cup: Pact with God or the Devil?" *The Guardian*. 26 March.

Juma, M. 2011a. "Tiba ya Loliondo yamtisha Kakobe." *Mwananchi*. 7 March.

———. 2011b. "Mchungaji Mwasapila apinga dawa yake iwe ya vidonge." *Mwananchi*. 1 May.

Juma, M., and C. Mshana. 2011. "Hospitali nne kuchunguza dawa ya Babu." *Mwananchi*. 30 April.

Justice, L. 2011. "Waganga wa jadi wanaojitangaza hawana uwezo wa kutibu." *Majira*. 26 May.

Kaigarula, W. 2011. "Tricky Balancing Between Secular Medicine, Divine Healing . . . ." *Guardian on Sunday*. 13 March.

Kalipeni, E., A. Muula, and O. Liveve. 2009. "HIV and Religion in Africa: The Politics of Treatment and Prevention in a Changing Religious Landscape." Prolonging Life, Challenging Religion Conference, Lusaka, 16 April 2009. Lusaka: International Research Network on Religion and HIV/AIDS in Africa.

Kalofonos, I. 2008. "'All I Eat Is ARVs': Living with HIV/AIDS at the Dawn of the Treatment Era in Central Mozambique." PhD diss., University of California.

———. 2010. "'All I Eat Is ARVs': The Paradox of AIDS Treatment Interventions in Central Mozambique." *Medical Anthropology Quarterly* 24, no. 3: 363–80.

Kasper, T., D. Coetzee, F. Louis, A. Boulle, and K. Hilderbrand. 2003. "Demystifying Antiretroviral Therapy in Resource-Poor Settings." *Essential Drugs Monitor* 32: 20–21.

Kates, K., A. Wexler, E. Lief, and UNAIDS. 2017. *Donor Government Funding for HIV in Low- and Middle-Income Countries in 2016*. Menlo Park, CA: The Henry J. Kaiser Family Foundation.

Katulanda, F. 2011. "Foundation Says Mwasapila Has Not Been Saying the Truth." *The Citizen*. 19 April.

Kayombo, E., F. Uiso, Z. Mbwambo, R. Mahunnah, M. Moshi, and Y. Mgonda. 2007. "Experience of Initiating Collaboration of Traditional Healers in Managing HIV and AIDS in Tanzania." *Journal of Ethnobiology and Ethnomedicine* 3, no. 1: 6.

Kelly, M. 2010. "International Biopolitics: Foucault, Globalisation and Imperialism." *Theoria* 57, no. 123: 1–26.

Kendall, C., and Z. Hill. 2010. "Chronicity and AIDS in Three South African Communities." In *Chronic Conditions, Fluid States: Chronicity and the Anthropology of Illness*. Edited by L. Manderson and C. Smith-Morris, 175–94. New Brunswick, NJ: Rutgers University Press.

Kenworthy, N., M. Thomann, and R. Parker. 2017. "From a Global Crisis to the 'End of AIDS': New Epidemics of Signification." *Global Public Health* 10: 1–12.

King, R. 2002. *Ancient Remedies, New Disease: Involving Traditional Healers in Increasing Access to AIDS Care and Prevention in East Africa*. Geneva: UNAIDS.

Kipp, W., D. Tindyebwa, E. Karamagi, and T Rubaale. 2006. "Family Caregiving to AIDS Patients: The Role of Gender in Caregiver Burden in Uganda." *Journal of International Women's Studies* 7, no. 4: 1–13.

Kipp, W., D. Tindyebwa, T. Rubaale, E. Karamagi, E. Bajenja. 2007. "Family Caregivers in Rural Uganda: The Hidden Reality." *Health Care for Women International* 28, no. 10: 856–71.

Kisembo, P. 2011. "'Babu' Cupful Gets Initial Nod." *The Guardian*. 29 March.

Kistner, U. 2009. "Adversities in Adherence: Paralogisms of 'Biological Citizenship' in South Africa." AEGIS 3rd European Conference on African Studies, Leipzig, 4–7 June 2009. Leipzig: Africa-Europe Group for Interdisciplinary Studies.

Klaits, F. 2010. *Death in a Church of Life: Moral Passion During Botswana's Time of AIDS*. Berkeley: University of California Press.

Kleinman, A. 1992. "Local Worlds of Suffering: An Interpersonal Focus for Ethnographies of Illness Experience." *Qualitative Health Research* 2, no. 2: 127–34.

———. 1994. "Pain and Resistance: The Deligitimation and Religitimation of Local Worlds." In *Pain as Human Experience: An Anthropological Perspective*. Edited by M.-J. DelVecchio Good, P. Brodwin, B. Good, and A. Kleinman, 169–97. Berkeley: University of California Press.

———. 1999. "Moral Experience and Ethical Reflection: Can Ethnography Reconcile Them? A Quandary for 'the New Bioethics.'" *Daedalus* 128, no. 4: 69–97.

Kleinman, A., V. Das, and M. Lock, eds. 1997. *Social Suffering*. Berkeley: University of California Press.

Kleinman, A., and J. Kleinman. 1991. "Suffering and Its Professional Transformation: Toward an Ethnography of Interpersonal Experience." *Culture, Medicine and Psychiatry* 15, no. 3: 275–301.

Kwansa, B. 2010. "Complex Negotiations: 'Spiritual' Therapy and Living with HIV in Ghana." *African Journal of AIDS Research* 9, no. 4: 449–58.

Kwesigabo, G., M. Mwangu, D. Kakoko, I. Warriner, C. Mkony, J. Killewo, S. Macfarlane, E. Kaaya, and P. Freeman. 2012. "Tanzania's Health System and Workforce Crisis." *Journal of Public Health Policy* 33: S35–44.

Kyakuwa, M. 2009. "More Hands in Complex ART Delivery: Experiences from the Expert Clients Initiative in Rural Uganda." *African Sociological Review* 13, no. 2: 143-67,

———. 2011. *Going the Extra Mile: An Ethnography of Care-Giving and Care Designing among Nurses in Uganda*. Amsterdam: University of Amsterdam.

Kyakuwa, M., A. Hardon, and Z. Goldstein. 2012. "The Adopted Children of ART: Expert Clients and Role Tensions in ART Provision in Uganda. *Medical Anthropology* 31, no. 2: 149–61.

Laing, R., and C. Hodgkin. 2006. "Overview of Antiretroviral Therapy, Adherence and Drug-Resistance." In *From Access to Adherence: The Challenges of Antiretroviral Treatment; Studies from Botswana, Tanzania and Uganda*. Edited by A. Hardon, S. Davey, and T. Gerrits, 21–31. Geneva: WHO.

Lamtey, G. 2012. "Government out to Set up AIDS Trust Fund." *The Guardian*. 18 February.

Langwick, S. 2006. "Geographies of Medicine: Interrogating the Boundary between 'Traditional' and 'Modern' Medicine in Colonial Tanganyika." In *Borders and Healers. Brokering Therapeutic Resources in Southeast Africa*. Edited by T. Luedke and H. West, 143–65. Bloomington: Indiana University Press.

———. 2011. *Bodies, Politics, and African Healing: The Matter of Maladies in Tanzania*. Bloomington: Indiana University Press.

Langwick, S., H. Dilger, and A. Kane. 2012. "Introduction: Transnational Medicine, Mobile Experts." In *Medicine, Mobility, and Power in Global Africa. Transnational Health and Healing*. Edited by H. Dilger, A. Kane, and S. Langwick, 1-27. Bloomington: Indiana University Press.

Lavers, M. 2017. "Pelosi: Trump Budget Would Hurt People with HIV/AIDS." Retrieved 7 February 2018 from https://www.washingtonblade.com/2017/09/07/pelosi-trump-budget-hurt-people-hivaids/.

Le Marcis, F. 2012. "Struggling with AIDS in South Africa: The Space of the Everyday as a Field of Recognition." *Medical Anthropology Quarterly* 26, no. 4: 486–502.

Lemke, T. 2002. "Foucault, Governmentality, and Critique." *Rethinking Marxism* 14, no. 3: 49–64.

Link, B., and J. Phelan. 2001. "Conceptualizing Stigma." *Annual Review of Sociology* 27: 363–85.

Lock, M., and V.-K. Nguyen. 2010. *An Anthropology of Biomedicine*. Malden, MA: Wiley-Blackwell.

Long, D., C. Hunter, and S. Van der Geest. 2008. "When the Field Is a Ward or a Clinic: Hospital Ethnography." *Anthropology & Medicine* 15, no. 2: 71–78.

Lugalla, J. 1995. "The Impact of Structural Adjustment Policies on Women's and Children's Health in Tanzania." *Review of African Political Economy* 22, no. 63: 43–53.

———. 2008. *Social Context of Disclosing HIV Test Results: HIV Testing in Tanzania*. Dar es Salaam: Center for Strategic Research and Development and Macro International Inc.

Luhwago, Rodgers. 2011. "This Is a Golden Chance—Shelukindo." *Guardian on Sunday*. 13 March.

Lunogelo, H., A. Mbilinyi, and M. Hangi. 2009. "The Global Financial Crisis and Tanzania: Effects and Policy Responses." Dar es Salaam: Economic and Social Research Foundation.

Lupton, D. 1995. *The Imperative of Health: Public Health and the Regulated Body*. London: Sage.

———. 1997. "Foucault and the Medicalization Critique." In *Foucault, Health and Medicine*. Edited by A. Petersen and R. Bunton, 94–110. London; New York: Routledge.

Mackenrodt, L. 2011. *Swahili Spirit Possession and Islamic Healing in Contemporary Tanzania: The Jinn Fly on Friday*. Hamburg: Kovač.

Maina, T., and D. Ngowi. 2011. *Draft Report on Tanzania's Programmatic and Financial Gap Analysis*. Unpublished document.

Makore, R. 2011. "Serikali kutolea tamko rasmi dawa ya Babu wa Loliondo." *Nipashe*. 31 August.

Malebo, H., and Z. Mbwambo. 2011. *Technical Report on Miracle Cure Prescribed Rev. Ambilikile Mwasupile in Samunge Village*. Dar es Salaam: National Institute for Medical Research.

Malpas, J. 2003. "Bio-Medical Topoi: The Dominance of Space, the Recalcitrance of Place, and the Making of Persons." *Social Science & Medicine* 56: 2343–51.

Manderson, L. 2015. "Telling Points." In *Disclosure in Health and Illness*. Edited by M. Davis and L. Manderson, 1–15. New York: Routledge.

Manderson, L., and C. Smith-Morris. 2010. "Introduction: Chronicity and the Experience of Illness." In *Chronic Conditions, Fluid States: Chronicity and the Anthropology of Illness*. Edited by L. Manderson and C. Smith-Morris, 1–18. New Brunswick, NJ: Rutgers University Press.

Marseille, E., P. Hofmann, and J. Kahn. 2002. "HIV Prevention before HAART in Sub-Saharan Africa." *The Lancet* 359, no. 9320: 1851–56.

Marsland, R. 2007. "The Modern Traditional Healer: Locating 'Hybridity' in Modern Traditional Medicine, Southern Tanzania." *Journal of Southern African Studies* 33, no. 4: 751–65.

———. 2012. "(Bio)Sociality and HIV in Tanzania: Finding a Living to Support a Life." *Medical Anthropology Quarterly* 26, no. 4: 470–85.

Marsland, R., and R. Prince. 2012. "What Is Life Worth? Exploring Biomedical Interventions, Survival, and the Politics of Life." *Medical Anthropology Quarterly* 26, no. 4: 453–69.

Marten, M. 2014. "Aid Withdrawal and Health Care Sustainability: Shifting Mandates in Health Institutions and HIV/AIDS Programs in Tanzania." PhD diss., University of South Florida.

Marwick, M., ed. 1990. *Witchcraft and Sorcery: Selected Readings*. London: Penguin.

Mattes, D. 2011. "'We Are Just Supposed to Be Quiet': The Production of Adherence to Antiretroviral Treatment in Urban Tanzania." *Medical Anthropology* 30, no. 2: 158–82.

———. 2012. "'I Am Also a Human Being!' Antiretroviral Treatment in Local Moral Worlds." *Anthropology & Medicine* 19, no. 1: 75–84.

———. 2014a. "Caught in Transition: The Struggle to Live a 'Normal' Life with HIV in Tanzania." *Medical Anthropology* 33, no. 4: 270–87.

———. 2014b. "'Life Is Not a Rehearsal, It's a Performance': An Ethnographic Enquiry into the Subjectivities of Children and Adolescents Living with Antiretroviral Treatment in Northeastern Tanzania." *Children and Youth Services Review* 45: 28–37.

———. 2014c. "The Blood of Jesus and CD4 Counts: Dreaming, Developing and Navigating Therapeutic Options for Curing HIV/AIDS in Tanzania." In *Religion and AIDS Treatment in Africa. Saving Souls, Prolonging Lives.* Edited by R. van Dijk, H. Dilger, M. Burchardt, and T Rasing, 169–93. Farnham: Ashgate.

Mattingly, C. 1994. "The Concept of Therapeutic 'Emplotment.'" *Social Science & Medicine* 38, no. 6: 811–22.

Mbembe, A. 2001. *On the Postcolony*. Berkeley: University of California Press.

Mbonea, E. 2011a. "Babu akana kuwa sangoma." *Mtanzania*. 17 May.

———. 2011b. "Wafanyabiashara wakimbia Samunge." *Mtanzania*. 13 July.

McFalls, L. 2010. "Benevolent Dictatorship: The Formal Logic of Humanitarian Government." In *Contemporary States of Emergency: The Politics of Military and Humanitarian Interventions*. Edited by D. Fassin and M. Pandolfi, 317–33. New York: Zone Books.

McGrath, J., M. Winchester, D. Kaawa-Mafigiri, E. Walakira, F. Nabutiibwa, J. Birungi, G. Ssendegye, A. Nalwoga, E. Kyarikunda, S. Kisakye, N. Ayebazidwe, and C. Rwabukwali. 2014. "Challenging the Paradigm: Anthropological Perspectives on HIV as a Chronic Disease." *Medical Anthropology* 33, no. 4: 303–17.

McMillen, H. 2004. "The Adapting Healer: Pioneering through Shifting Epidemiological and Sociocultural Landscapes." *Social Science & Medicine* 59, no. 5: 889–902.

McNeil, D. "Global AIDS Fund Will Pause New Grants and Seek New Manager." *New York Times*. 23 November.

Meinert, L., H. Mogensen, and J. Twebaze. 2009. "Tests for Life Chances: CD4 Miracles and Obstacles in Uganda." *Anthropology & Medicine* 16, no. 2: 195–209.

Meinert, L. 2013. "Regimes of Homework in AIDS Care Questions of Responsibility and the Imagination of Lives in Uganda." In *Making and Unmaking Public Health in Africa: Ethnographic and Historical Perspectives.* Edited by R. Prince and R. Marsland, 119–39. Athens: Ohio University Press.

Merson, M. H., J. O'Malley, D. Serwadda, and C. Apisuk. 2008. "The History and Challenge of HIV Prevention." *The Lancet* 372, no. 9637: 475–88.

Mesaki, S. 1993. "Witchcraft and Witch-Killings in Tanzania." PhD diss., University of Minnesota.

Messac, L., and K. Prabhu. 2013. "Redefining the Possible: The Global AIDS Response." In *Reimagining Global Health: An Introduction.* Edited by P. Farmer, J. Y. Kim, A. Kleinman, and M. Basilico, 111–32. Berkeley: University of California Press.

Mfecane, S. 2011. "Negotiating Therapeutic Citizenship and Notions of Masculinity in a South African Village." *African Journal of AIDS Research* 10, no. 2: 129–38.

Mgamba, R. 2011. "The Magic Man, the Tree and a Cup of Life." *Guardian on Sunday.* 27 March.

Mhala, J. 2011. "Babu wa Loliondo apewa cheti maalumu." *Habari Leo.* 11 May.

Middleton, J. 1992. *The World of the Swahili: An African Mercantile Civilization.* New Haven, CT: Yale University Press.

Middleton, J., and E. Winter. 1963. *Witchcraft and Sorcery in East Africa.* London: Routledge.

Mikaili, J. 2011. "Loliondo's New Billionaires." *Guardian on Sunday.* 27 March.

Miller, P., and N. Rose. 2008. *Governing the Present: Administering Economic, Social and Personal Life.* Cambridge, MA: Polity.

Mlekani, K. 2011. "Madaktari: Tiba ya Babu imeleta maafa Cosmas Mlekani." *Nipashe.* 25 August.

Moatti, J. P., I. N'Doye, S. Hammer, J. Hale, and M. Kazatchkine. 2003. "Antiretroviral Treatment for HIV Infection in Developing Countries: An Attainable New Paradigm." *Nature Medicine* 9, no. 12: 1449–52.

Moen, K., P. Aggleton, M. Leshabari, and A.-L. Middelthon. 2013. "Situating Condoms in Sexual Lives: Experiences of Same-Sex-Attracted Men in Tanzania." *International Journal of Sexual Health* 25, no. 3: 185–97.

Mogensen, H. 1995. *AIDS Is a Kind of Kahungo That Kills: The Challenge of Using Local Narratives When Exploring AIDS among the Tonga of Southern Zambia.* Oslo: Scandinavian University Press.

———. 2009. "Surviving AIDS? The Uncertainty of Antiretroviral Treatment." In *Dealing with Uncertainty in Contemporary Africal Lives.* Edited by L. Haram and C. Bawa Yamba, 179–93. Uppsala: Nordiska Afrikainstitutet.

———. 2010. "New Hopes and New Dilemmas: Disclosure and Recognition in the Time of Antiretroviral Treatment." In *Morality, Hope, and Grief. Anthropologies of AIDS in Africa.* Edited by H. Dilger and U. Luig, 61–79. New York; Oxford: Berghahn Books.

Mol, A. 2008. *The Logic of Care: Health and the Problem of Patient Choice.* New York: Routledge.

Molotsky, I. 1987. "US Approves Drug to Prolong Lives of AIDS Patients." *New York Times.* 21 March.

Mosoba, T. 2011. "Woman Who Set Off the Rush for the 'Drink.'" *The Citizen.* 13 March.

———. 2012. "Fruits of Babu's Cup." *The Citizen.* 24 November.

Moyer, E. 2012. "Faidha Gani? What's the Point: HIV and the Logics of (Non)-Disclosure among Young Activists in Zanzibar." *Culture, Health & Sexuality* 14, suppl. 1: S67–79.

———. 2013. "The Duty to Disclose in Kenyan Health Facilities: A Qualitative Investigation of HIV Disclosure in Everyday Practice." *Journal of Social Aspects of HIV/AIDS* 10, S1: S60–72.

———. 2015. "The Anthropology of Life After AIDS: Epistemological Continuities in the Age of Antiretroviral Treatment." *Annual Review of Anthropology* 44, no. 1: 259–75.

Moyer, E., M. Burchardt, and R. van Dijk. 2013. "Editorial Introduction: Sexuality, Intimacy and Counselling: Perspectives from Africa." *Culture, Health & Sexuality* 15, suppl. 4: S431–39.

Moyer, E., and A. Hardon. 2014. "A Disease Unlike Any Other? Why HIV Remains Exceptional in the Age of Treatment." *Medical Anthropology* 33, no. 4: 263–9.

Moyer, E., and E. K. Igonya. 2014. "When Families Fail: Shifting Expectations of Care among People Living with HIV in Nairobi, Kenya." *Anthropology & Medicine* 21, no. 2: 136–48.

MSF (Médecins Sans Frontières). 2012a. *Losing Ground: How Funding Shortfalls and the Cancellation of the Global Fund's Round 11 Are Jeopardizing the Fight against HIV and TB.* Geneva: MSF.

———. 2012b. *Progress under Threat: Perspectives on the HIV Treatment Gap.* Geneva: MSF.

———. 2013. *Untangling the Web of Antiretroviral Price Reductions.* Geneva: MSF.

MSF (Médecins Sans Frontières), Department of Public Health at the University of Cape Town, and the Provincial Administration of the Western Cape. 2003. *Antiretroviral Therapy in Primary Health Care: Experience of the Khayelitsha Programme in South Africa.* Geneva: World Health Organization.

MSF (Médecins Sans Frontières), Western Cape Province Department of Health, City of Cape Town Department of Health, and University of Cape Town, Centre for Infectious Disease Epidemiology and Research. 2011. *Kayelitsha 2001–2011: 10 Years of HIV/TB Care at Primary Health Care Level.* Cape Town: MSF.

Mshana, G., M. Plummer, J. Wamoyi, Z. Shigongo, D. Ross, and D. Wight. 2006. "'She Was Bewitched and Caught an Illness Similar to AIDS': AIDS and Sexually Transmitted Infection Causation Beliefs in Rural Northern Tanzania." *Culture, Health & Sexuality* 8, no. 1: 45–58.

Msikula, A. 2017. ATF: Funding Anti-AIDS Activities to Avoid Donor Dependency. *Daily News.* 14 December.

Mtullu, S., B. Olekawanara, M. Karata, S. Omar, Z. Tittee, and R. Kombo. 2009. *Annual Progress Report TAN 07-01 HIV.* Tanga: Tanga AIDS Working Group.

Mundell, J., M. Visser, J. Makin, B. Forsyth, and K. Sikkema. 2012. "Support Group Processes: Perspectives from HIV-Infected Women in South Africa." *Qualitative Research in Psychology* 9, no. 2: 173–87.

Mvungi, A. 2011. "Babu aitaka serikali kujiandaa kupokea wageni wengi toka nje." *Nipashe.* 7 May.

Mwachali, A. 2011. "Kulola sasa adai Babu katumwa na jini." *Nyakati.* 19–25 June.

Mwilolezi, C. 2016. "Babu Loliondo ajiandaa kwa mafuriko mapya." *Nipashe Jumapili.* 21 February.

NACP (National AIDS Control Programme). 2003a. *Health Sector HIV/AIDS Strategy for Tanzania 2003-2006.* Dar es Salaam: NACP.

———. 2003b. *HIV/AIDS Care and Treatment Plan 2003-2008.* Dar es Salaam: NACP.

———. 2008. *National Guidelines for the Management of HIV and AIDS.* 3rd ed. Dar es Salaam: NACP.

———. 2011a. *HIV/AIDS/STI Surveillance Report Report Number 22.* Dar es Salaam: NACP.

———. 2011b. *Implementation of HIV/AIDS Care and Treatment Services in Tanzania. Report No. 2. March 2011.* Dar es Salaam: NACP.

———. 2012. *National Guidelines for the Management of HIV and AIDS.* 4th ed. Dar es Salaam: NACP.

———. 2013. *Third Health Sector HIV and AIDS Strategic Plan (HSHSP III) 2013–2017.* Dar es Salaam: NACP.

———. 2017. *National Guidelines for the Management of HIV and AIDS.* 6th ed. Dar es Salaam: NACP.

National Bureau of Statistics and Tanga Regional Commissioner's Office. 2008. *Tanga Regional Socio-Economic Profile.* Dar es Salaam: Ministry of Planning, Economy and Empowerment.

Nattrass, N. 2007. *Mortal Combat: AIDS Denialism and the Struggle for Antiretrovirals in South Africa.* Scottsville, South Africa: University of KwaZulu-Natal Press.

Nettleton, S. 1997. "Governing the Risky Self How to Become Healthy, Wealthy, and Wise." In *Foucault, Health and Medicine.* Edited by A. Petersen and R. Bunton, 207–22. London: Routledge.

Nguyen, V.-K. 2005. "Antiretroviral Globalism, Biopolitics, and Therapeutic Citizenship." In *Global Assemblages: Technology, Politics, and Ethics as*

Anthropological Problems. Edited by A. Ong and S. Collier, 124–44. Malden, MA: Blackwell.

———. 2009a. "Government-by-Exception: Enrolment and Experimentality in Mass HIV Treatment Programmes in Africa." *Social Theory & Health* 7, no. 3: 196–217.

———. 2009b. "Therapeutic Evangelism—Confessional Technologies, Antiretrovirals and Biospiritual Transformation in the Fight against AIDS in West Africa." In *AIDS and Religious Practice in Africa.* Edited by F. Becker and P. W. Geissler, 359–78. Leiden: Brill.

———. 2010. *The Republic of Therapy: Triage and Sovereignty in West Africa's Time of AIDS; Body, Commodity, Text.* Durham, NC: Duke University Press.

Nguyen, V.-K., C. Yapo Ako, P. Niamba, A. Sylla, and I. Tiendrébéogo. 2007. "Adherence as Therapeutic Citizenship: Impact of the History of Access to Antiretroviral Drugs on Adherence to Treatment." *AIDS* 21, suppl. 5: S31–35.

Nichter, M. 2002. "The Social Relations of Therapy Management." In *New Horizons in Medical Anthropology.* Edited by M. Nichter and M. Lock, 81–110. New York: Routledge.

Nkwame, M. 2011. "No child yet? Go to 'Babu.'" *Daily News.* 20 June.

Nyenyembe, C. 2011. "Babu wa taifa waokoe watanzania wanaumwa." *Tanzania Daima.* 11 March.

Ogden, J., and L. Nyblade. 2005. *Common at Its Core: HIV-Related Stigma across Contexts.* Washington, DC: International Center for Research on Women.

Oosthuizen, G. 1992. *The Healer-Prophet in Afro-Christian Churches.* Leiden: Brill.

Otiso, Kefa. 2013. *Culture and Customs of Tanzania.* Santa Barbara, CA: Greenwood.

Parker, R., and P. Aggleton. 2002. *HIV/AIDS-Related Stigma and Discrimination: A Conceptual Framework and an Agenda for Action.* New York: The Population Council New York. Retrieved 7 December 2018 from http://eldis.org/vfile/upload/1/document/0708/DOC13171.pdf.

———. 2003. "HIV and AIDS-Related Stigma and Discrimination: A Conceptual Framework and Implications for Action." *Social Science & Medicine* 57, no. 1: 13–24.

Parkin, D. 2014. "Pathways to Healing: Curative Travel among Muslims and Non-Muslims in Eastern East Africa." *Medical Anthropology* 33, no. 1: 21–36.

Patten, P. 2011. "Samunge Is Not It . . . But There Are Many Reasons to Promote a Lie." *Guardian on Sunday.* 29 June.

Patterson, A. 2010. "Church Mobilisation and HIV/AIDS Treatment in Ghana and Zambia: A Comparative Analysis." *African Journal of AIDS Research* 9, no. 4: 407–18.

PEPFAR (The U.S. President's Emergency Plan for AIDS Relief). 2009. "About PEPFAR." Retrieved 4 September 2016 from http://www.pepfar.gov/about/.

———. 2010. *Five-Year Partnership Framework in Support of the Tanzania National Response to HIV and AIDS 2009–2013*. Washington, DC: PEPFAR.

———. 2013. *Tanzania Operational Plan Report FY 2013*. Retrieved 25 July 2016 from http://www.pepfar.gov/documents/organization/222184.pdf.

———. 2017a. *Tanzania Country Operational Plan (COP) 2017: Strategic Summary*. Washington, DC: PEPFAR.

———. 2017b. *Strategy for Accelerating HIV/AIDS Epidemic Control (2017-2020)*. Washington, DC: PEPFAR.

Persson, A., C. Newman, L. Mao, and J. de Wit. 2016. "On the Margins of Pharmaceutical Citizenship: Not Taking HIV Medication in the "Treatment Revolution" Era: HIV and Pharmaceutical Citizenship." *Medical Anthropology Quarterly* 30, no. 3: 359–77.

Petersen, A., and D. Lupton. 1996. *The New Public Health: Discourses, Knowledges, Strategies*. London: Sage.

Petryna, A., and A. Kleinman. 2006. "The Pharmaceutical Nexus." In *Global Pharmaceuticals. Ethics, Markets, Practices*. Edited by A. Petryna, A. Lakoff, and A. Kleinman, 1–32. Durham, NC: Duke University Press.

Pew Forum on Religion and Public Life. 2010. *Tolerance and Tension: Islam and Christianity in Sub-Saharan Africa*. Washington, DC: Pew Research Center.

Pfaff-Czarnecka, J. 2011. "From 'Identity' to 'Belonging' in Social Research: Plurality, Social Boundaries, and the Politics of the Self." Working Papers in Development Sociology and Social Anthropology. No. 368. Retrieved 23 June 2015 from http://www.unibielefeld.de/(en)/tdrc/ag_sozanth/publica tions/working_papers/WP368.pdf.

Pfeiffer, J. 2013. "The Struggle for a Public Sector PEPFAR in Mozambique." In *When People Come First. Cricital Studies in Global Public Health*. Edited by J. Biehl and A. Petryna, 166–81. Princeton, NJ: Princeton University Press.

Philemon, L. 2011. "Retired pastor suspends services to new patients." *The Guardian*. 28 March.

———. 2012. "Babu: God Has Given Me New Miracle Cure." *The Citizen*. 21 February.

Poku, N., and A. Whiteside. 2004. *The Political Economy of AIDS in Africa*. Aldershot: Ashgate.

Prince, R. 2009. "Christian Salvation and Luo Tradition: Arguments of Faith in a Time of Death in Western Kenya." In *AIDS and Religious Practice in Africa*. F. Becker and P. W. Geissler, 49–83. Leiden: Brill.

———. 2014a. "Navigating 'Global Health' in an East African City." In *Making and Unmaking Public Health in Africa. Ethnographic and Historical Perspectives*. Edited by R. Prince and R. Marsland, 208–29. Athens: Ohio University Press.

———. 2014b. "Introduction: Situating Health and the Public in Africa. Historical and Anthropological Perspectives." In *Making and Unmaking Public Health in Africa. Ethnographic and Historical Perspectives*. Edited by R. Prince and R. Marsland, 1–51. Athens: Ohio University Press.

Probst, P. 1999. "Mchape '95, or, the Sudden Fame of Billy Goodson Chisupe: Healing, Social Memory and the Enigma of the Public Sphere in Post-Banda Malawi." *Africa* 69, no. 01: 108–38.

Rabinow, P. 1996. "Artificiality and Enlightenment: From Sociobiology to Biosociality." In *Essays on the Anthropology of Reason*, 234–52. Princeton, NJ: Princeton University Press.

Ranger, T. 1992. "Plagues of Beasts and Men; Prophetic Responses to Epidemics in Eastern and Southern Africa." In *Epidemics and Ideas. Essays on the Historical Perception of Pestilence*. Edited by T. Ranger and P. Slack, 241–68. Cambridge, UK: Cambridge University Press.

Rasmussen, L. M. 2013. "Counselling Clients to Follow 'the Rules' of Safe Sex and ARV Treatment." *Culture, Health & Sexuality* 15, suppl. 4: S537–52.

Reddi, A. 2010. "Truth and Reconciliation: President Obama's Global Health Initiative and HIV/AIDS. Raising the Bar." *Huffington Post*. 27 July. Retrieved 13 June 2014 from http://www.huffingtonpost.com/anand-reddi/truth-and-reconciliation_b_660586.html.

Reihling, P. 2013. "Vulnerable Men: Gender and Sentiment at the Margins of Cape Town." PhD diss., Freie Universität Berlin.

Richey, L. A. 2006. "Gendering the Therapeutic Citizen: ARVs and Reproductive Health." University of Cape Town, Center for Social Science Research, Working Paper no. 175.

———. 2012. "Counselling Citizens and Producing Patronage: AIDS Treatment in South African and Ugandan Clinics." *Development and Change* 43, no. 4: 823–45.

Robins, S. 2004. "'Long Live Zackie, Long Live': AIDS Activism, Science and Citizenship after Apartheid." *Journal of Southern African Studies* 30, no. 3: 651–72.

———. 2006. "From 'Rights' to 'Ritual': AIDS Activism in South Africa." *American Anthropologist* 108, no. 2: 312–23.

———. 2009. "Foot Soldiers of Global Health: Teaching and Preaching AIDS Science and Modern Medicine on the Frontline." *Medical Anthropology* 28, no. 1: 81–107.

Rödlach, A. 2006. *Witches, Westerners, and HIV: AIDS and Cultures of Blame in Africa*. Walnut Creek, CA: Left Coast Press.

Root, R. 2012. "Being HIV Positive A Phenomenology of HIV Disclosure in Swaziland." In *Disclosure in Health and Illness*. Edited by M. Davis and L. Manderson, 36–55. New York: Routledge.

Rösch, P.-G. 1995. *Der Prozess der Strukturanpassung in Tansania*. Hamburg: Institut für Afrika-Kunde.

Rose, N. 2007. *The Politics of Life Itself: Biomedicine, Power, and Subjectivity in the Twenty-First Century*. Princeton, NJ: Princeton University Press.

Rosenbrock, R., F. Dubois-Arber, M. Moers, P. Pinell, D. Schaeffer, and M. Setbon. 2000. "The Normalization of AIDS in Western European Countries." *Social Science & Medicine (1982)* 50, no. 11: 1607–29.

Rottenburg, R. 2009. "Social and Public Experiments and New Figurations of Science and Politics in Postcolonial Africa." *Postcolonial Studies* 12, no. 4: 423–440.

Rottenburg, R., S. Merry, S. Park, and J. Mugler, eds. 2015. *The World of Indicators: The Making of Governmental Knowledge through Quantification.* Cambridge, UK: Cambridge University Press.

Roura, M., M. Urassa, J. Busza, D. Mbata, A. Wringe, and B. Zaba. 2009. "Scaling up Stigma? The Effects of Antiretroviral Roll-out on Stigma and HIV Testing Early Evidence from Rural Tanzania." *Sexually Transmitted Infections* 85, no. 4: 308–12.

Russell, S., and J. Seeley. 2010. "The Transition to Living with HIV as a Chronic Condition in Rural Uganda: Working to Create Order and Control When on Antiretroviral Therapy." *Social Science & Medicine* 70, no. 3: 375–82.

Sangaramoorthy, T. 2018. "Chronicity, Crisis, and the 'End of AIDS.'" *Global Public Health* 13, no. 8: 982–96.

Sarna, A., M. Chersich, J. Okal, S. Luchters, K. Mandaliya, N. Rutenberg, and M. Temmerman. 2009. "Changes in Sexual Risk Taking with Antiretroviral Treatment: Influence of Context and Gender Norms in Mombasa, Kenya." *Culture, Health & Sexuality* 11, no. 8: 783–97.

Scandlyn, J. 2000. "When AIDS Became a Chronic Disease." *The Western Journal of Medicine* 172, no. 2: 130–33.

Scheinman, D. 2002. *Traditional Medicine in Tanga Today: The Ancient and Modern Worlds Meet* (No. 51), IK Notes. Washington, DC: Africa Region's Knowledge and Learning Center, 1–4.

Scheper-Hughes, N. 1995. "The Primacy of the Ethical: Propositions for a Militant Anthropology." *Current Anthropology* 36, no. 3: 409–40.

Scheper-Hughes, N., and M. Lock. 1987. "The Mindful Body: A Prolegomenon to Future Work in Medical Anthropology." *Medical Anthropology Quarterly* 1, no. 1: 6–41.

Schoepf, B. 2001. "International AIDS Research in Anthropology: Taking a Critical Perspective on the Crisis." *Annual Review of Anthropology* 30: 335–61.

Schoffeleers, M. 1999. "The Aids Pandemic, the Prophet Billy Chisupe, and the Democratization Process in Malawi." *Journal of Religion in Africa* 29, no. 4: 406–41.

Schwartländer, B., I. Grubb, and J. Perriëns. 2006. "The 10-Year Struggle to Provide Antiretroviral Treatment to People with HIV in the Developing World." *Lancet* 368, no. 9534: 541–6.

Seckinelgin, H. 2012. "The Global Governance of Success in HIV/AIDS Policy: Emergency Action, Everyday Lives and Sen's Capabilities." *Health & Place* 18, no. 3: 453–60.

Seeley, J., S. Russell, K. Khana, E. Ezati, R. King, and R. Bunnell. 2009. "Sex after ART: Sexual Partnerships Established by HIV-Infected Persons Taking Anti-Retroviral Therapy in Eastern Uganda." *Culture, Health & Sexuality* 11, no. 7: 703–16.

Setel, P. 1999. *A Plague of Paradoxes: AIDS, Culture, and Demography in Northern Tanzania*. Chicago: University of Chicago Press.

Shekighenda, L. 2011. "COSTECH: Trademark for 'Babu' cure on the way." *The Guardian*. 1 April.

———. 2012. "Not the Long Awaited HIV Cure." *The Guardian*. 31 July.

Silla, A., and M. Juma. 2011. "Kiongozi wa Anglikana akunwa na tiba ya Babu." *Mwananchi*. 23 April.

Skovdal, M., C. Campbell, C. Madanhire, Z. Mupambirei, C. Nyamukapa, and S. Gregson. 2011. "Masculinity as a Barrier to Men's Use of HIV Services in Zimbabwe." *Global Health* 7, no. 1: 1–13.

Smith, D. J., and B. Mbakwem. 2010. "Antiretroviral Therapy and Reproductive Life Projects: Mitigating the Stigma of AIDS in Nigeria." *Social Science & Medicine* 71, no. 2: 345–52.

Smith, J. H., and A. Whiteside. 2010. "The History of AIDS Exceptionalism." *Journal of the International AIDS Society* 13, no. 1.

Smith, L., and A. Kleinman. 2010. "Emotional Engagements: Acknowledgement, Advocacy, and Direct Action." In *Emotions in the Field. The Psychology and Anthropology of Fieldwork Experience*. Edited by J. Davies and D. Spencer, 171–87. Stanford, CA: Stanford University Press.

Smith, R., and P. Siplon. 2006. *Drugs into Bodies: Global AIDS Treatment Activism*. Westport, CT: Praeger.

Smith-Morris, C. 2010. "The Chronicity of Life, the Acuteness of Diagnosis." In *Chronic Conditions, Fluid States: Chronicity and the Anthropology of Illness*. Edited by L. Manderson and C. Smith-Morris, 21–37. New Brunswick, NJ: Rutgers University Press.

Spirig, R. 1998. "Support Groups for People Living with HIV/AIDS: A Review of Literature." *Journal of the Association of Nurses in AIDS Care* 9, no. 4: 43–55.

Ssewaya, A. 2011. "Sustaining Adherence to Antiretroviral Therapy among HIV/AIDS Patients in Uganda." PhD diss., University of Amsterdam.

Steuer, N. 2012. *Krankheit und Ehre: Über HIV und soziale Anerkennung in Mali*. Bielefeld: Transcript.

Stoczkowski, W. 2008. "The 'Fourth Aim' of Anthropology Between Knowledge and Ethics." *Anthropological Theory* 8, no. 4: 345–56.

Strauss, A. 1984. *Chronic Illness and the Quality of Life*. St. Louis: Mosby.

Stroeken, K. 2012. *Moral Power: The Magic of Witchcraft*. New York: Berghahn Books.

Sullivan, N. 2011a. "Mediating Abundance and Scarcity: Implementing an HIV/AIDS-Targeted Project Within a Government Hospital in Tanzania." *Medical Anthropology* 30, no. 2: 202–21.

———. 2011b. "Negotiating Abundance and Scarcity: Health Sector Reform, Development Aid, and Biomedical Practice in a Tanzanian Hospital." PhD diss., University of Florida.

Svensson, J. 2009. "'Muslims Have Instructions': HIV/AIDS, Modernity, and Islamic Religious Education in Kisumu, Kenya." In *AIDS and Religious*

Practice in Africa. Edited by F. Becker and P. W. Geissler, 189–219. Leiden: Brill.

Swidler, A. 2009. "Dialectics of Patronage Logics of Accountability at the African AIDS-NGO Interface." In *Globalization, Philanthropy, and Civil Society. Projecting Institutional Logics Abroad.* Edited by D. Hammack and S. Heydemann, 192–220. Bloomington: Indiana University Press.

TACAIDS (Tanzania Commission for HIV/AIDS). 2002. *National Multi-Sectoral Strategic Framework on HIV/AIDS 2003-2007.* Dar es Salaam: TACAIDS.

———. 2012a. *Country Progress Reporting: Part A. Tanzania Mainland.* Dar es Salaam: TACAIDS.

———. 2012b. *Public Expenditure Review, 2011 HIV and AIDS: Tanzania Mainland.* Dar es Salaam: TACAIDS.

———. 2013a. *Tanzania HIV/AIDS and Malaria Indicator Survey 2011–12.* Dar es Salaam: TACAIDS, ZAC, NBS, OCGS, ICF International.

———. 2013b. *Tanzania Third National Multi-Sectoral Strategic Framework for HIV and AIDS (2013/14–2017/18).* Dar es Salaam: TACAIDS.

———. 2014. *National HIV and AIDS Response Report 2013: Tanzania Mainland.* Dar es Salaam: TACAIDS.

Tanga City Council. 2007. *Socio-Economic Profile for Tanga City Council.* Tanga: Tanga City Council.

Tawfik, Y., S. Kinoti, G. Chad Blain. 2002. *Introducing Antiretroviral Therapy (ART) on a Large Scale: Hope and Caution; Program Planning Guidance Based on Early Experiences from Resource-Limited and Middle-Income Countries.* Washington, DC: AED Global Health, Population and Nutrition Group.

Tenga, M. G. 2008. *Sisal Industry in Tanzania since Colonial Era: Uncovered Modern Slavery to Liberation.* Bloomington, IN: Xlibris.

Ter Haar, G. 1992. *Spirit of Africa: The Healing Ministry of Archbishop Milingo of Zambia.* Trenton, NJ: C. Hurst & Co.

Tesha, G. 2011. "Wataalamu: Kikombe cha 'Babu' ni kinga bomba." *Habari Leo.* 6 May.

Theilgaard, Z., T. Katzenstein, M. Chiduo, C. Pahl, I. Bygbjerg, J. Gerstoft, M. Lemnge, and B. Tersbøl. 2011. "Addressing the Fear and Consequences of Stigmatization—a Necessary Step towards Making HAART Accessible to Women in Tanzania: A Qualitative Study." *AIDS Research and Therapy* 8: 28.

Tibandebage, P., and T. Kida. 2013. "The Gendered Impact of the Global Economic Crisis on Financing and Access of Health Care in Tanzania." ESRF Discussion Paper no. 37. Dar es Salaam: Economic and Social Research Foundation.

Tocco, J. U. 2014. "Prophetic Medicine, Antiretrovirals, and the Therapeutic Economy of HIV in Northern Nigeria." In *Religion and AIDS Treatment in Africa: Saving Souls, Prolonging Lives.* Edited by R. Van Dijk, H. Dilger, M. Burchardt, and T. Rasing, 119–45. Burlington, VT: Ashgate.

Togarasei, L. 2010. "Christian Theology of Life, Death and Healing in an Era of Antiretroviral Therapy: Reflections on the Responses of Some Botswana Churches." *African Journal of AIDS Research* 9, no. 4: 429–35.

Trostle, J. 1988. "Medical Compliance as an Ideology." *Social Science & Medicine* 27, no. 12: 1299–308.

Tsing, A. L. 2005. *Friction: An Ethnography of Global Connection*. Princeton, NJ: Princeton University Press.

Turner, V. 1968. *The Drums of Affliction*. Oxford: Clarendon.

Turshen, M. 1999. *Privatizing Health Services in Africa*. New Brunswick, NJ: Rutgers University Press.

Uiso, F., E. Kayombo, Z. Mbwambo, Y. Mgonda, R. Mahunnah, and M. Moshi. 2007. "Traditional Healer's Knowledge and Implications to the Management and Control of HIV/AIDS in Arusha, Tanzania." *Tanzania Journal of Health Research* 8, no. 2: 95–100.

UNAIDS (Joint United Nations Programme on HIV/AIDS). 1997. *Counselling and HIV/AIDS. Technical Update*. Geneva: UNAIDS.

———. 2012. *Together We Will End AIDS*. Geneva: UNAIDS.

———. 2014. *Fast Track: Ending the AIDS Epidemic by 2030*. Geneva: UNAIDS.

———. 2015. *How AIDS Changed Everything. MDG 6: 15 Years, 15 Lessons of Hope from the AIDS Response*. Geneva: UNAIDS.

———. 2017a. *Country Fact Sheet United Republic of Tanzania 2016*. Geneva: UNAIDS.

———. 2017b. *Fact Sheet—World AIDS Day 2017*. Geneva: UNAIDS.

———. 2017c. *UNAIDS Data 2017*. Geneva: UNAIDS.

United Nations General Assembly. 2016. "Political Declaration on HIV and AIDS: On the Fast Track of the Fight against HIV and to Ending the AIDS Epidemic by 2030." New York: UNGASS.

The United Republic of Tanzania. 2001. *National Policy on HIV/AIDS*. Dar es Salaam: Prime Minister's Office.

———. 2002. *The Traditional and Alternative Medicines Act*. Dar es Salaam: Government Printer.

———. 2008. *Human Resource for Health Strategic Plan 2008–2013*. Dar es Salaam: Ministry of Health and Social Welfare.

———. 2013. *2012 Population and Housing Census*. Dar es Salaam: National Bureau of Statistics.

———. 2017. *Summary Sheet: Preliminary Findings—Tanzania HIV Impact Survey (THIS) 2016–2017*. Dar es Salaam: National Bureau of Statistics.

Van de Bruinhorst, G. 2007. *"Raise Your Voices and Kill Your Animals": Islamic Discourses on the Idd El-Hajj and Sacrifices in Tanga (Tanzania); Authoritative Texts, Ritual Practices and Social Identities*. ISIM diss., Amsterdam University Press.

Van der Geest, S., and K. Chamberlain. 2011. "Researching the Life Stages of Medicines." *Medische Antropologie* 23, no. 1994: 231–42.

Van der Geest, S., and K. Finkler. 2004. "Hospital Ethnography: Introduction." *Social Science & Medicine* 59, no. 10: 1995–2001.

Van der Geest, S., and A. Hardon. 2006. "Social and Cultural Efficacies of Medicines: Complications for Antiretroviral Therapy." *Journal of Ethnobiology and Ethnomedicine* 2, no. 1: 48.

Van der Geest, S., S. R. Whyte, and A. Hardon. 1996. "The Anthropology of Pharmaceuticals: A Biographical Approach." *Annual Review of Anthropology* 25: 153–78.

Van Dijk, R. 2009. "Gloves in Times of AIDS: Pentecostalism, Hair and Social Distancing in Botswana." In *AIDS and Religious Practice in Africa*. Edited by F. Becker and P. W. Geissler, 283–306. Leiden: Brill.

Vaughan, M. 1991. *Curing Their Ills: Colonial Power and African Illness.* Stanford, CA: Stanford University Press.

Wallace, A. 1956. "Revitalization Movements." *American Anthropologist* 58, no. 2: 264–81.

Waning, B., E. Diedrichsen, and S. Moon. 2010. "A Lifeline to Treatment: The Role of Indian Generic Manufacturers in Supplying Antiretroviral Medicines to Developing Countries." *Journal of the International AIDS Society* 13, no. 1: 35.

Wendland, C. 2010. *A Heart for the Work: Journeys through an African Medical School.* Chicago: University of Chicago Press.

West, H., and T. Luedke. 2006. "Introduction: Healing Divides: Therapeutic Border Work in Southeast Africa." In *Borders and Healers. Brokering Therapeutic Resources in Southeast Africa.* Edited by T. Luedke and H. West, 1–20. Bloomington: Indiana University Press.

Westerhaus, M., and A. Castro. 2006. "How Do Intellectual Property Law and International Trade Agreements Affect Access to Antiretroviral Therapy?" *PLoS Medicine* 3, no. 8: 1230–36.

WHO (World Health Organization). 2002a. "A Commitment to Action for Expanded Access to HIV/AIDS Treatment." Geneva: WHO.

———. 2002b. *Scaling up Antiretroviral Therapy in Resource-Limited Settings: Guidelines for a Public Health Approach.* Geneva: WHO.

———. 2003. *Treating 3 Million by 2005: Making It Happen. The WHO Strategy.* Geneva: WHO.

———. 2005. *United Republic of Tanzania: Summary Country Profile for HIV/ AIDS Treatment Scale-Up.* Geneva: WHO.

———. 2006. *Antiretroviral Therapy for HIV Infection in Adults and Adolescents: Recommendations for a Public Health Approach. 2006 Revision.* Geneva: WHO.

———. 2010a. *Antiretroviral Therapy for HIV Infection in Adults and Adolescents: Recommendations for a Public Health Approach. 2010 Revision.* Geneva: WHO.

———. 2010b. *Towards Universal Access: Scaling up Priority HIV/AIDS Interventions in the Health Section: Progress Report 2010.* Geneva: WHO.

———. 2013. *Consolidated Guidelines on the Use of Antiretroviral Drugs for Treating and Preventing HIV Infection: Recommendations for a Public Health Approach.* Geneva: WHO.

———. 2015. *Guideline on When to Start Antiretroviral Therapy and Pre-Exposure Prophylaxis for HIV.* Geneva: WHO.

———. 2017. *Fact Sheet—Treat All: Policy Adoption and Implementation Status in Countries.* Geneva: WHO.

Whyte, S. R. 1997. *Questioning Misfortune: The Pragmatics of Uncertainty in Eastern Uganda*. Cambridge, UK: Cambridge University Press.

———. 2005. "Going Home? Belonging and Burial in the Era of AIDS." *Africa* 75, no. 02: 154–72.

———. 2009. "Epilogue." In *Dealing with Uncertainty in Contemporary African Lives*. Edited by L. Haram and C. B. Yamba, 213–6. Uppsala: Nordiska Afrikainstitutet.

———. 2012. "Chronicity and Control: Framing 'Noncommunicable Diseases' in Africa." *Anthropology & Medicine* 19, no. 1: 63–74.

Whyte, S. R., E. Alber, and S. Van der Geest. 2008. "Generational Connections and Conflicts in Africa: An Introduction." In *Generations in Africa. Connections and Conflicts*. Edited by E. Alber, Sjaak Van der Geest, and S. R. Whyte, 1–23. Münster: LIT.

Whyte, S. R., D. Kyaddondo, and L. Meinert. 2014. "Children." In *Second Chances: Surviving AIDS in Uganda*. Edited by S. R. Whyte, 152–66. Durham, NC: Duke University Press.

Whyte, S. R., L. Meinert, and H. Mogensen. 2014. "Bodies." In *Second Chances: Surviving AIDS in Uganda*. Edited by S. R. Whyte, 223–63. Durham, NC: Duke University Press.

Whyte, S. R., L. Meinert, and J. Twebaze. 2014. "Clientship." In *Second Chances: Surviving AIDS in Uganda*. Edited by S. R. Whyte, 56–69. Durham, NC: Duke University Press.

Whyte, S. R., H. Mogensen, and L. Meinert. 2014. "Life." In *Second Chances: Surviving AIDS in Uganda*. Edited by S. R. Whyte, 268–83. Durham, NC: Duke University Press.

Whyte, S. R., H. Mogensen, and J. Twebaze. 2014. "Families." In *Second Chances: Surviving AIDS in Uganda*. Edited by S. R. Whyte, 104–17. Durham, NC: Duke University Press.

Whyte, S. R., S. Van der Geest, and A. Hardon, eds. 2002. *Social Lives of Medicines*. Cambridge, UK: Cambridge University Press.

Whyte, S. R., M. Whyte, and D. Kyaddondo. 2010. "Health Workers Entangled: Confidentiality and Certification." In *Morality, Hope, and Grief: Anthropologies of AIDS in Africa*. Edited by H. Dilger and U. Luig, 80–101. New York: Berghahn Books.

Whyte, S. R., M. Whyte, L. Meinert, and B. Kyaddondo. 2006. "Treating AIDS: Dilemmas of Unequal Access in Uganda." In *Global Pharmaceuticals: Ethics, Markets, Practices*. Edited by A. Petryna, A. Lakoff, and A. Kleinman, 240–62. Durham, NC: Duke University Press.

Whyte, S. R., M. Whyte, L. Meinert, and J. Twebaze. 2013. "Therapeutic Clientship: Belonging in Uganda's Projectified Landscape of AIDS Care." In *When People Come First: Critical Studies in Global Public Health*. Edited by J. Biehl and A. Petryna, 140–65. Princeton, NJ: Princeton University Press.

Wind, G. 2008. "Negotiated Interactive Observation: Doing Fieldwork in Hospital Settings." *Anthropology & Medicine* 15, no. 2: 79–89.

Wolf, A. 2001. "AIDS, Morality and Indigenous Concepts of Sexually Transmitted Diseases in Southern Africa." *Africa Spectrum* 36, no. 1: 97–107.

———. 2010. "Orphan's Ties Belonging and Relatedness in Child-Headed Households in Malawi." In *Morality, Hope, and Grief: Anthropologies of AIDS in Africa*. Edited by H. Dilger and U. Luig, 292–311. New York: Berghahn Books.

Wolfe, W., S. Weiser, K. Leiter, W. Steward, F. Percy-de-Korte, N. Phaladze, V. Iacopino, and M. Heisler. 2008. "The Impact of Universal Access to Antiretroviral Therapy on HIV Stigma in Botswana." *American Journal of Public Health* 98, no. 10: 1865–71.

WTO (World Trade Organization). 2001. *Declaration on the TRIPS Agreement and Public Health*. Geneva: WTO.

Yamba, C. B. 1997. "Cosmologies in Turmoil: Witchfinding and AIDS in Chiawa, Zambia." *Africa: Journal of the International African Institute* 67, no. 2: 200–23.

Yang, A., P. Farmer, and A. McGahan. 2010. "'Sustainability' in Global Health." *Global Public Health* 5, no. 2: 129–35.

Zola, I. K. 1972. "Medicine as an Institution of Social Control." *The Sociological Review* 20, no. 4: 487–504.

Zuniga, J., A. Whiteside, A. Ghaziani, and J. Bartlett, eds. 2008. *A Decade of HAART: The Development and Global Impact of Highly Active Antiretroviral Therapy*. Oxford: Oxford University Press.

Index